Pediatrics: Medical Care of Children

Pediatrics: Medical Care of Children

Edited by **Larry Stone**

hayle medical

New York

Published by Hayle Medical,
30 West, 37th Street, Suite 612,
New York, NY 10018, USA
www.haylemedical.com

Pediatrics: Medical Care of Children
Edited by Larry Stone

International Standard Book Number: 978-1-63241-409-0 (Hardback)

Printed in the United States of America.

Contents

Preface

In my initial years as a student, I used to run to the library at every possible instance to grab a book and learn something new. Books were my primary source of knowledge and I would not have come such a long way without all that I learnt from them. Thus, when I was approached to edit this book; I became understandably nostalgic. It was an absolute honor to be considered worthy of guiding the current generation as well as those to come. I put all my knowledge and hard work into making this book most beneficial for its readers.

Pediatrics is the branch of medicine that deals with prevention, diagnosis and treatment of diseases related to infants and children. According to medical science the anatomy and structure of children is considerably different from that of adults and they cannot be treated with same strong dosages of drugs. Neonates require specialized attention and milder medicines during their early stages of life. This book aims to provide a fair idea about this discipline and help develop a better understanding of the latest advances within this field. Most of the topics introduced herein cover new diagnostic techniques and treatment strategies in pediatrics. This book presents researches and studies performed by experts across the globe. It is meant for students, doctors and for those who are looking for an elaborate reference text on medical care of children.

I wish to thank my publisher for supporting me at every step. I would also like to thank all the authors who have contributed their researches in this book. I hope this book will be a valuable contribution to the progress of the field.

Editor

1

The Difficulties of Congenital Syphilis Diagnosis about 3 Cases at Libreville, Gabon

C. M. Essomo Megnier-Mbo[1,2,3], S. Mayi[2], Y. Vierin[3], A. Ndjoyi Biguino[4], J. Koko[3], A. Moussavou[3]

[1]Service de Réanimation Néonatale et Néonatologie HIAOBO, Libreville, Gabon
[2]Departement Mère Enfant HIAOBO, Libreville, Gabon
[3]Département de Pédiatrie, Faculté de Médecine, Libreville, Gabon
[4]Laboratoire de Microbiologie, Faculté de Médecine, Libreville, Gabon
Email: owonomegniermbo@yahoo.fr

Abstract

First described embryo fetopathy, congenital syphilis remains a public health problem mostly in developing countries. The diagnosis mainly based on bacteriological and immunological evidence of mother-child couple is not always easy, as it is shown in our three clinical cases. Those three clinical observations demonstrate the difficulties encountered in the diagnosis of congenital syphilis in our country where only the TPHA (*Treponema Pallidum* Haemaglutination Assay) and VDRL (Venereal Disease Research Laboratory) tests are the only ones to be routinely carried out. Actually, these tests can be negative at the earliest stage of the syphilis or in case of zonal phenomenon. In addition, maternal antibodies could be found in child blood, even if the baby is in good health. At last, the child could have been contaminated belatedly while tests were negative at the third month of pregnancy. Congenital syphilis still exists in our developing countries and, in order to better manage this pathology, a proposition of an efficient algorithm is submitted.

Keywords

Congenital Syphilis, Diagnosis, Difficulties, Libreville, Gabon

1. Introduction

Congenital syphilis is a public health problem mostly in developing countries where its prevalence remains high [1]-[5]. After having practically disappeared in industrialized countries, we are witnessing a resurgence of the disease since 2001, mostly in women from marginalized populations for cultural reasons such as "gens du voyage" (Gypsy group) or those living in social and economic precariousness [6]-[9].

In Gabon, the presence of a remaining high number of unattended pregnancies despite of free medical care in mother-and-child healthcare centers and the high seroprevalence of the illness (13.3%) could explain the found cases [10] [11].

The diagnosis, which relies essentially on bacteriological and immunological evidences, is not always easy as illustrated in our cases. Thus, it was done by combining together the anamnesis, the maternal history and the newborn biology (*i.e.*, blood count, CRP, TPHA, VDRL) at birth along with skeleton's X-rays. The goal of this study was to display the difficulties inherent in that diagnosis and to propose a therapeutically management algorithm for patients.

2. Observations

2.1. Case 1

It was about a male baby born at the right term (38 weeks of amenorrhea). The pregnancy was unattended. The syphilitic serology realized at the second trimester of pregnancy had shown a positive TPHA test along with positive VDRL. The mother was not treated. The delivery took place at home. The baby cried immediately as recommended, and the newborn was transferred at the hospital for examination and medical care management. At the entry, it presented intrauterine harmonious growth retardation with a body weight of 2000 grams (gr), a size of 46 centimeters (cm) and a cranial perimeter of 31 centimeters (cm). The clinical examination revealed a seropurulent nasal discharge obstructing the nostrils in places, a dermatosis made of post-blistered sweating in places, located in lower limbs (from knees to ankles), back of hand, nose rim, upper lip, umbilical region along with palmo-plantar desquamation (**Figure 1**). We also noticed an incurvation of the four limbs, mostly pronounced in the lower ones, a hepatomegaly (HSMG) during the abdominal auscultation, and a slight decrease of

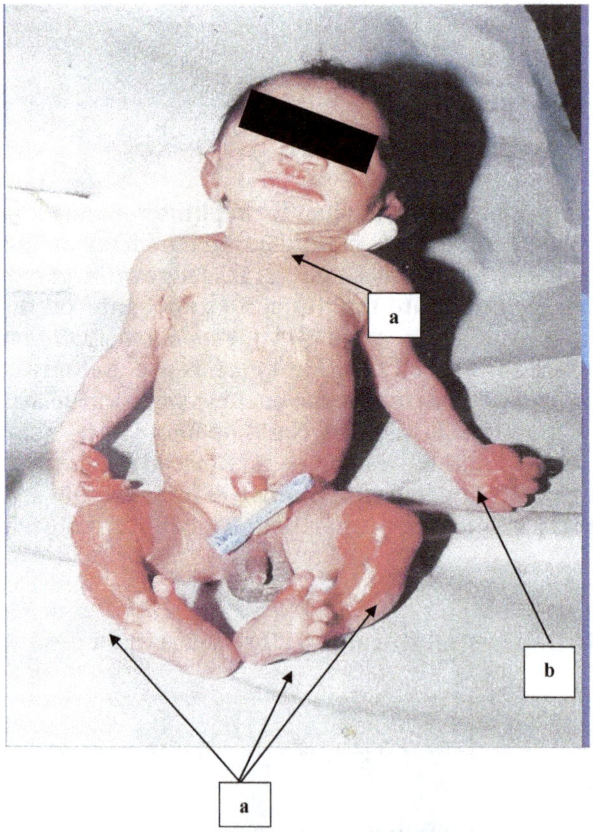

Figure 1. Illustration of a newborn suffering from cutaneo-mucous membrane lesions (Case 1): a) post-blistered sweating and b) Palmo-plantar desquamation.

spontaneous motility. Cardio-pulmonary auscultation was normal along with the all the remaining tests. The newborn was hospitalized.

Facing that severe neonatal infectious overall clinical picture, triple anti-biotherapy (ampicillin-cefotaxim-netilmicin) was prescribed, while awaiting bacteriological tests results.

Complementary tests results were the following: Leucocytes: 27,500 with 60% of polynuclear neutrophils; hemoglobin at 14 g/dL; platelets at 160,000/mm^3; C-reactive protein (CRP) dosage at 165 mg/L. Syphilitic serology of the baby was negative. Cutaneous lesions swabbing was negative especially with the absence of *Treponema pallidum*. Skeleton radiographs displayed metaphysary affection made of light bands predominant in lower limbs long bones, and the presence of metaphysary notches at both tibia upper-inner extremities, evocating a Wimberger positive syndrome (**Figure 2**).

A treatment made of Penicillin G was installed during ten days under the cover of a corticotherapy. The evolution was favorable with regression of the above-described clinical radiological signs.

2.2. Case 2

We dealt with a four weeks premature male newborn (34 WA). The pregnancy was unattended. No ultrasound has been performed. Syphilitic serology realized at the first trimester has shown negative TPHA and VDRL tests.

The delivery took place at home. The baby had cried immediately. APGAR score could not be determined. At birth, the baby presented harmonious intrauterine growth retardation with a body weight of 1500 gr, a size of 40 cm and a cranial perimeter of 29 cm. The clinical examination at birth showed a purulent conjunctivitis, hepatic overwhelming and a discreet incurvation of the four limbs mostly pronounced in the lower ones with decrease of spontaneous motility. All the remaining clinical tests were uninfluential, with absence of cutaneo-mucous membrane lesions.

The paraclinical check-up showed white blood cells rate at 25,000 with predominant polynuclear neutrophils, red blood cells at 3.3 × 10^6/mm^3; hemoglobin rate at 12.3 g/dL, platelets at 160,000/mm^3; The C-reative protein was at 145 mg/L and the syphilitic serology was positive (for both TPHA and VDRL).

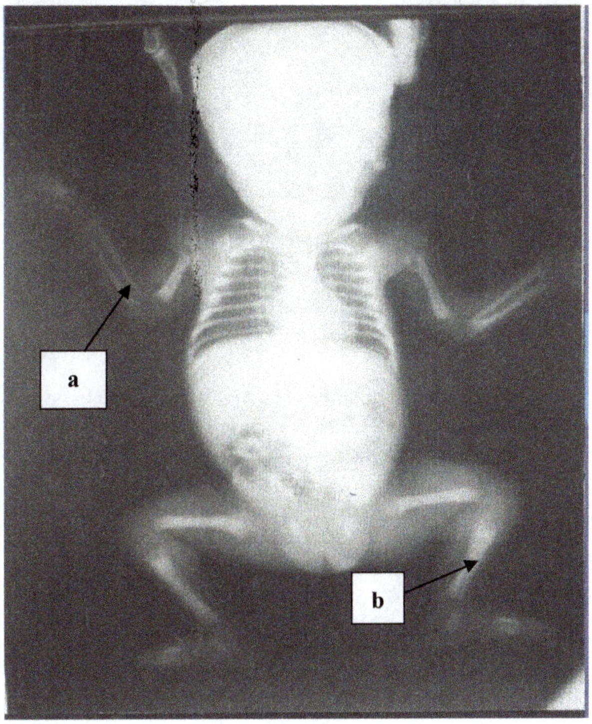

Figure 2. X-rays diagram displaying osteo-articular lesions (Case 1): The metaphysico-diaphysary affection appears easily (a and b).

Skeleton's X-rays showed predominant metaphyso-diaphysary affection in long bones with positive Wimberger test typical of syphilitic osteochondritis (**Figure 3**). The newborn was placed under antibiotics treatment based on penicillin G at the posology of 100,000 U/kg/day during ten days. The evolution was favorable.

2.3. Case 3

It was about a male baby born at the right term (39 WA). The pregnancy was mismanaged. The serology performed at the last trimester was positive at the TPHA and VDRL tests. The mother was not treated. The delivery occurred in a hospital. At birth, the baby was presenting signs of hypotrophy (weight: 2100 gr; size: 44 cm; and cranial perimeter of 31.3 cm). The clinical exam at birth was normal. The baby's syphilitic serology was positive (TPHA and VDRL, without any precision of mentioned titration). The radiography of skeleton was absolutely normal along with all the biological check-up.

Therapeutically management issues had come up while facing the absence of an irrefutable diagnosis. After discussion, a treatment based on penicillin G had been recommended following the posology of 100,000 U/kg/day during ten days. We lost the track of the newborn because the parents have checked-out without leaving no information or medical advice.

3. Discussion

Those three observations perfectly illustrated the difficulties encountered when it comes to deal with congenital syphilis diagnosis and came up with the problem of the therapeutically management (**Table 1**).

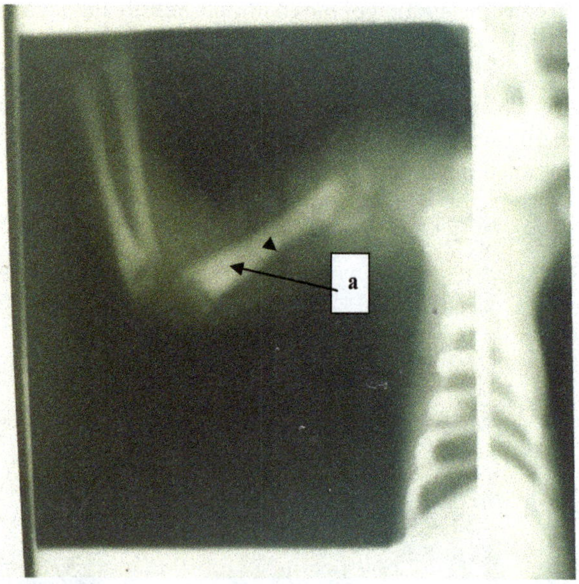

Figure 3. Right antero-brachial X-rays showing osteo-articular lesions (Case 2). The mataphysico-diapdysary affection (a) appears clearly.

Table 1. Summary of clinical information.

	Case 1	Case 2	Case 3
Mismanaged pregnancy	+	+	+
Maternal syphilis serology	+	-	+
Newborn	RCIU	RCIU	RCIU
Cutaneous lesions	+	-	-
HSMG	+	+	-
Bone lesions	+	+	-
Newborn syphilis serology	-	+	+
Conclusion	Congenital syphilis?	Congenital syphilis?	Congenital syphilis?

In fact, congenital syphilis remains a worrying form of syphilis [12]. Its increasing frequency is parallel to the recrudescence of adult primary and secondary syphilis. It is mostly evoked in cases of untreated or badly managed maternal syphilis. According to the World Health Organization (WHO), two millions of pregnant women are concerned by the illness every year, and only 17% undergo a serological check-up at the beginning of their pregnancy [13]. About 25% of pregnancies have a pathological evolution (in utero death, spontaneous abortion…), 60% of newborns are asymptomatic at birth, and 25% of those are underweighted. The agent responsible of the disease is a spirochete, the *Treponema pallidum* [14].

The fetus contamination is possible at any moment of the pregnancy but mostly after the fourth month (protector effect of Langherans' cells). That mother-to-child transmission is almost ranging from 70% up to 100% if the maternal syphilis is not treated; it is about 40% if it is precociously latent (<1 year), and it is about 10% if it is belatedly latent (>1 year) [15]-[17].

The diagnosis is not always easy. It is evoked while facing an untreated maternal positive syphilitic serology associated to cutaneous and bone lesions along with a hepatosplenomegaly at birth [5] [16] [18]. It can be suspected *in utero* by using ultrasound that displays non-specific signs such as hypotrophy, oligoamnios and other signs leading towards an infectious fetopathy such as fetal hydrops or the fetoplacental anasarca, microcephaly, hyperechogene intestine, hepatosplenomegaly and the increasing of placental thickness [15]. **Table 2** displays precocious congenital syphilis clinical signs frequencies registered by Chawla in Zimbabwe in 1986 [18].

The irrefutable diagnosis is based on the finding of the treponema by using immunofluorescent or black-tinted microscopy preparations of placental or cutaneo-mucous membrane lesions along with serological tests [3] [15] [19] [20]. Placental histological affection by treponema corresponds to a villus hypertrophy, an obturating endovascular proliferation or an acute or chronic villus inflammation. Those lesions are not specific, but their association strongly suggests the diagnosis [21] [22].

However, that direct test has a low output for multiple reasons (local or general antibiotics treatment previously applied, bad smear test, inconsistent lesions) and is almost no longer used [23]. Serological tests, currently used are divided in two groups: non-treponemic tests (Venereal Disease Research Laboratory) and treponemic tests (*Treponema Pallidum* Haemagglutination Assay along with the Fluorescent Treponemal Assay) [24]. The VDRL uses a cardiolipidic antigen. Based on a single sampling, it does not allow reaching a conclusion between a progressive syphilis and a passive crossing of maternal antibodies. Meanwhile, a rate four-time superior to that of the mother in the newborn is likely in favor of the infection. The TPHA test uses a treponemic antigen and is more specific than the VDRL test. When they are combined, VDRL and TPHA have a good sensitivity, but still under that of immunofluorescence.

The FTA-abs-IgM is a highly sensitive method but it is costly and difficult to realize. It is based on a serological reaction between inactive treponema and specific seral IgM. The method helps to confirm the diagnosis of congenital syphilis.

Table 2. Frequency of congenital syphilis clinical signs registered in Zimbabwe (Chawla *et al.*, 1986).

	Number of cases	Percentage (%)
Low weight at birth	41	77
Hepatomegaly	28	53
Splenomegaly	27	51
Hepatosplenomegaly	26	49
Icterus	25	47
Cutaneous lesions	20	38
Thrombopeny	12	38
Respiratory failure	10	19
Anasarca	3	6
Pseudo paralysis	2	4
Coryza	2	4
Anemia[a]	16	50

a. Blood formula numerations could be performed only for 32 newborns.

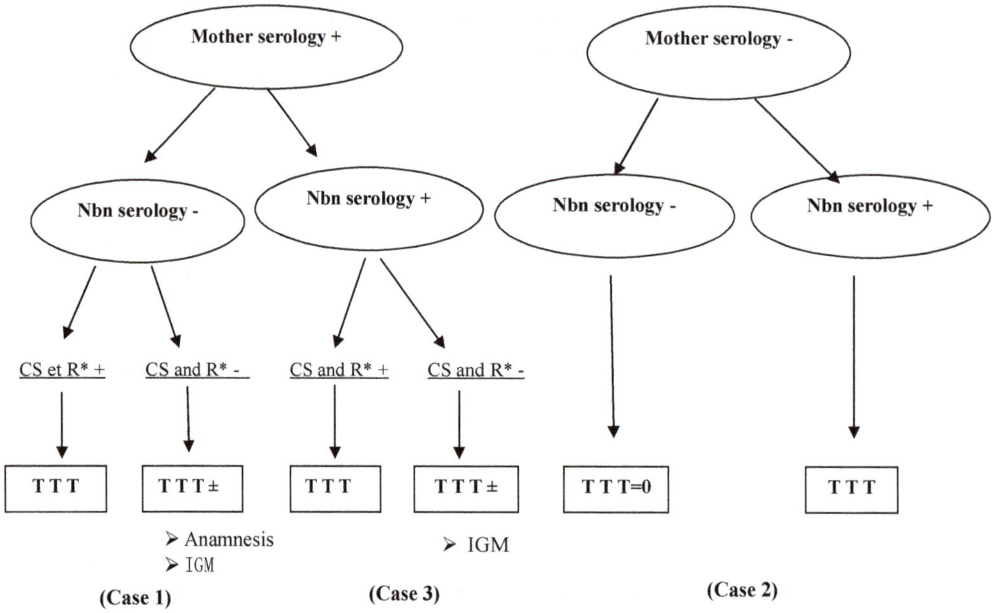

Figure 4. Congenital syphilis medical management's Algorithm. Abbreviations list: Nbn: newborn; CS: clinical signs; R*: Rx; TTT: treatment; IGM: immunoglobulins.

In addition, antibodies (IgG) could be searched in the cebrospinal fluid (CSF) by using immunofluorescence reaction (FTA-abs) or TPHA reaction. That research does not allow differentiating between central nervous system affection and simple antibodies passing if cytology and CSF chemistry are normal. Searching IgM in the CSF is possible, but it is technically difficult to realize in routine. When it is positive, it asserts central affection, but it does not elude the diagnosis.

In industrialized countries, other techniques such as the polymerase chain reaction (PCR) are realized on amniotic liquid sampling, placenta or umbilical chord, and using the solid phase hemabsorption assay (SPHA) by dosage of IgM through immunocaptation on blood and CSF sampling. The results are good.

Those three clinical observations demonstrate the difficulties of congenital syphilis diagnosis in our country wherein only the TPHA and VDRL tests are available. In fact, both tests can be negative at the precocious stage of syphilis or in case of zonal phenomenon (false negative due to excessive antibodies). In that case, it is better to dilute the serum in order to get the positive reaction (Case 1) [25]. In addition, maternal antibodies can be found in the newborn blood, even if it is uncontaminated when the mother is treated at the beginning of the pregnancy. Those antibodies are decreasing during the first year. Conversely, the child may have been contaminated lately (eighth month of pregnancy for example) while the tests were negative at the third month of pregnancy. Serological reactions may in this case be negative at birth and become positive later (Case 3) [26] [27].

In addition, congenital syphilis may be asymptomatic or paucisymptomatic in one third of case, but generally signs appear before the second month after birth (Case 2) [28]. In this case, bone lesions which are found in 80% of congenital syphilis are uplifting either alone or associated to cutaneous forms and they must rule out other congenital affections such as rubella, hyperparathyroidism, hemoglobinopathies, septicemias, neonatal leukemia, Silverman or Ambroise Tardieu syndrome (termed "Beaten children Disease") [29].

In the second clinical observation, we did the penicillin test and the clinical status along with radiological signs has improved markedly. This treatment can be combined with corticosteroids to prevent Herxheimer reaction due to the sudden lysis of treponemas. The Anglo-Saxons immediately use high doses of penicillin G 50,000 - 100,000 U/kg by intramuscular or intravenous way for 15 to 20 days [18]. Benzathine Penicillin in the dosage of 50,000 U/kg by IM injection is reserved for newborns at risk of clinical signs who are asymptomatic [1] [30] [31].

In our study, all three patients were treated with penicillin G at a dose of 100,000 U/kg/day or two infusions of 50,000 U/kg per day for a period of 10 days associated with corticosteroid treatment 2 mg/kg/d, despite the lack of diagnostic certainty in the third case. We have not used Benzathine Penicillin. The outcome was favorable in the first two cases and the third patient on treatment was lost.

This study shows the difficulty that may arise in the diagnosis of congenital syphilis especially in our situation where we cannot do efficiently all syphilis serology. In this case, the overall clinical study, maternal history and syphilis serology of the mother and child determine the therapeutic management hence our proposed scheme that we termed congenital syphilis medical management's Algorithm (**Figure 4**) takes into account maternal syphilis serology, clinical status and child syphilis serology.

4. Conclusion

The congenital syphilis still exists in Gabon. Its diagnosis must be evoked based on irrefutable clinical and radiological signs and, if there is any subsisting doubt serology and bacteriological sampling should be performed on both mother and newborn. Thus, it is utterly important to detect maternal syphilis during pregnancy, which would allow a simultaneous treatment of both the mother and the fetus.

References

[1] Walker, D.G. and Walker, G.J. (2002) Forgotten but Not Gone: The Continuing Scourse of Congenital Syphilis. *Lancet Infect Disease*, **7**, 433-436.

[2] Hoareau, C., Ranivoharimina, V., Chavet-Quéru, M.S., *et al.* (1999) Syphilis Congénitale. Mise au Point et Perspectives. *Cahiers*, **9**, 38-45.

[3] Morshed, M.G. (2014) Current Trend on Syphilis Diagnosis: Issues and Challenges. *Advances in Experimental Me- dicine and Biology*, **808**, 51-64.

[4] Araùjo, M.A., de Freita, S.C., de Moura, H.J., *et al.* (2013) Prevalence and Factors Associated with Syphilis in Parturient Woman in Northeast, Brazil. *BMC Public Health*, **13**, 206.

[5] Gupta, R. and Vora, R.V. (2013) Congenital Syphilis, Still a Reality. *Indian Journal of Sex Transm Disease*, **34**, 50-52.

[6] Dobson, S. (2004) Congenital Syphilis Resurgent. *Advances in Experimental Medicine and Biology*, **549**, 35-40.

[7] Su, J.R., Berman, S.M., Davis, D., *et al.* (2010) Centers for Disease Control and Prevention (CDC). Congenital Syphilis-United States, 2003-2008. *MMWR Morbidity and Mortality Weekly Report*, **59**, 413-417.

[8] Hussey, J., Mitchell, L., Hew, Y., *et al.* (2013) Preventing Congenital Syphilis—A Regional Audit of Syphilis in Pregnant Women Seen in Genitourinary Medecine Services. *International Journal of STD AIDS*, **2013**, 27.

[9] Qin, J.B., Feng, T.J., Yang, T.B., *et al.* (2014) Risk Factors for Congenital Syphilis and Adverse Pregnancy Outcomes in Offspring of Women with Syphilis in Shenzen, China: A Prospective Nested Case-Control Study. *Sex Transm Disease*, **41**, 13-23.

[10] Aplogan Ongotha, D.J.C. (2001) Santé de la mère et de l'enfant. Enquête démographique et de santé Gabon 2000: Direction Générale de la Statistique et des Etudes Economiques-Fonds des Nations Unis pour la Population-ORC Macro.

[11] Carles, G., Lochet, S., Youssef, M., *et al.* (2008) Syphilis et grossesse. Etude de 85 cas en Guyane française. *Journal of Obstetrics & Gynecology and Reproductive Biology*, **37**, 353-357.

[12] Simms, I. and Broulet, N. (2008) Congenital Syphilis Reemerging. *Journal of Dtsch*, **6**, 269-272.

[13] Organisation mondiale de la santé (OMS) (2009) L'élimination mondiale de la syphilis congénitale: Raison et stratégie 2009. OMS, Genève, 48.

[14] Chaudhary, M., Kashyap, B. and Bhalla, P. (2007) Congenital Syphilis, Still a Reality in 21st Century: A Case Report. *Journal of Medical Case Reports*, **1**, 90.

[15] Narducci, F., Switala, I., Rajabally, R., *et al.* (1998) Syphilis maternelle et congénitale. *Journal of Obstetrics & Gynecology and Reproductive Biology*, **27**, 150-160.

[16] Stoll, B. (1994) Congenital Syphilis: Evaluation and Management of Neonates Born to Mothers with Reactive Serologic Test for Syphilis. *Pediatric Infectious Disease Journal*, **13**, 845-853. http://dx.doi.org/10.1097/00006454-199410000-00001

[17] Gomez, G.B., Kamb, M.L., Newman, L.M., *et al.* (2013) Untread Maternel Syphilis and Adverse Outcomes of Pregnancy: A Systematic Review and Meta-Analysis. *Bull World Health Organ*, **91**, 217-226. http://dx.doi.org/10.2471/BLT.12.107623

[18] Patterson, M.J. and Davies, H.D. (2011) Syphilis (*Treponema pallidum*). In: Kliegman, R.M., Behrman, R.E., Jenson, H.B. and Stanton, B.F., Eds., *Nelson Textbook of Pediatrics*, Chap. 210, 19th Edition, Saunders Elsevier, Philadelphia.

[19] Chwala, V., Bandit, P.B. and Nkrumah, F.K. (1989) Congenital Syphilis in the Newborn. *Archives of Disease in Childhood*, **143**, 916-921.

[20] Maleville, J., Larregue, M. and Ball, M. (1991) Les divers aspects de la syphilis congénitale. *Bulletin of the Exotic*

Pathology Society, **84**, 609-613.

[21] Genest, D.R., Choi-Hong, S.R., Tate, J.E., *et al.* (1996) Diagnosis of Congenital Syphilis from Placental Examination: Comparison of Histopathology, Steiner Stain, and Polymerase Chain Reaction for *Treponema pallidum* DNA. *Human Pathology*, **27**, 366-372. http://dx.doi.org/10.1016/S0046-8177(96)90110-0

[22] Walker, D.G. and Walker, G.J. (2002) Forgotten but Not Gone: The Continuing Scourge of Congenital Syphilis. *The Lancet Infectious Diseases*, **2**, 432-436. http://dx.doi.org/10.1016/S1473-3099(02)00319-5

[23] Ray, J.G. (1995) Lues-Lues: Maternel and Fetal Considerations of Syphilis. *Obstetrical & Gynecological Survey*, **50**, 845-849. http://dx.doi.org/10.1097/00006254-199512000-00003

[24] Basse-Guerineau, A.L. and Assous, M.V. (2004) Syphilis: Les sérologies d'interprétation délicate. *La revue du praticien*, **54**, 387-391.

[25] Jurado, P.D.R., Campbell, J. and Martin, P.D. (1993) Prozone Phenomenon in Secondary Syphilis. Has Its Time Arrived? *Archives of Internal Medicine*, **153**, 2496-2498. http://dx.doi.org/10.1001/archinte.1993.00410210124014

[26] Herremans, T., Kortbeek, L. and Notermans, D.W. (2010) A Review of Diagnostic Tests for Congenital Syphilis in Newborns. *European Journal of Clinical Microbiology & Infectious Diseases*, **29**, 495-501. http://dx.doi.org/10.1007/s10096-010-0900-8

[27] Peterman, T.A., Newman, D.R., Davis, D. and Su, J.R. (2013) Do Women with Persistently Negative Nontreponemal Test Results Transmit Syphilis during Pregnancy? *Sexually Transmitted Diseases*, **40**, 311-315. http://dx.doi.org/10.1097/OLQ.0b013e318285c5a7

[28] Gendrel, D., Moussavou, A., Engohan, E., *et al.* (1987) Syphilis congenitale paucisymptomatique et automedication pendant la grossesse. *Médecine d'Afrique Noire*, **34**, 11-13.

[29] Ghadouane, M., Benjelloun, B.S. and Elharim-Roudies, L. (1995) L'atteinte osseuse de la syphilis congénitale précoce (à propos de 86 cas). *REVUE DU RHUMATISME*, **62**, 457-461.

[30] Paryani, S.G., Vaughan, A.J., Crosby, M. and Lawrence, S. (1994) Treatment of Asymptomatic Congenital Syphilis: Benzathine versus Procaine Penicillin G Therapy. *The Journal of Pediatrics*, **125**, 471-475. http://dx.doi.org/10.1016/S0022-3476(05)83300-1

[31] Lakdar, I.M., Ismaili, L. and Bouharrou, A. (2011) La syphilis congénitale révélée par une fracture spontanée. *The Pan African Medical Journal*, **10**, 42-47.

2

Follow-Up Profile and Outcome of Preterms Managed with Kangaroo Mother Care

Wubishet Lakew[1], Bogale Worku[2]

[1]Department of Pediatrics and Child Health, University of Gondar, Gondar, Ethiopia
[2]Department of Pediatrics and Child Health, Addis Ababa University Medical Faculty, Addis Ababa, Ethiopia
Email: wubishet@gmail.com

Abstract

Background: Kangaroo mother care (KMC) is effective in preventing hypothermia, establishing breastfeeding, and reducing nosocomial infection in preterm babies in resource-limited areas. Relatively little is known about long-term morbidity and mortality outcomes among Ethiopian infants managed with KMC. Aims: To describe the follow up profiles and outcome of infants managed with KMC and discharged alive. Methods: This cross-sectional descriptive study examined outcomes among infants who were 1) managed by KMC at Black Lion Hospital, 2) discharged alive, and 3) available for follow-up. Structured, pretested questionnaires were administered to mothers. Results: Of the 110 infants included in the study, 9.1% died over the study period and 60% of the deaths occurred at home. Mortality was 100% in those babies with mothers aged less than 18 years. Thirty five percent of the deaths occurred in those from rural location. Common medical problems identified in study subjects were respiratory infections (10%), gastroenteritis (7%), rickets (7%), and anemia (6%). About 20% of infants were readmitted to hospital at least once. KMC initiation within one week was not found to be significantly associated with survival, but continued KMC after discharge significantly decreased mortality in our sample. Conclusion: Frequent follow up is very important especially those with teenage mothers and coming from a rural location. Follow up should be frequent in the first 2 months after discharge. Further research is needed to explore the determinants of mortality and morbidity after hospital discharge.

Keywords

Preterm, Very Low Birth Weight, Kangaroo Mother Care, Follow Up Profile

1. Introduction

Survival among neonates is directly related to birth weight, with approximately 20% surviving among those between 500 and 600 g and 90% among those between 1250 and 1500 g. In the US, where life-support technology is readily available, VLBW infants account for >50% of neonatal deaths and 50% of disabled infants [1]. A study done in hospital setting in Ethiopia showed 32.8% mortality for low birth weight infants and many had hypothermia as a related cause of death [2]. Considering the high mortality related to hypothermia and prematurity, KMC is started as a way of reducing low birth weight mortality in black lion hospital. KMC is one of the interventions proven to be a safe alternative to conventional neonatal care in resource-limited settings [3]. However, little is known about long-term outcomes.

KMC is a package of care including skin-to-skin contact, exclusive breastfeeding, support to the mother child dyad, and avoiding mother-child separation [4]. Some centers also include early discharge in the definition but this approach is only warranted where good community support can be guaranteed. These activities are important to the medical, emotional, psychological, and physical well being of both the mother and the child [5] [6].

Black lion specialized general hospital is a tertiary level referral and teaching hospital which delivers comprehensive care to sick neonates. It has a 40-bed neonatal and 10 bed KMC unit. All preterm neonates weighing <1500 grams born in black lion hospital or in other district hospitals will be sent to KMC unit. KMC consisted of skin-to-skin contact on the mother's chest 24 hours/day, nearly exclusive breastfeeding, and early discharge, with close ambulatory monitoring.

The neonates are discharged once they are able to breast feed and show persistent increment in weight for 3 consecutive days. During discharge process, address and important data will be entered into a computer and appointment will be given to high-risk infant clinic at the same hospital.

Little research has explored how KMC affects the health and well being of infants after discharge from hospital. This study will assess the clinical condition, follow up profile and determinants of morbidity and mortality of infants treated with KMC and discharged alive from Black lion specialized hospital neonatal unit.

2. Methods

A descriptive cross sectional study was conducted. Children treated with KMC at Black Lion hospital from July 2009 to May 2010 and discharged alive were included in the study. We had managed 140 VLBW neonates in the neonatal unit through the study period. The neonates were referred from black lion maternity unit and other hospitals and health centers. Twelve neonates died before discharged from KMC. About 128 VLBW neonates were discharged alive. We were able to contact and retrieve 110 neonates who were discharged alive from the hospital. Eighteen children whose caretakers were not willing to come to the follow up clinic, or not willing to participate in the study were excluded.

Data about live infants were collected by using an interview based questionnaire and physical examination. Information about weight at KMC initiation, duration of KMC, and address, were extracted from a computerized registry and patient charts. Parents who were not bringing their children for follow up were contacted by phone and follow up was arranged. Senior paediatrician interviewed mothers at high-risk infant clinic after verbal consent was obtained. Parents of the study subjects were asked about and evaluated for presence of medical problems, history of health institution visit, type of feeding, and hospital admission. Delay in KMC initiation was calculated from the time of hospital admission to the first date of KMC. Type of feeding practiced during hospital admission and discharge was analyzed in relation to medical problems encountered during the study. Sick children who came to the follow up clinic at the time of the study were treated.

Parents whose infants had died were interviewed by phone after verbal consent was taken. Data were collected by a structured verbal autopsy questionnaire. Demographics, clinical problems and presumed causes of death as described by the parents are mentioned.

Data were processed with a Statistical package SPSS version 16 (SPSS Inc., 233 South Wacker Drive, 11th Floor, Chicago, IL 60606-6412). Measures of central tendency and dispersion with graphical presentation of data were used for summarising descriptive findings. Statistical associations between different variables and outcome were checked using chi-square and fisher's exact tests. A p-value of 5% was used for the statistical analyses used in this study.

Ethical clearance was obtained from department of Pediatrics and child health research and publication committee and from Addis Ababa University Medical Faculty, Institution Review Board, Addis Ababa, Ethiopia.

3. Results

A total of 110 infants and toddlers were included in this study. 57 (51.8%) study subjects were females. The mean age at evaluation was 12.4 months with a standard deviation of 7.1. 96 (87.3%) study subjects lived in urban areas. 101 (92%) mothers were between 18 and 35 years of age. 3.6% of infants had mothers aged less than 18 years.

Spontaneous vaginal delivery accounted for 52.7% of the cases. The rest were delivered either by assisted vaginal delivery or caesarean section. Most of the babies were delivered at between gestational ages of 32 - 36 weeks (51%). The mean birth weight of the study subjects was 1336.2 grams with standard deviation (SD) of 211.5 grams. The mean duration of KMC given in the neonatal ward was 14 days with standard deviation (SD) 9. The mean delay in initiation of kangaroo mother care was 11 days.

KMC was continued at home for an average of 2 weeks in 83.6% of infants. Out of 110 infants, only 79 (71.8%) returned back to the follow up clinic at least once. The continuation of KMC after discharge was associated with reduced mortality (6.5% vs. 23.5%, P = 0.046) (**Table 1**). Non-significant increases in mortality were noted among children that failed to follow-up after discharge. After discharge, 12.7% of them were on exclusive breast-feeding, 15.5% on formula feeding, 34.5% on mixed feeding and 37.3% were on family diet. Age appropriate feeding was seen only in 40% of infants.

Out of 110 infants, 36.4% had a history of unscheduled hospital visit, and 20% have history of hospital admissions. The most common medical problems encountered in live infants during the study were respiratory infections (10%), rickets (7%), gastroenteritis (7%), anaemia (6%) and other problems account for 14% of the study subjects (**Table 2**).

Nine percent of the study subjects died. No difference in deaths existed between sexes (5 vs. 5, P = 0.090). Mortality after discharge was 100% in infants whose mothers were aged less than 18 years (4, P = 0.01). Mortality was found to be high (90%) within the first 2 months of age, which abruptly decrease after the age of 4 months. Out of the 10 deaths encountered, 60% of them were witnessed at home while the rest have died in health institutions. Higher percentage of deaths (35.7%) was encountered in those living in rural areas.

Respiratory problems were mentioned as possible causes of death by caretakers in 6 (60%) of the cases while sudden unexpected death in 3 (30%) of them. Mortality rates have shown to be higher in infants who were on feeding other than exclusive breastfeeding at discharge (OR 5.7, CI 1.05, 41.5. P = 0.02) (**Table 3**).

4. Discussion

The demographics of our population were comparable to those described in the African literature. Since our

Table 1. KMC continued at home and outcome during follow up of neonates who were admitted, managed with KMC, and discharged alive from Black lion specialized general hospital, neonatal unit from July 2008 and May 2010 G.C. (OR = 4.462, CI = 1.108 to 17.965, P = 0.046).

	Died during follow up period
KMC continued at home	6/93 (6.5%)
KMC not continued at home	4/17 (23.5%)
Total	10/110 (9.1%)

Table 2. Table showing type of feeding at discharge versus medical problems identified during the study of neonates who were admitted, managed with KMC, and discharged alive from black lion specialized general hospital neonatal unit from July 2009 and May 2011 G.C. (This table excludes dead subjects).

Types of medical problems	Number of patients	Percentage
Gastroenteritis	7	7%
Respiratory problems	10	10%
Anaemia	6	6%
Rickets	7	7%
Others	14	14%
No problems documented or reported	56	56%

Table 3. Table showing type of feeding at discharge of neonates who were admitted, managed with KMC, and discharged alive from black lion specialized general hospital neonatal unit from July 2009 and May 2011 G.C. (OR 5.7, CI 1.05, 41.5, P = 0.02).

Type of feeding at discharge	Died during follow-up period
Breastfed	2/61 (3.3%)
Formula fed or mixed	8/49 (16.3%)
Total	10/110 (9.1%)

hospital is located in the centre of a city, however, most of our patients originated from urban or per-urban areas.

Almost 84% of infants in our study continued KMC at home, and those that continued KMC were more likely to survive. Our study adds to the fact that KMC is still very important intervention survival after discharge in the low-income country setting. A longitudinal study done in Kumasi, Ghana showed that infants who were on either continuous or intermittent KMC at home showed an optimal increase in weight [7]. There is lack of adequate researches to compare our findings and see how KMC affects infants when it is done at home.

Our study described the common medical problems encountered after hospital discharge. Respiratory infections, rickets, gastroenteritis, anaemia were identified as main medical problems in these infants. Other problems like central nervous system disorders, surgical problems, and congenital heart diseases were also seen in the study subjects.

We have also shown that rickets was one of the problems encountered in these infants. To our knowledge this association has not been reported elsewhere in the literature concerning infants managed with KMC. The result in our study could be low because of missed-diagnosis, higher age range of the study subjects and lack of other diagnostic modalities like radiography. Rickets at a very early age is less likely to be associated with lack of sunlight exposure and subsequent Vitamin D deficiency. When premature babies are fed human milk, the supply of both calcium and phosphorus is low, but the critical factor leading to rickets is the lack of phosphorus. Serum phosphate levels decrease and there is not enough substrate for incorporation into the organic bone matrix [8].

This study also examined the rate of hospital visits and re-admissions. LBW infants have high risk of readmission shortly after discharge mainly related to the underlying medical problems they have. In a study done in Zimbabwe, rate of hospital readmission in infants who had been managed and discharged after KMC is 22.9%, which is comparable to our finding [8].

Nine percent of infants in our study died after discharge, and most deaths occurred at home. Careful follow up of infants born to mothers form a rural area and those born to teenage mothers should be prioritized.

There are several limitations in this study. The generalizability of the study may be affected as many study subjects were from Addis Ababa, the capital city of Ethiopia. In Addis Ababa, health care service is better accessed than other regions. We also have a lower sample size to do some statistical analysis like logistic regression. Further research with a larger sample size may allow for such calculations.

5. Conclusion and Recommendation

Among infants discharged from our hospital that have received KMC, 9.1% died before 2 years of age. Teenage mothers, rural origin, and lack of KMC continuation were associated with death. Particularly high rates of respiratory infection, gastroenteritis, rickets, and anemia were appreciated over a period of follow up. We recommend frequent follow up for babies after discharge from our center, especially those with teenage mothers. Further researches like case control studies are needed to explore the determinants of mortality and morbidity after hospital discharge.

Authors' Contribution

Wubishet Lakew was involved in all phases of the study and BogaleWorku was involved in supervision and data cleaning.

WubishetLakew, MD is an assistant professor of pediatrics at University of Gondar and Bogale Worku, MD is a professor of Pediatrics at Addis Ababa University Medical faculty.

Acknowledgements

We would like to thank the study participants and family for their cooperation. We also want to acknowledge the support and cooperation of the staffs at Addis Ababa University Medical faculty neonatal unit. We also want to thank Dr David Gordon and Dr Getahun Asres for their important comments about the data analysis.

References

[1] Barbara, J. (2004) Overview of Morbidity and Mortality. In: Kliegman, Behrman, Jensen and Stanton, Eds., *Nelson Textbook of Pediatrics*, Elsevier, New York, 550-558.

[2] Bogale, W. (1999) The Low Birth Weight Infant in the Ethio-Swedish Children's Hospital, Addis Ababa. *Ethiopian Medical Journal*, **37**, 111-119.

[3] Conde-Agudelo, A., Belizán, J.M. and Diaz-Rossello, J. (2011) Kangaroo Mother Care to Reduce Morbidity and Mortality in Low Birthweight Infants. John Wiley & Sons, Ltd. http://dx.doi.org/10.1002/14651858.CD002771.pub2

[4] Charpak, N., Riuz, J.G. and Zupan, J. (2005) Kangaroo Mother Care: 25 Years after. *Acta Pediatrica*, **94**, 514-522. http://dx.doi.org/10.1080/08035250510027381

[5] Tessier, R., Cristo, M., Velez, S., Girón, M., de Calume, Z.F. and Ruiz-Paláez (1998) Kangaroo Mother Care and the Bonding Hypothesis. *Pediatrics*, **102**, e17-e17. http://dx.doi.org/10.1542/peds.102.2.e17

[6] Ludington-Hoe, S.M., Ferreira, C.N. and Goldstein, M.R. (1999) Kangaroo Care with a Ventilated Preterm Infant. *Acta Paediatrica*, **87**, 711-771. http://dx.doi.org/10.1111/j.1651-2227.1998.tb01539.x

[7] Nguah, S.B., Wobil, P.N., Obeng, R., Yakubu, A., Kerber, K.J. and Lawn, J.E. (2011) Perception and Practice of Kangaroo Mother Care after Discharge from Hospital in Kumasi, Ghana. *BMC Pregnancy Childbirth*, **11**, 99. http://dx.doi.org/10.1186/1471-2393-11-99

[8] Rauch, F. and Schoenau, E. (2002) Skeletal Development in Premature Infants. *A Review of Bone Physiology beyond Nutritional Aspects. Archives of Diseases in Childhood Fetal and Neonatal Edition*, **86**, F82-F85. http://dx.doi.org/10.1136/fn.86.2.F82

[9] Kambarami, R.A., Chidede, O. and Pereira, N. (2003) Long-Term Outcome of Preterm Infants Discharged Home on Kangaroo Care in a Developing Country. *Annals of Tropical Paediatrics*, **23**, 55-59. http://dx.doi.org/10.1179/000349803125002931

3

Alcohol Drinking Habits and Negative Experiences among Adolescents in Greece

Konstantinos Tsoumakas[1], Marsela Tanaka[1], Konstantinos Petsios[1], Georgios Fildisis[1], Athanasios Gkoutzivelakis[2], Ioanna Pavlopoulou[1]

[1]Faculty of Nursing, National and Kapodistrian University of Athens, Athens, Greece
[2]University General Hospital of Alexandroupoli, Alexandroupoli, Greece
Email: mtanaka@nurs.uoa.gr

Abstract

Introduction: Alcohol use during adolescence remains a prominent public health problem with short- and long-term consequences. The study aims at investigating the epidemiological characteristics of alcohol use among Greek adolescents. Important parallel aims were to identify alcohol-related problems and its consequences experienced by the adolescence. Methods: The study population was a convenience sample of 1100 students of secondary education (junior and senior high school) from 12 public and private schools in Athens. 573 boys and 527 girls aged 12 to 19 years old [mean age 15.3 (±1.7)] answered a specially structured anonymous questionnaire. Results: Recent alcohol consumption was reported by more than the half of students (57.3%) and was more prevalent among adolescents over 15 years old (67.3%) and among boys (59.3%). Beer was the most popular type of alcoholic beverage (65.9%) at all ages. On average, both males and females stated the onset of alcohol at the age of 12 years. Boys reported being drunk more often than girls (25.7% versus 14.9%). However, more girls reported being drunk at least once a year than boys (27.1% versus 17.6%). The vast majority of the participants stated that they were informed about the possible addiction to alcohol (86.2%) and its negative consequences. A statistically significant correlation was found between age and hangover ($p < 0.001$). Conclusion: Alcohol consumption remains a serious problem among adolescents. There is a need to implement preventive measures and counseling approaches in school. The study will contribute to the public awareness concerning adolescent's drinking behavior in Greece.

Keywords

Adolescents, Alcohol, Epidemiology, Characteristics, Consequences

1. Introduction

Adolescents' alcohol consumption is an international phenomenon, related to the health and welfare of population that has shown a small but continuous increase during the last decade and is associated with many health risks and social problems [1]-[3]. Alcohol still remains the most widely used substance among adolescents [4]-[7], exceeding the use of tobacco and illicit drugs. However, alcohol consumption and its consequences may differ significantly between countries [1] [8]. European Union (EU) is the region with the highest alcohol consumption in the world, since 87% of the European adolescents have drunk alcohol at least once during their lifetime, in addition to 70.8% of the American adolescents [3] [9] [10].

A number of recent studies have linked early alcohol use to various problems, not only due to the immediate consequences of intoxication and its possible somatic complications, but also due to long-term developmental and well-being consequences [1] [11]-[13]. Even low consumption is associated with greater risk for accidents and injuries, violent behavior, use of psychotropic drugs, tobacco use and risky behavior including unsafe sex [13]-[17]. Literature suggests three types of influence on adolescent alcohol use: social (parental characteristics, family model, parenting style and parental status), attitudinal (culture, general values, media influence, school environment and peers' drinking habits) and intrapersonal (personal traits, biological dispositions and emotional instability) [18]-[20]. Younger age at initiation of alcohol use and younger age at first intoxication are strong predictors of later alcohol abuse and are associated with higher risk of alcohol-related injuries [21]-[23]. Moreover, adolescence is the period when lifestyles and habits develop and future attitudes are established [24]. Interestingly, the age of first alcohol consumption has decreased during last decade in both genders [25].

Levels of alcohol use change over time, only studies that compare the adolescents of different ages at a single point in time can assess age and trends. According to a recent report of the European School Survey Project on Alcohol and Other Drugs (ESPAD), Greece holds one of the highest rates concerning adolescents' alcohol use among other European countries [26].

The main aim of this study was to investigate the epidemiological characteristics of alcohol use among Greek adolescents. Important parallel aims were to identify alcohol-related problems and its consequences experienced by the adolescence.

2. Methodology

The study population was a convenience sample of 1100 students of secondary education (junior and senior high school) from public and private schools in Athens. The sample was selected from 5 representative geographical area of Attica. In particular, we randomly selected 10 public and two private schools from official list of schools. The study was approved by the Committee on Health Promotion of the Ministry of National Education and Religions. Parents were informed by a letter sent in advance of the survey, asked to give consent for researchers to contact their children, and then the students provided verbal assent. Confidentiality and anonymity were assured.

2.1. Data Collection

Data collection was performed via a 20-item structured, multiple-choice questionnaire. This was the main tool for our study and was constructed based on literature and authors' clinical expertise. More specifically, the questionnaire included questions concerning alcohol consumption habits, high-risk drinking, drunkenness, experienced alcohol-related problems, negative consequences that had experienced after or under alcohol use, along with questions concerning parental smoking and drinking habits as well as supplementary socio-demographic data. Moreover, a pilot test was performed in a sample from two public schools in advance of the study.

The questionnaires were distributed during the school year 2010-2011, with the knowledge and support of the responsible officers of the schools and distributed in each classroom by a member of the research team. The forms were handed to each student, were asked to complete them in 20 - 25 minutes and to return them. Teachers were allowed to stay in the classroom during the completion of the form. To preserve a rigorously anonymous management of the data, while keeping the link with individual information collected on subsequent surveys, the questionnaires were labeled with an 8-digit individual code generated by the student.

2.2. Statistics

Absolute and relative frequencies were used to describe qualitative variables. The average values (mean) and standard deviations (SD) were used to describe quantitative variables. The proportions were compared using the chi-square (×2) test or Fisher's exact test. The Benforri correction was used to control the Type I error and the significance level was set at 0.05/k (k = number of comparisons). Adjusted odds ratios (OR) 95% confidence intervals (95% CI) were computed from the results of the logistic regression analyses. For the analysis, the statistical software SPSS was used (Version 17.0).

2.3. Glossary

1) *Recent alcohol consumption*: Drinking alcohol at least once during the past 30 days before the study; 2) *Systematic or regular drinking*: 6 - 35 times during the past 30 days before the study; 3) *Early alcohol use*: Drinking alcohol before the age of 12 years old; 4) *Lifetime alcohol use*: Drinking alcohol at least once during their lifetime; 5) *Heavy episodic drinking*: Having five or more drinks on one occasion.

3. Results

A total of 1100 students (573 boys and 527 girls) from private and public schools with a mean age of 15.3 (±1.7) participated the study. On average, both males and females stated onset of alcohol at the age of 12 years old. 239 boys (41.7%) and 108 girls (20.4%) reported systematic drinking. A total of 97 (13.7%) reported intoxication during the past 30 days. The mean age of the parents was 43.2 years and more than the half were highly educated (49.7% of mothers and 52.8% of fathers). Systematic use of alcohol (20.6% - 36.6%) was stated by both parents along with active smoking (39.3% - 49.3%). Recent alcohol consumption was reported by more than the half of students (57.3%). It was more prevalent among students over 15 years old (67.3%) and among boys than girls (59.3% versus 55.4%). Beer was the most popular type of alcoholic beverage (65.9%) consumed among all age groups followed by wine (61.3%) and spirits (49.5%), with a statistical significant prevalence especially in adolescents over 15 years old.

The participants stated their preference to drink with friends at home (29.3%), during parties (34.3%) or in night clubs (30.0%), rather than alone (6.4%). In addition, pleasure was the main reason for drinking alcohol (79.1%), whereas sensation/novelty seeking (9.9%), peers impression (4.3%) or drinking as a coping strategy for emotional or family problems (6.7%), were less frequent reasons for alcohol use.

Among drinkers, 21.8% reported being drunk at least once during the past year prior to the study, 13.7% during the past 30 days prior to the study, and 5.9% of them more than once a week prior to the study. More boys than girls (25.7% versus 14.9%) reported being drunk once in two months or more often. By contrast, more girls than boys (27.1% versus 17.6%) reported being drunk at least once a year. The association between recent alcohol consumption, type of alcohol and frequency of drunkenness with age and sex is presented in **Table 1** and **Table 2**.

Table 1. Alcohol consumption among different age groups.

Alcohol Use Parameters		Age (yrs) 12 - 13 N		14 - 15 N		>15 N		p chi-square (χ^2) test
		N	%	N	%	N	%	
Recent[1] alcohol use	No	107	69.5	128	45.2	159	32.7	<0.001
	Yes	47	30.5	155	54.8	327	67.3	
Beer consumption during the past year	None or 1 - 3 times a year	156	76.8	205	59.2	253	45.9	<0.001
	>1 - 3 times a year	47	23.2	141	40.8	298	54.1	
Wine consumption during the past year	1 - 3 times a year	147	72.4	212	61.3	265	48.1	<0.001
	>1 - 3 times a year	56	27.6	134	38.7	286	51.9	
Spirits consumption during the past year	1 - 3 times a year	169	83.3	259	74.9	284	51.5	<0.001
	>1 - 3 times a year	34	16.7	87	25.1	267	48.5	
Drunkenness incident during the past year	No	31	86.1	97	61.0	203	53.0	0.001
	One time in two months or more frequently	3	8.3	35	22.0	83	21.7	
	One time a year	2	5.6	27	17.0	97	25.3	

[1]During the month prior to the study.

Table 2. Alcohol consumption and gender.

Alcohol Use Parameters		Gender				p chi-square (χ^2) test
		Boys		Girls		
		N	%	N	%	
Recent[1] alcohol use	No	187	40.7	207	44.6	0.234
	Yes	272	59.3	257	55.4	
Beer consumption during the past year	1 - 3 times a year	256	44.7	358	67.9	<0.001
	>1 - 3 times a year	317	55.3	169	32.1	
Wine consumption during the past year	1 - 3 times a year	283	49.4	341	64.7	<0.001
	>1 - 3 times a year	290	50.6	186	35.3	
Spirits consumption during the past year	1 - 3 times a year	349	60.9	363	68.9	0.006
	>1 - 3 times a year	224	39.1	164	31.1	
Drunkenness incident during the past year	No	183	56.7	148	58.0	0.001
	One time in two months or frequently	83	25.7	38	14.9	
	One time a year	57	17.6	69	27.1	

[1]During the month prior to the study.

We applied a logistic regression model having alcohol consumption in the past month as dependent variable and the variable adolescent's gender as independent. There was found no significant difference in the likelihood of boys having consumed more alcohol than girls in the past month prior to the study (OR = 1.17, 95% CI: (0.90 - 1.52), p = 0.35). Similarly, we applied a logistic regression model having the variable alcohol consumption in the past month as dependent and age as the independent. We found that 14- to 15-year-old adolescents had 2.76 times higher chance of consuming alcohol than did 12- to 13-year-old adolescents [Cl: (1.82 - 4.17), p < 0.001]. Moreover, adolescents >15 years had 4.68 times higher probability of consuming alcohol in the past month than those of 12- to 13-year-old adolescents [CI: (3.16 - 6.93), p < 0.001].

In our study, 24.9% of adolescents were encouraged to stop drinking, 12.7% had drunk alcohol in the morning after waking up, 15.6% had been criticized by others because of alcohol usage, and an even smaller proportion (14.1%) had felt guilty because of alcohol use (**Table 3**). Moreover, a significant correlation was found between adolescents' age and driving under the influence of alcohol (p = 0.035) (**Table 4**). Specifically, we found a higher prevalence of 14- to 15-year-old adolescents that drove while drunk (p = 0.012). In addition, as age increases so does the proportion of adolescents who experience hangover (p = 0.001) or nausea (p = 0.05) after consuming alcohol (**Table 4**). However, the vast majority of the participants stated that they were informed about the possible addiction to alcohol (86.2%) and the negative consequences from its consumption (85.5%) such as hangover, nausea, vomiting etc. According to their responses, main sources of information were any member of their family (51.9%), their friends (11.0%) or the media (26.5%) (TV, radio etc.).

4. Discussion

According to our findings the majority of the adolescents (57.3%) stated recent alcohol consumption. Our findings are comparable to data from international studies that took place in 36 European countries in 2011 as a part of ESPAD study [9]. Recent alcohol consumption was more prevalent among older adolescents and among boys compared to girls. Comparing our results with those reported earlier we noticed a decreasing trend in alcohol consumption [27]. These findings are in line with other studies indicating a decline in alcohol consumption in many countries with previously high alcohol consumption, particularly in the traditional wine-producing and wine-drinking countries in Europe [28] [29]. According to Simons-Morton *et al*, this decrease is a result of the anti alcohol marketing and targeted country-level policies [29]. Therefore, strategies targeted to youth and also to entire population should be implemented.

Consistent with prior research, we found that rates of adolescent alcohol use increases with age [5] [9] [26] [30] [31]. Specifically, as age increases, so does the prevalence of adolescents having drunk alcohol during the

Table 3. Experienced problems caused due to alcohol consumption among different age groups.

Consequences		Age Group (yrs)						p chi-square (χ^2) test
		12 - 13		14 - 15		>15		
		N	%	N	%	N	%	
Fight	No	24	72.7	117	83.0	312	86.0	0.117
	Yes	9	27.3	24	17.0	51	14.0	
Relationship problems	No	26	86.7	121	87.1	318	88.1	0.935
	Yes	4	13.3	18	12.9	43	11.9	
Argue	No	24	77.4	109	77.9	305	85.0	0.125
	Yes	7	22.6	31	22.1	54	15.0	
Trouble with the police	No	27	90.0	128	92.1	340	95.8	0.149
	Yes	3	10.0	11	7.9	15	4.2	
Drove the car	No	29	96.7	125	86.8	334	93.3	0.035
	Yes	1	3.3	19	13.2	24	6.7	
Attending class	No	29	96.7	117	81.3	294	81.0	0.097
	Yes	1	3.3	27	18.8	69	19.0	
Missing class	No	28	93.3	122	84.7	313	87.2	0.425
	Yes	2	6.7	22	15.3	46	12.8	

Table 4. Negative consequences caused by alcohol consumption among different age groups.

Consequences		Age Group (yrs)						p chi-square (χ^2) test
		12 - 13		14 - 15		>15		
		N	%	N	%	N	%	
Hangover	No	20	55.6	62	41.1	105	28.7	<0.001
	Yes	16	44.4	89	58.9	261	71.3	
Nausea/vomiting	No	29	82.9	97	69.8	223	63.9	0.050
	Yes	6	17.1	42	30.2	126	36.1	
Lack of energy	No	24	70.6	86	59.7	218	61.9	0.502
	Yes	10	29.4	58	40.3	134	38.1	
Fatigue/weakness	No	24	70.6	86	60.1	190	53.2	0.080
	Yes	10	29.4	57	39.9	167	46.8	
Insomnia	No	28	82.4	108	75.5	238	68.2	0.087
	Yes	6	17.6	35	24.5	111	31.8	
Decreased appetite	No	27	79.4	98	69.0	238	68.4	0.412
	Yes	7	20.6	44	31.0	110	31.6	
Sleepy	No	25	69.4	93	66.4	207	59.1	0.201
	Yes	11	30.6	47	33.6	143	40.9	
Dyspepsia/disorders stools	No	30	88.2	117	84.8	289	84.3	0.827
	Yes	4	11.8	21	15.2	54	15.7	
Chills	No	28	82.4	119	85.6	278	80.8	0.459
	Yes	6	17.6	20	14.4	66	19.2	
Tachycardia	No	29	85.3	115	82.7	286	83.4	0.937
	Yes	5	14.7	24	17.3	57	16.6	
Sweating	No	29	82.9	121	87.1	280	81.4	0.325
	Yes	6	17.1	18	12.9	64	18.6	
Respiratory distress	No	28	80.0	125	90.6	312	91.0	0.115
	Yes	7	20.0	13	9.4	31	9.0	

past 30 days before the study and who got drunk at least once during the past year prior to the study.

On average, both males and females stated onset of alcohol at the age of 12 years according to our findings. Earlier age of drinking onset is strongly related to experiencing alcohol dependence during one's life [32]. According to ESPAD findings, nearly six in ten of the European students had consumed at least one glass of alcohol and 12% had been drunk at the age of 13 or younger [9]. Tsiligianni *et al.* reported that 15% of elementary school students in Crete under the age of 10 had already experimented with alcohol [33]. These findings reveal once more the cultural effect, since alcohol consumption in Greece is a mean of socializing and is integrated into the ceremonial, social, and religious structures, along with the influence from the alcohol industry, since Greece is a producer and exporter of alcohol beverages. Drinking alcohol at a younger age has been associated with the three leading causes of death among youth (unintentional injury, homicide, and suicide) [6] [13]. On the other hand, close family and community relationships in Greece provide a control against overconsumption [27]. However, early alcohol onset (≤12 years old) in Greece has not decreased despite the fact that the sale of alcoholic beverages to children under eighteen has been prohibited. This is in accordance to findings from other countries [34].

The participants stated that they prefer to drink with friends at home or out rather than alone. Therefore, our study supports the belief that alcohol consumption is related to friends' influences. Dick *et al.* stated that gender of friends moderate the associations between friends' behaviour and adolescents' alcohol use, with evidence that girls, and those with opposite sex friends, are more susceptible to friends' influence [35]. There might be a strong affinity among adolescents sharing the same habits and certain alcohol behaviours may be linked to the characteristics of alcohol use [36].

Beer was the most popular type of alcoholic beverage among all ages, in our study and this is in accordance to previous findings since beer is reported to be the main alcoholic beverage consumed among adolescents worldwide [25]. A possible explanation for that was that beer is much cheaper than spirits and access to beer is easier for younger adolescents [37]. Whereas, the preference for beer and spirits is more likely to be related to heavy drinking than is the preference for wine [38].

Based on the literature, there are four categories of drinking motives: Enhancement, Social, Coping, and Conformity Motives. Motives are strongly related to drinking in situations where heavy drinking is condoned (e.g. with same-sex friends, and in bars), drinking in response to pleasant emotional states, and drinking in response to urges and temptations [39]. Heavy episodic drinking is positively associated with extraversion-defined as gregariousness, sociability, and high levels of activity and excitement-seeking [40]. In our study participants stated that pleasure was the main reason for drinking alcohol. Novelty seeking, peers impression or drinking as a coping strategy for emotional or family problems, were less frequent reasons for alcohol use.

Our findings revealed a significant association between recent alcohol consumption, type of alcohol and frequency of drunkenness with age and sex. Literature has addressed gender differences in biological and psychosocial risk factors for emerging alcohol problems through the course of adolescence [41]. Similarly, the prevalence of lifetime alcohol use increases as teens get older [42]. In general, risk behaviours are often initiated during early adolescence and the frequency of engagement in behaviours rises with increasing age during the teenage years, often continuing into early adulthood [43].

Participants were randomly selected from areas with different socioeconomic status. However, there was found no correlation between the living area and frequency of alcohol intake, quantity of alcohol intake and drunkenness in our study. In the literature it's not clear whether area level is associated to adolescents drinking behaviour, since many studies have found no association [24] [44] [45].

Adolescents in our study stated a number of negative experienced problems due to alcohol consumption (**Table 4**). Negative criticism and feelings of guilt because of alcohol use were acknowledged by adolescents. A significant correlation was found between age and hangover. Specifically, as age increases so does the proportion of adolescents who experience hangover after consuming alcohol. This last finding is in accordance with previous studies concluding that hangover is the most usual negative consequence experienced by adolescents [9] [46].

However, a significant correlation was found between adolescents' age and driving under the influence of alcohol. This study prospectively replicates findings that early drinking onset is associated with driving under the influence of alcohol, and putting themselves in risky situations after drinking, which are strong predictors of experiencing alcohol-related injuries. Driving under alcohol influences increases the risk of a road traffic accident [23]. In Greece, according to a WHO report (2011) road death rates due to alcohol use in ages >15 years old was

31.3% for males and 7.5% for females [47]. In the USA, 50% of all head injuries in adolescents were associated with alcohol consumption [15].

5. Limitations

There are several limitations. All prevalence estimates were obtained by self-reports. Therefore, prevalence of consumption may have been underestimated as this is a stigmatizing habit. The vast majority of 12- to 19-year-old adolescents attend regular public and private schools, and therefore a greater number of participants from private schools (higher socio-economical status) may influence the results, although there was not noticed such a trend. The impact of co-consumption of tobacco and other illicit drugs in adolescent substance use were not examined in this study. Moreover, the influence of peers on adolescent substance use was not analyzed. Also, the sample was derived only from Attica and due to the huge diversity of other areas in Greece; the results should be interpreted with caution since the sample cannot represent the whole country.

6. Conclusions

The prevalence of recent alcohol consumption among Greek adolescents remains one of the highest in Europe (4th place, between 36 European countries) and has reached alarming prevalence [9]. Alcohol intake showed high prevalence in both genders and began at an early stage. In addition, rates of adolescent alcohol use and drunkenness increase with age, thus confirming previous studies [5] [9] [26] [30]. The persistence of adolescents' drinking problems underscores an urgent need to implement preventions and counseling approaches targeting at younger adolescents by health providers, teachers, family member and by all professionals and other people that are in contact with children. These efforts should be directed on changing drinking behaviour and on reducing risk factors for problematic drinking. Regular monitoring, effective policy measures and health education are essential in order to prevent further increases in adolescents' alcohol consumption.

Therefore, cultural sensitive interventions, addressing the cultural effect of family interaction and focusing on common risk factors with differentiated strategies for each gender, including the 11- to 15-year age group, should be implemented to prevent alcohol consumption and the adverse health and social consequences resulting from this behaviour.

Acknowledgements

The authors gratefully thank all the students and their parents who participated in the study for their valuable contribution to this study.

Competing Interest

The authors declare that they have no competing interests.

References

[1] Danielsson, A.K., Wennberg, P., Hibell, B. and Romelsjö, A. (2012) Alcohol Use, Heavy Episodic Drinking and Subsequent Problems among Adolescents in 23 European Countries: Does the Prevention Paradox Apply? *Addiction*, **107**, 71-80. http://dx.doi.org/10.1111/j.1360-0443.2011.03537.x

[2] Visser, L., de Winter, A.F. and Reijneveld, S.A. (2012) The Parent-Child Relationship and Adolescent Alcohol Use: A Sytematic Review of Longitudinal Studies. *BMC Public Health*, **12**, 886. http://dx.doi.org/10.1186/1471-2458-12-886

[3] WHO Regional Office for Europe (2012) Alcohol in the European Union Consumption, Harm and Policy Approaches. WHO Regional Office for Europe, Copenhagen. http://www.euro.who.int/data/%20assets/pdf_file/0003/160680/%20e96457.pdf

[4] Johnston, L., O'Malley, P.M., Bachman, J.G. and Schulenberg, J.E. (2011) Monitoring the Future National on Results on Adolescent Drug Use: Overview of Key Findings, 2010. Ann Arbor: Institute for Social Research, The University of Michigan. http://radar.boisestate.edu/radar/pdfs/mtf-overview 2010.pdf

[5] Johnston, L.D., O'Malley, P.M., Bachman, J.G. and Schulenberg, J.E. (2012) Monitoring the Future National Results on Adolescent Drug Use: Overview of Key Findings, 2011. Ann Arbor: Institute for Social Research, The University of Michigan. http://files.eric.ed.gov/fulltext/ED529133.pdf

[6] Department of Health and Human Services (2007) The Surgeon General's Call to Action to Prevent and Reduce Un-

derage Drinking. Department of Health and Human Services, Office of the Surgeon General. http://www.ncbi.nlm.nih.gov/books/NBK44360/pdf/TOC.pdf

[7] American Academy of Pediatrics (2010) Policy Statement. Alcohol Use by Youth and Adolescents: A Pediatric Concern. *Pediatrics*, **125**, 185. http://dx.doi.org/10.1542/peds.2010-0438

[8] Plant, M.A, Plant, M.L., Miller, P., Gmel, G. and Kuntsche, S. (2009) The Social Consequences of Binge Drinking: A Comparison of Young Adults in Six European Countries. *Journal of Addictive Diseases*, **28**, 294-308. http://dx.doi.org/10.1080/10550880903182978

[9] Hibell, B., *et al.* (2012) The 2011 ESPAD Report—Substance Use Among Students in 36 European Countries. The Swedish Council for Information on Alcohol and other Drugs (CAN). Stockholm, Sweden. http://www.can.se/PageFiles/2619/The_2011_ESPAD_Report_FULL.pdf?epslanguage=sv

[10] Eaton, D.K., *et al.* (2012) Youth Risk Behavior Surveillance—United States (2011) Morbidity and Mortality Weekly Report (MMWR), **61**, 1-162. http://www.cdc.gov/mmwr/preview/ mmwrhtml/ss6104a1.htm

[11] Eaton, D.K., *et al.* (2010) Youth Risk Behavior Surveillance—United States, 2009. *Morbidity and Mortality Weekly Report* (*MMWR*), **59**, 1-142. http://www.cdc.gov/mmwr/pdf/ss/ss5905.pdf

[12] Hingson, R.W. and Winter, M. (2003) Epidemiology and Consequences of Drinking and Driving. *Alcohol Research Health*, **27**, 63-78. http://pubs.niaaa.nih.gov/publications/arh27-1/63-78.pdf

[13] Miller, J.W., Naimi, T.S., Brewer, R.D. and Jones, S.E. (2007) Binge Drinking and Associated Health Risk Behaviors among High School Students. *Pediatrics*, **119**, 76-85. http://dx.doi.org/10.1542/peds.2006-1517

[14] Strauch, E.S., Pinheiro, R.T., Silva, R.A. and Horta, B.L. (2009) Alcohol Use among Adolescents: A Population-Based Study. *Revista de Saúde Pública*, **43**, 647-655. http://dx.doi.org/10.1590/S0034-89102009005000044

[15] Stolle, M., Sack, P.M. and Thomasius, R. (2009) Binge Drinking in Childhood and Adolescence: Epidemiology, Consequences and Interventions. *Deutsches Ärzteblatt International*, **106**, 323-328.

[16] National Research Council and Institute of Medicine (2004) Reducing Underage Drinking: A Collective Responsibility. In: Richard, J., Bonnie and O'Connell, M.E., Eds., Committee on Developing a Strategy to Reduce and Prevent Underage Drinking, Board on Children, Youth and Families, *Division of Behavioral and Social Sciences and Education*, The National Academies Press, Washington DC. http://www.ncbi.nlm.nih.gov/books/NBK37589/pdf/TOC.pdf

[17] Kraus, L., Baumeister, S.E., Pabst, A. and Orth, B. (2009) Association of Average Daily Alcohol Consumption, Binge Drinking and Alcohol-Related Social Problems: Result from the German Epidemiology Surveys of Substance Abuse. *Alcohol & Alcoholism*, **44**, 314-320. http://dx.doi.org/10.1093/alcalc/agn110

[18] Chun, J. and Chung, I.J. (2013) Gender Differences in Factors Influencing Smoking, Drinking and Their Co-Occurrence among Adolescents in South Korea. *Nicotine & Tobacco Research*, **15**, 542-551. http://dx.doi.org/10.1093/ntr/nts181v

[19] Poelen, E.P.A., *et al.* (2007) Drinking by Parents, Siblings and Friends as Predictors of Regular Alcohol Use in Adolescents and Young Adults: A Longitudinal Twin-Family Study. *Alcohol and Alcoholism*, **42**, 362-369. http://dx.doi.org/10.1093/alcalc/agm042

[20] Scholte, R.H.J., *et al.* (2008) Relative Risks of Adolescent and Young Adult Alcohol Use: The Role of Drinking Fathers, Mothers, Siblings and Friends. *Addictive Behaviors*, **33**, 1-14. http://dx.doi.org/10.1016/j.addbeh.2007.04.015

[21] Donovan, J.E. (2009) Estimated Blood Alcohol Concentrations for Child and Adolescent Drinking and Their Implications for Screening Instruments. *Pediatrics*, **123**, e975-e981. http://dx.doi.org/10.1542/peds.2008-0027

[22] Hingson, R.W., Heeren, T. and Winter, M.R. (2006) Age of Alcohol-Dependence Onset: Associations with Severity of Dependence and Seeking Treatment. *Pediatrics*, **118**, e755-e763. http://dx.doi.org/10.1542/peds.2006-0223

[23] Hingson, R.W., Edwards, E.M., Heeren, T. and Rosenbloom, D. (2009) Age of Drinking Onset and Injuries, Motor Vehicle Crashes and Physical Fights after Drinking and When Not Drinking. *Alcoholism*: *Clinical and Experimental Research*, **33**, 783-790. http://dx.doi.org/10.1111/j.1530-0277.2009.00896.x

[24] Vinther-Larsen, M., Huckle, T., You, R. and Casswell, S. (2013) Area Level Deprivation and Drinking Patterns among Adolescents. *Health & Place*, **19**, 53-58. http://dx.doi.org/10.1016/j.healthplace.2012.09.014

[25] Verho, A., Laatikainen, T., Vartiainen, E. and Puska, P. (2012) Changes in Alcohol Behaviour among Adolescents in North-West Russia between 1995 and 2004. *Journal of Environmental and Public Health*, **2012**, Article ID: 736249.

[26] Kokkevi, A., Richardson, C., Olszewski, D., Matias, J., Monshouwer, K. and Bjarnason, T. (2012) Multiple Substance Use and Self-Reported Suicide Attempts by Adolescents in 16 European Countries. *European Child & Adolescent Psychiatry*, **21**, 443-450. http://dx.doi.org/10.1007/s00787-012-0276-7

[27] Hibell, B., *et al.* (2009) The 2007 ESPAD Report: Substance use among Students in 35 European Countries. Swedish Council for Information on Alcohol and Other Drugs, Stockholm. http://www.espad.org/Uploads/ESPAD_reports/2007/The_2007_ESPAD_Report-FULL_091006.pdf

[28] Arvanitidou, M., *et al.* (2007) Decreasing Prevalence of Alcohol Consumption among Greek Adolescents. *The American Journal of Drug and Alcohol Abuse*, **33**, 411-417. http://dx.doi.org/10.1080/00952990701315384

[29] Simons-Morton, B.G., *et al.* (2009) Gender Specific Trends in Alcohol Use: Cross-Cultural Comparisons from 1998 to 2006 in 24 Countries and Regions. *International Journal of Public Health*, **54**, 199-208. http://dx.doi.org/10.1007/s00038-009-5411-y

[30] Melchior, M., Chastang, J.F., Goldberg, P. and Fombonne, E. (2008) High Prevalence Rates of Tobacco, Alcohol and Drug Use in Adolescents and Young Adults in France: Results from the GAZEL Youth Study. *Addictive Behaviours*, **33**, 122-133. http://dx.doi.org/10.1016/j.addbeh.2007.09.009

[31] Johnston, L.D., O'Malley, P.M., Bachman, J.G. and Schulenberg, J.E. (2012) Monitoring the Future National Survey Results on Drug Use, 1975-2011: Volume I, Secondary School Students. Ann Arbor: Institute for Social Research, The University of Michigan. www.monitoringthefuture.org/ pubs/monographs/mtf-vol2_2011.pdf

[32] Hingson, R.W. and Zha, W. (2009) Age of Drinking Onset, Alcohol Use Disorders, Frequent Heavy Drinking and Unintentionally Injuring Oneself and Others after Drinking. *Pediatrics*, **123**, 1477-1484. http://dx.doi.org/10.1542/peds.2008-2176

[33] Tsiligianni, *et al.* (2012) The Association between Alcohol and Tobacco Use among Elementary and High School Students in Crete, Greece. *Tobacco Induced Diseases*, **10**, 15. http://dx.doi.org/10.1186/1617-9625-10-15

[34] Filhol, V.C.B., de Campos, W. and da Silva Lopes, A. (2012) Prevalence of Alcohol and Tobacco Use among Brazilian Adolescents: A Systematic Review. *Revista de Saúde Pública*, **46**, 901-917. http://dx.doi.org/10.1590/S0034-89102012000500018

[35] Dick, D.M., Pagan, J.L., Viken, R., Purcell, S., Kaprio, J., Pulkkinen, L. and Rose, R.J. (2007) Changing Environmental Influences on Substance Use Across Development. *Twin Research and Human Genetics*, **10**, 315-326. http://dx.doi.org/10.1375/twin.10.2.315

[36] Whiteman, S.D., Jensen, A.C. and Maggs, J.L. (2013) Similarities in Adolescent Siblings' Substance Use: Testing Competing Pathways of Influence. *Journal of Studies on Alcohol and Drugs*, **74**, 104-113.

[37] Bellis, M.A., Phillips-Howard, P.A., Hughes, K., Hughes, S., Cook, P.A., Morleo, M., Hannon, K., Smallthwaite, L. and Jones, L. (2009) Teenage Drinking, Alcohol Availability and Pricing: A Cross-Sectional Study of Risk and Protective Factors for Alcohol-Related Harms in School Children. *BMC Public Health*, **9**, 380. http://dx.doi.org/10.1186/1471-2458-9-380

[38] Graziano, F., Bina, M., Giannotta, F. and Ciairano, S. (2012) Drinking Motives and Alcoholic Beverage Preferences among Italian Adolescents. *Journal of Adolescence*, **35**, 823-831. http://dx.doi.org/10.1016/j.adolescence.2011.11.010

[39] Stewart, S.H. and Devine, H. (2000) Relations between Personality and Drinking Motives in Young Adults. *Personality and Individual Differences*, **29**, 495-511. http://dx.doi.org/10.1016/S0191-8869(99)00210-X

[40] Kuntsche, E., Von Fischer, M. and Gmel, G. (2008) Personality Factors and Alcohol Use: A Mediator Analysis of Drinking Motives. *Personality and Individual Differences*, **45**, 796-800. http://dx.doi.org/10.1016/j.paid.2008.08.009

[41] Schulte, M.T., Ramo, D. and Brown, S.A. (2009) Gender Differences in Factors Influencing Alcohol Use and Drinking Progression among Adolescents. *Clinical Psychology Review*, **29**, 535-547. http://dx.doi.org/10.1016/j.cpr.2009.06.003

[42] Eaton, D.K., Kann, L., Kinchen, S., Shanklin, S., Ross, J., Hawkins, J., *et al.* (2008) Youth Risk Behavior Surveillance —United States, 2007. *Morbidity and Mortality Weekly Report* (*MMWR*), **57**, 1-131.

[43] MacArthur, G.J., Smith, M.C., Melotti, R., Heron, J., Macleod, J., Hickman, M., Kipping, R.R., Campbell, R. and Lewis, G. (2012) Patterns of Alcohol Use and Multiple Risk Behaviour by Gender during Early and Late Adolescence: The ALSPAC Cohort. *Journal of Public Health*, **34**, i20-i30. http://dx.doi.org/10.1093/pubmed/fds006

[44] Breslin, F.C. and Adlaf, E.M. (2005) Part-Time Work and Adolescent Heavy Episodic Drinking: The Influence of Family and Community Context. *Journal of Studies on Alcohol and Drugs*, **66**, 784-794.

[45] Karriker-Jaffe, K.J. (2011) Areas of Disadvantage: A Systematic Review of Effects of Area-Level Socioeconomic Status on Substance Use Outcomes. *Drug and Alcohol Review*, **30**, 84-95. http://dx.doi.org/10.1111/j.1465-3362.2010.00191.x

[46] Hibell, B., *et al.* (2004) The ESPAD Report 2003: Alcohol and Other Drug Use among Students in 35 European Countries. The Swedish Council for Information on Alcohol and Other Drugs (CAN) and the Pompidou Group at the Council of Europe, Stockholm. http://www.espad.org/Uploads/ESPAD_reports/2003/The_2003_ESPAD_report.pdf

[47] WHO (2011) Global Status Report on Alcohol and Health. World Health Organization, Geneva. http://www.who.int/substance_abuse/publications/global_alcohol_report/msbgsruprofil. pdf

4

Hospitalization Can Correct Behavioral Feeding Disorders in Children by Resetting the Pedagogic Climate

Ellen van der Gaag, Miriam Münow

Department of Pediatrics, Hospital Group Twente, Hengelo, The Netherlands
Email: e.gaagvander@zgt.nl

Abstract

Background: Behavioral feeding disorders are common among children, which sometimes become progressive, and consequently, children may refuse to eat anything. Parents have lots of difficulties to reset such a disturbed eating pattern. The aim of this study was to perform an analysis of clinical intervention in behavioral feeding disorders in young children. Methods: We conducted a retrospective analysis of data of 28 children aged 1 - 9 years with behavioral feeding disorders. A pediatrician and pediatric social worker conducted the training in two groups: outpatient or inpatient setting. Both groups were treated with parental education and guidance. The inpatient group also had a temporarily (2 weeks) resetting of the pedagogic climate in a pediatric ward of a general hospital under guidance of a pediatric social worker. Results: Almost all parents were inconsistent in applying appropriate behavioral contingencies during meals. Eleven patients followed 8 months of outpatient treatment and 25 patients followed 2 weeks of inpatient treatment. The overall success rate of outpatient treatment after 2 weeks was 18%, and that of inpatient treatment after 8 months was 88%. The corrected relapse rates are 18% and 56% respectively after 6 months. Conclusion: Short clinical intervention in a structured pedagogic environment is a successful treatment in behavioral feeding disorders. Herewith, pediatricians have a powerful tool for treating behavioral feeding disorders by temporarily resetting and changing the pedagogic climate.

Keywords

Behavioral Feeding Disorder, Hospitalisation, Behavioral Contingencies, Pediatrics

1. Introduction

Behavioral feeding disorders, such as eating low quantities, delay in self-feeding, or restricted food preferences are common among children, and up to 25% of the normally developing children and up to 80% of atypical developing children experience some type of feeding problem [1]-[4]. Determination of the difference between physical and psychological factors is difficult, because behavioral feeding problems may persist even after organic difficulties have been resolved [5]. Environmental and parental factors may interact to influence and maintain the problem [5]. Though this subject is not a field for innovative treatments, the need for solutions among parents is very high. General pediatricians frequently encounter parents and give advice about the minimum required dietary intake. They also evaluate the children's physical condition and advice them with ways to deal with the feeding disorder. When the child is really threatened, they can admit the child to their hospital for tube feeding or in a feeding clinic for further treatment. But is there a place for a general hospital to improve feeding techniques by the parents, to improve the pedagogic climate for the parents and to teach them how to manage the feeding problem of their child?

Sporadic information is available on clinical treatment of behavioral feeding disorders. The only described clinical treatments are about prematurely born infants. These studies performed in the 1980s only focused on the weight gain of the children, and concluded that hospitalization leads to appropriate weight gain [6]-[9]. They did not study to reset or manage the feeding disorder. Nowadays, studies mostly focus on treating behavioral feeding disorders in outpatient setting, using multidisciplinary teams and video equipment, which is time-consuming and takes a long time to observe the result of the treatment.

We presume that it would be useful to shorten the duration of treatment of behavioral feeding disorder. Not only because of the fact that it is a very unpleasant condition for the child and his/her family, but also because the feeding problems can persist for 4 - 6 years [10] [11] and that it is believed [12] [13] that childhood feeding disorders are related to (symptoms of) adolescent and adult eating disorders. It can also have influence on the development of behavioral problems [14]-[16] and cognitive development [17].

Our hypothesis is that short and intensive inpatient treatment is a good replacement of outpatient treatment, especially in more severe behavioral feeding disorders.

2. Methods

2.1. Participants

We conducted a retrospective analysis of the data available on the treatment of children with behavioral feeding disorders according to Burklow [18] during the last five years in our general hospital, Hospital Group Twente, location Hengelo, The Netherlands.

For evaluation, 28 children were available, 8 children overlapped in treatments and followed both inpatient and outpatient treatment. We collected data from charts made by their pediatricians and pediatric social workers on family structure, presence of behavioral or psychological child factors, parents with psychological or psychiatric problems, and inconsistencies in parental approach of the child.

The inclusion of behavioral feeding disorders in sub classifications is still open to debate [19], but our patients could be categorized into five types of feeding disorders: feeding disorder of infancy or early childhood, rumination disorder and pica (according to DSM-IV-TR), selective eating [20] [21], and refusal to eat [22]. Sensory food aversion [23] was not evaluated as an individual group, and the children with sensory food aversion experienced more than the aversion alone. The type of feeding disorder was determined from the description of the parents and observations made by our pediatric social worker.

2.2. Treatment Groups

The children were enrolled in inpatient or outpatient behavioral therapy. Inclusion for inpatient or outpatient treatment was based on the estimated severity of the feeding disorder and the burden of the parents (both judged by pediatric social workers). Children who clinically deteriorated badly were enrolled in inpatient treatment. Children whose parents still had energy to try home treatment were enrolled in outpatient treatment. The outpatient group underwent the program at home and the inpatient group was hospitalized in a structured pedagogic climate in a general hospital. In this setting, the patients could be medically observed and a hospital has the ability to temporarily put children in another environment with a medical staff and pediatric social workers. Behavioral therapy is based on the idea that eating is a normal daily habit and that there should be a neutral atmosphere surrounding feeding moments.

2.3. Inpatient Treatment

A day schedule was made with 2 hours of school, 2 hours of playtime, resting hours, 4 hours of visiting time for parents, and 3 mealtimes. The children ate two meals together with our pediatric social worker and other children and one meal in a one to one interaction with a pediatric nurse in the absence of parents. Children over 2 - 3 years of age ate themselves, below 2 - 3 years were "spooned" by the pediatric social worker. No snacks or sweets were given to the children in between the meals, to prevent them from having a feeling of satiety before mealtimes. To ensure a neutral atmosphere during feeding moments, the pediatric social worker ate with the inpatient-trained children in a group with all hospitalized children; they were not pushed to eat everything in their plate, and were not praised for eating well. If necessary, the pediatric social worker prompts a few times; "Dylan, you can take one bite, you are a big boy" or "Mind the time Dylan, you only have 10 minutes left" etc. If the child did not eat at all, the mealtime passed and we started again at the next mealtime. Inappropriate mealtime behavior was corrected: "No Dylan, we do not allow throwing food from this table" or "we do not allow gagging at this table". In the beginning, we start with small amounts, so the child can finish its meal in 20 minutes. At that stage in the training the mealtimes takes 20 minutes. In the course of the training, the amounts of food are increased to age-appropriate portions. The staff determines the amount of food, not the child. When the quantity is too much, the pediatric social worker says how much bites the child has to take in the 20 minutes. At the end of the training, mealtime was ended when the child ate an age appropriate portion, with a maximum of 30 minutes.

Between the meals, the parents are updated and explained what we do. When the child showed an improved pattern of eating, based upon their particular problem for which they were admitted to the hospital, the parents were allowed to watch a meal through a one-way screen and slowly take over the lead of the meals from the pediatric social worker. They start with the meal that is most easy for the child. A video recording is made from the mealtime through the one-way screen, and the interaction in relation to mealtime behavior is discussed afterwards with the parents. When both the parents and pediatric social worker became satisfied with the meals, the child was discharged from the hospital.

Back at home, the parents were asked to fill out an intake list. After 1 week, the situation at home was evaluated with the pediatric social worker. The families were invited for regular (usually monthly) outpatient follow-up during the next 6 months, or longer, if needed. The follow-up was conducted by the pediatric social worker and a pediatrician.

2.4. Outpatient Treatment

During outpatient treatment, there was individual guidance during 30 minute visits at the outpatient clinic by our pediatric social worker. The rules during treatment were the same as those for the inpatient program. So, no in between snacks, no inappropriate mealtime behavior, 20 minute meals, clear prompting, the parents determine the portion-size. The pediatric social worker provided the parents with guidelines for a normal feeding situation as well as advices in changing the particular problems the family experienced. The parents had to make the changes themselves in their own home situation, without direct supervision of a pediatric social worker. Once every 2 weeks, the parents and the child had an appointment with the pediatric social worker in the hospital to evaluate the progress. If necessary, the guidance was adjusted to the new situation. If the treatment had no or little effect, a switch to inpatient treatment could be made. The major difference with inpatient treatment was; no temporarily resetting of the pedagogic climate, no detachment from their parents, and only supervision on a distance.

After successful treatment, the families were invited for regular (usually monthly) outpatient follow-up during the next 6 months, or longer, if needed. The follow-up was conducted by the pediatric social worker and a pediatrician.

2.5. Evaluation

Growth was calculated on the basis of measurements of height and weight during the visits to the clinic. These measurements were compared with the normal growth curves of the Dutch children (using Growth Analyser 3.5, Dutch Growth Foundation, The Netherlands, 2006, available on http://www.growthanalyser.org/) to calculate the standard deviation of weight and height. We analyzed the amount of additional problems that the children experienced, based on parental reports. The problems that we analyzed were recurrent infections, constipation, incontinence (for both urine and feces), sleeping problems, tiredness, and behavioral problems.

Success was defined when the volume of foods consumed during the meals were increased to age appropriate portions (according to the Dutch Center of Food) [24], together with a consistent manner of handling future (feeding) problems by the parent. The slow eating or selectively refusing to eat one or two items were tolerated. The pediatric social worker determined whether the feeding disorder was sufficiently treated and whether the child had gained a normal pattern of eating.

Relapses were defined as (partial) regaining their old feeding disorder, based on the findings of our pediatric social worker and parental reports of the child's feeding behavior at home.

Statistical analysis were made with SPSS version 13.0 (SPSS Inc. Chicago, IL, USA) for windows.

3. Results

3.1. Descriptives

In the last 5 years, 33 patients were referred by their general practitioner because of behavioral feeding disorders. For evaluation, we excluded five of them for having either a present medical problem or a medical history that could explain the feeding disorder.

Initially, 8 of the 28 evaluated participants were enrolled in our outpatient program; 20 were immediately enrolled as inpatients owing to the estimated severity of their feeding disorder. After evaluation of the initial treatment, 5 participants of the outpatient group were transferred to the inpatient group after failing the outpatient program and 3 patients of the originally inpatient group were transferred to the outpatient group after failing the inpatient program. Children who received both the treatments were evaluated in the results of both the groups, because the effect of the treatment program was the main outcome of the study. The group characteristics are described in **Table 1**. The age of the children at which they enrolled the program did not differ between the two groups, and ranged from 1 to 9 years.

In the outpatient group, mean height at presentation was −0.96 SD (SD = 0.67) with a mean weight for height of −1.35 SD (SD = 1.09). In the inpatient group, the measurements at presentation were −0.69 SD (SD = 0.76) and −0.96 SD (SD = 1.05) for height and weight for height, respectively.

Children could suffer from one or more additional problems. All additional problems were equally spread over both groups. Three children experienced no additional problems. Nine children had recurrent infections. Seventeen children suffered from constipation and 6 had incontinence for either urine or feces. Furthermore, sleeping problems were reported in 6 participants and tiredness was a problem for 12 children. Parents complained of having a child with behavioral problems in 13 cases.

Twenty-four families consisted of two parents with one or more children, 2 families were formed by a single parent with two or more children, while 2 families consisted of one biological parent, one stepparent, the patient, and the children of the stepparent.

Table 1. Group characteristics.

Characteristics	Groups	
	Outpatients N = 11	Inpatients N = 25
Male:Female	5:6	12:13
Age in years (SD)	3.28 (2.7)	3.25 (2.2)
Selectivity	4 (22%)	9 (36%)
Food refusal	7 (64%)	17 (68%)
Feeding disorder of childhood	1 (9%)	1 (4%)
Rumination	0 (0%)	2 (8%)
Pica	0 (0%)	1 (4%)
Sensory abnormalities	2 (18%)	5 (20%)

Three children were diagnosed with a DSM-IV-diagnosis (e.g. ADHD, conduct disorder, and anxiety disorder) and 19 showed some kind of non-diagnosed behavioral problem as reported by the parents (e.g. aggressive behavior, bad listening to the parents, oppositional problems etc.). Most parents ($n = 24$) turned out to have behavioral mismanagement (e.g. inconsistencies in the parental approach to the child), which could explain why their child showed behavioral problems.

In addition, in only one family both the parents were consistent in applying appropriate behavioral contingencies during meals, while in three families one of the parents was consistent and the other parent was not. In all the other 24 of the 28 families both parents were inconsistent in applying behavioral contingencies during meals. Complementary, in 6 families, one of the parents was known with psychological or psychiatric problems themselves.

3.2. Outcomes

Two children were treated successfully in the initial outpatient group. Of the 6 who were not, 5 were enrolled in the inpatient program. All 5 were treated successfully in the additional inpatient program. With the 20 patients who started initially with the inpatient program, 17 patients succeeded, while 3 failed the treatment. These 3 were subsequently enrolled in an outpatient program, where they also failed treatment. The results of the per protocol analysis are shown in **Table 2**.

None of the children who were treated successfully in the outpatient group relapsed. In the inpatient group, 8 of the 22 successfully treated children relapsed. Of these 8 children, 4 children did not relapse completely, but partially fell back into their old behavior. When corrected for relapse rate, outpatient treatment was successful for 18.2% of the patients and inpatient treatment was successful for 56% of the patients.

3.3. Measurements

There were no significant differences in growth in neither height nor weight for height during the follow-up period. Children in the outpatient group showed a bend in the growth curve for height with a growth of −0.20 SD (SD = 0.42). They had a growth in weight of 0.19 SD (SD = 0.69), while those in the inpatient group grew 0.02 SD (SD = 0.30) in height and 0.14 SD (SD = 0.59) in weight.

We tried to determine a predictive factor for the success or relapse rate, but found no relation with the type of eating disorder, height and weight for height at presentation, age at presentation, additional problems, or pedagogic environment.

4. Discussion

From this study, we confirmed our hypothesis that hospitalization can be a therapeutic intervention in the treatment of behavioral feeding disorders. Short clinical intervention with a structured pedagogic environment and a behavioral treatment program proved to be a successful single treatment or continuation of failed outpatient treatment in behavioral feeding disorders.

In the literature, the effect of inpatient treatment was also proven for children with obesity; a cognitive behavioral non-diet approach was found to be promising, even though this program lasted for 14 months [25]. The

Table 2. Success and relapse rates.

Characteristics	Groups	
	Outpatients N = 11	Inpatients N = 25
Duration of treatment (days)	72	13
Initial success rate	2 (18.2%)	22 (88%)**
Relapse rate in follow up	0 (0%)	8 (32%)**
Final success rate	2 (18.2%)	14 (56%)*
Change in length after treatment in SD	−0.20 (0.4)	0.02 (0.3)
Change in weight for height after treatment in SD	0.19 (0.17)	0.14 (0.6)

*$p < 0.05$, students' t-test; **$p < 0.01$, students' t-test.

effect of the treatment is probably owing to temporary resetting of the pedagogic environment and guidance to the parents to continue this at home. The negative home situation is broken through and the parents and children are put in another direction. However, owing to the inability of the parents because of their inconsistency, this is unlikely to succeed in the home situation. Low success rates of outpatient treatment support this theory. Nevertheless, all the children return to their old home situations and the chances of falling back into old habits for both parents and children do exist, as is shown by the relapse rates.

Neither the type of feeding disorder nor the additional problems or the family structure from where the children came had any influence on the success of treatment or relapse rate. Children in our study group came from similar environments as those in the regional population. The main difference between our study group and the regional population could be that most of the parents in our study were inconsistent in applying appropriate behavioral contingencies during meals.

Our results oppose those of Singer, who found that extended hospitalization with a mean duration of 17 weeks was most successful [6]. This is probably owing to the fact that Singer's study group consisted of infants with a mean age of 5.4 months, while ours consisted of children with a mean age of 3.25 years. Goldstein *et al.* found data similar to our data, with an increase in weight during inpatient treatment of 15.9 days on an average [9]. However, this study focused on infants with a mean age of 8.4 months, which is younger than our study group.

In recent studies, behavioral feeding disorders are mostly treated in outpatient setting. Good results have been achieved with outpatient treatment, but the mean duration of treatment is usually longer than the inpatient treatment in our study.

There are some limitations to this retrospective study that need to be mentioned. The sample size of this study is small, therefore limiting the significance of our results. Hence, it may be possible that we did not find any predictive factors for failure of treatment and relapse after successful treatment. Second, children in both the groups were not randomized. The distribution between the groups was based on the severity of the feeding disorder, making it difficult to compare both the groups.

Even though there are limitations to this study, we are certain that it can be used in designing future treatment plans for behavioral feeding disorders. Even in a small sample like ours, it seems clear that behavioral feeding disorders are better treated in an inpatient rather than an outpatient setting, not only because the percentage of successful treatment is higher, but also because the duration of treatment is shorter. To prevent relapse and intervene if it occurred, it is wise to have a period of outpatient follow-up.

Obviously, in all the behavioral feeding disorders a behavioral component is present. However, we did not investigate that component, but only the parental approach and to place the child outside its comfort zone. Our study shows that the parental strategy plays a big contribution to the existence and persistence of these feeding disorders. When the parents learn how to cope with their child's feeding disorder, the need for direct investigation of the behavioral component disappears because the child starts to eat again. We did not investigate further implications of the behavioral component. Nevertheless, this is one of the first studies in which a hospital admission can serve as a pedagogic tool with medical guidance for a medical/behavioral problem. However, by looking at the favorable results, it is worth investigating it further.

5. Conclusion

Short clinical intervention in a pedagogic structured environment and a behavioral program is an effective treatment for resetting behavioral feeding disorders in children. Our study group showed that most of the parents in our study were inconsistent in applying appropriate behavioral contingencies during meals. With the clinically resetting of the pedagogic environment, disturbed eating patterns can be normalized. Herewith, general pediatricians have a powerful tool for resetting behavioral feeding disorders in an early or advanced stage.

Acknowledgements

EvdG thanks Greg Reed PhD, NCSP (Associate Professor, Howard University, Washington DC, USA) for his clarifying remarks on our study.

References

[1] Linscheid, T.R., Budd, K.S. and Rasnake, L.K. (2003) Pediatric Feeding Disorders. In: Robberts, M.C., Ed., *Handbook*

of Pediatric Psychology, The guilford Press, New York, 481-498.

[2] Ramsay, M., Gisel, E.G., McCusker, J., Bellavance, F. and Platt, R. (2002) Infant Sucking Ability, Non-Organic Failure to Thrive, Maternal Characteristics, and Feeding Practices: A Prospective Cohort Study. *Developmental Medicine & Child Neurology*, **44**, 405-414. http://dx.doi.org/10.1111/j.1469-8749.2002.tb00835.x

[3] Lindberg, L., Bohlin, G., Hagekull, B. and Thurnstrom, M. (1994) Early Food Refusal: Infant and Family Characteristics. *Infant Mental Health Journal*, **15**, 262-277. http://dx.doi.org/10.1002/1097-0355(199423)15:3<262::AID-IMHJ2280150303>3.0.CO;2-Q

[4] Satter, E. (1990) The Feeding Relationship: Problems and Interventions. *Journal of Pediatrics*, **117**, S181-S189. http://dx.doi.org/10.1016/S0022-3476(05)80017-4

[5] Manikam, R. and Perman, J.A. (2000) Pediatric Feeding Disorders. *Journal of Clinical Gastroenterology*, **30**, 34-46. http://dx.doi.org/10.1097/00004836-200001000-00007

[6] Singer, L. (1986) Long-Term Hospitalization of Failure-to-Thrive Infants: Developmental Outcome at Three Years. *Child Abuse & Neglect*, **10**, 479-486. http://dx.doi.org/10.1016/0145-2134(86)90052-9

[7] Singer, L. (1987) Long-Term Hospitalization of Nonorganic Failure-to-Thrive Infants: Patient Characteristics and Hospital Course. *Journal of Developmental & Behavioral Pediatrics*, **8**, 25-31. http://dx.doi.org/10.1097/00004703-198702000-00006

[8] Field, M. (1984) Follow-Up Developmental Status of Infants Hospitalized for Nonorganic Failure to Thrive. *Journal of Pediatric Psychology*, **9**, 241-256. http://dx.doi.org/10.1093/jpepsy/9.2.241

[9] Goldstein, S. and Field, T. (1985) Affective Behavior and Weight Changes among Hospitalized Failure-to-Thrive Infants. *Infant Mental Health Journal*, **6**, 187-193. http://dx.doi.org/10.1002/1097-0355(198524)6:4<187::AID-IMHJ2280060402>3.0.CO;2-2

[10] Dahl, M., Rydell, A.M. and Sundelin, C. (1994) Children with Early Refusal to Eat: Follow-Up during Primary School. *Acta Paediatrica*, **83**, 54-58. http://dx.doi.org/10.1111/j.1651-2227.1994.tb12952.x

[11] Dahl, M. and Sundelin, C. (1992) Feeding Problems in an Affluent Society. Follow-Up at Four Years of Age in Children with Early Refusal to Eat. *Acta Paediatrica*, **81**, 575-579. http://dx.doi.org/10.1111/j.1651-2227.1992.tb12303.x

[12] Marchi, M. and Cohen, P. (1990) Early Childhood Eating Behaviors and Adolescent Eating Disorders. *Journal of the American Academy of Child and Adolescent Psychiatry*, **29**, 112-117. http://dx.doi.org/10.1097/00004583-199001000-00017

[13] Kotler, L.A., Cohen, P., Davies, M., Pine, D.S. and Walsh, B.T. (2001) Longitudinal Relationships between Childhood, Adolescent, and Adult Eating Disorders. *Journal of the American Academy of Child and Adolescent Psychiatry*, **40**, 1434-1440. http://dx.doi.org/10.1097/00004583-200112000-00014

[14] Galler, J.R., Ramsey, F., Solimano, G., Lowell, W.E. and Mason, E. (1983) The Influence of Early Malnutrition on Subsequent Behavioral Development. I. Degree of Impairment in Intellectual Performance. *Journal of the American Academy of Child and Adolescent Psychiatry*, **22**, 8-15. http://dx.doi.org/10.1097/00004583-198301000-00002

[15] Galler, J.R., Ramsey, F., Solimano, G., Kucharski, L.T. and Harrison, R. (1984) The Influence of Early Malnutrition on Subsequent Behavioral Development. IV. Soft Neurologic Signs. *Pediatric Research*, **18**, 826-832. http://dx.doi.org/10.1203/00006450-198409000-00004

[16] Galler, J.R., Bryce, C.P., Waber, D., Hock, R.S., Exner, N., Eaglesfield, D., Fitzmaurice, G. and Harrison, R. (2010) Early Childhood Malnutrition Predicts Depressive Symptoms at Ages 11-17. *Journal of Child Psychology and Psychiatry*, **51**, 789-798. http://dx.doi.org/10.1111/j.1469-7610.2010.02208.x

[17] Reif, S., Beler, B., Villa, Y. and Spirer, Z. (1995) Long-Term Follow-Up and Outcome of Infants with Non-Organic Failure to Thrive. *The Israel Medical Association Journal*, **31**, 483-489.

[18] Burklow, K.A., Phelps, A.N., Schultz, J.R., McConnell, K. and Rudolph, C. (1998) Classifying Complex Pediatric Feeding Disorders. *Journal of Pediatric Gastroenterology and Nutrition*, **27**, 143-147. http://dx.doi.org/10.1097/00005176-199808000-00003

[19] Bryant-Waugh, R., Markham, L., Kreipe, R.E. and Walsh, B.T. (2010) Feeding and Eating Disorders in Childhood. *International Journal of Eating Disorders*, **43**, 98-111.

[20] Timimi, S., Douglas, J. and Tsiftsopoulou, K. (1997) Selective Eaters: A Retrospective Case Note Study. *Child Care Health Development*, **23**, 265-278. http://dx.doi.org/10.1111/j.1365-2214.1997.tb00968.x

[21] Gentry, J.A. and Luiselli, J.K. (2008) Treating a Child's Selective Eating through Parent Implemented Feeding Intervention in the Home Setting. *Journal of Developmental and Physical Disabilities*, **20**, 63-70. http://dx.doi.org/10.1007/s10882-007-9080-6

[22] Chatoor, I. and Ganiban, J. (2003) Food Refusal by Infants and Young Children: Diagnosis and Treatment. *Cognitive and Behavioral Practice*, **10**, 138-146. http://dx.doi.org/10.1016/S1077-7229(03)80022-6

[23] Chatoor, I. (2002) Feeding Disorders in Infants and Toddlers: Diagnosis and Treatment. *Child & Adolescent Psychiatric Clinics of North America*, **11**, 163-183. http://dx.doi.org/10.1016/S1056-4993(01)00002-5

[24] The Dutch Nutrition Centre Foundation (2013) Age Appropriate Portions for Toddlers and Pre-Schoolers. https://www.voedingscentrum.nl/nl/schijf-van-vijf/schijf.aspx

[25] Braet, C., Tanghe, A., Decaluwe, V., Moens, E. and Rosseel, Y. (2004) Inpatient Treatment for Children with Obesity: Weight Loss, Psychological Well-Being, and Eating Behavior. *Journal of Pediatric Psychology*, **29**, 519-529. http://dx.doi.org/10.1093/jpepsy/jsh054

5

Replacing Missing Teeth with Dental Implants in Pubescent Patients—A Case Report

Wendy C. W. Wang, Loana Tovar Suinaga, Klenise S. Paranhos, Sang-Choon Cho

Ashman Department of Periodontology and Implant Dentistry, New York University College of Dentistry, New York, USA

Email: wcw251@nyu.edu

Abstract

Tooth loss due to traumatic dental injury or congenital absence can cause functional and social-psychological consequences in youth. Pubescent children with missing teeth are often targets for school bullying. The treatment modality chosen can impact their well-being during their formative years. Despite the high success rate in adult patients, implant placement in young patients is not common due to its ankylosed nature and concerns with possible infra-occlusion in the future. However, skeletal growth and remodeling is a continuous process throughout life and postponement of dental implant placement does not necessary prevent future complication or need for replacement. Dental implant placement should be considered as a viable treatment option for pubescent patients if all other conventional alternatives fail to alleviate patients' concerns both functionally and psychologically. This case report evaluates the considerations required to place dental implants in pubescent patients, as well as its advantages and disadvantages.

Keywords

Dental Implants, Pubescent, Social-Psychological, Bullying

1. Introduction

Tooth loss due to traumatic dental injury or congenital absence is a common and significant problem in youth [1]-[3]. Not only does it cause functional impairment, it may also lead to social-psychological consequences [3] [4]. Missing teeth in young patients has been shown to have a negative impact on their emotional status, social relationship, speaking, smiling and carrying out work [3].

A National Center for Education Statistics (NCES) survey (2009) showed that one third of teens reported being bullied while at school; about twenty percent of teens had been made fun because of their physical appearance [5]. Several studies have looked at the impact of dento-facial features on bullying in schools [6] [7]. Dental features have been found to be targets for nicknames, harassment, and teasing among schoolchildren [6] [7]. Moreover, comments about teeth were received more negatively than comments regarding other physical features [6]. The dento-facial features most commonly bullied were found to be spaced or missing teeth, shape and color of teeth, and prominent maxillary anterior teeth [8].

Furthermore, the treatment modality chosen has an impact on the quality of life of the young patient [3]. Often times, a removable prosthesis is prescribed for its ease of construction and low cost, however its removable naturemay not be welcomed by the patient [3]. A resin-bonded bridge may be recommended as a long-term interim prosthesis to replace the missing tooth. It is a conservative method and has been reported to have good survival rates but debonding can be a concern [9].

Dental implant placement to replace missing teeth has been documented to be a predictable treatment modality with high success rates [10] [11]. For adult patients, the use of osseointegrated dental implants is often the treatment of choice due to their independence from adjacent teeth, which are spared for preparation as bridge abutments. However, implant placement in young patients involves risks due to the "ankylosed" nature of the implant. As a result, the implant does not follow the dento-alveolar development. This nature could lead to infra-occlusion of the ankylosed implant with potential periodontal, occlusal and esthetic consequences in the future [12]-[14]. On the other hand, studies have demonstrated that alveolar remodeling and growth does not cease at puberty and vertical discrepancy between a single dental implant and its adjacent natural teeth continue to occur in adulthood [15] [16]. Therefore, postponement of dental implant placement in young patients does not necessarily exclude further complication.

The use of dental implant in pubescent patients can offer both functional and psychological benefits. The ankylosed implant is fixed into the alveolar bone and therefore feels more natural to the patient. Most importantly, the security offered by a fixed prosthesis has tremendous psychological benefits for the patient.

2. Case Report

A 14-year-old Asian American boy accompanied by his mother was referred to the private clinic in December 2011. The patient was healthy with unremarkable medical history. Clinical examination revealed a congenitally missing maxillary left lateral incisor (tooth #10). The patient had been receiving orthodontic treatment to redistribute his spaces and had been wearing a removable partial denture to replace the missing tooth (**Figure 1**).

The patient appeared withdrawn and uninvolved during the initial clinical examination. It was disclosed that the patient had been subjected to repeated bullying in school for his missing tooth and inability to pronounce certain words. The removable prosthesis required frequent removal for cleaning after food consumption and he was often teased for the act. The lack of psychological security of the denture also prevented the patient from participating in active sports in fear of denture swallowing or dislodgement, which further isolated him from his peers. The combination of verbal bullying and isolation has led to a negative impact on his academic achievement and interest in attending school. Following discussion of the various treatment options available and risks involved, both the patient and his mother felt that a more permanent solution to replace his missing tooth was the best option to improve the patient's self-esteem and social confidence.

A root form titanium dental implant (EBI Inc., Kyungsan, South Korea) of 3.25 mm in diameter and 13 mm in length was inserted under local anesthesia in a two-stage surgical procedure. After crestal and sulcular incisions of the adjacent teeth, a full-thickness flap was reflected to expose the alveolar bone. The drilling protocol was performed according to the manufacturer's specification. Primary stability of 35 N cm was achieved and a cover screw was placed (**Figure 2**). The implant was uncovered following three months of undisturbed healing and animplant-supported porcelain fused to metal crown was delivered (**Figure 3**). The patient was followed up for three years and no apparent vertical discrepancy between his implant and natural teeth were noted despite his skeletal growth. The patient reported a positive psychosocial consequence following the implant restoration.

3. Discussion

Bullying is a common experience for many children and adolescents and its prevalence is highest during middle

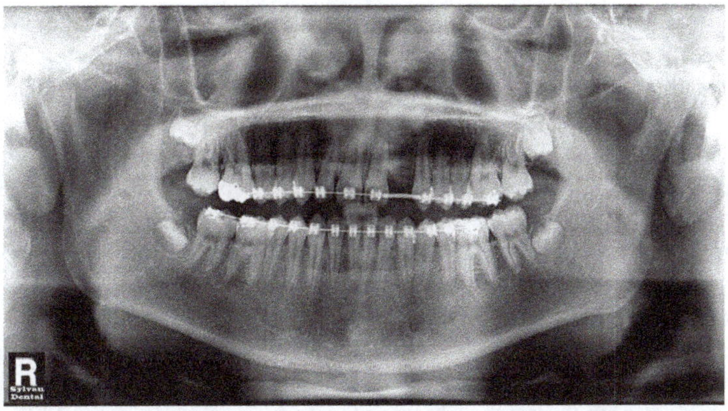

Figure 1. An orthopantomogram showing orthodontic redistribution.

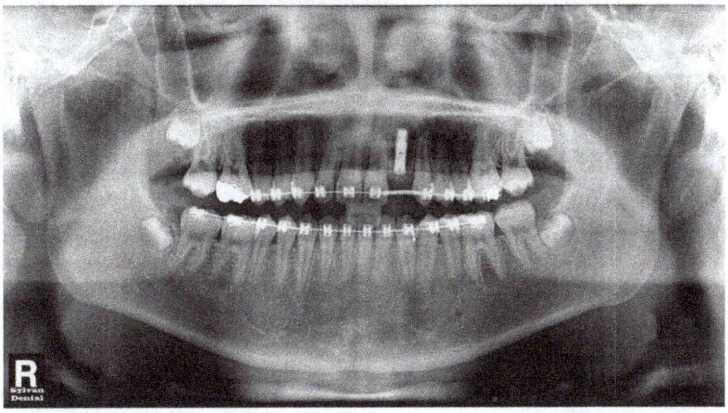

Figure 2. An orthopantomogram showing a titanium implant placed at #10 site at the time of implant placement.

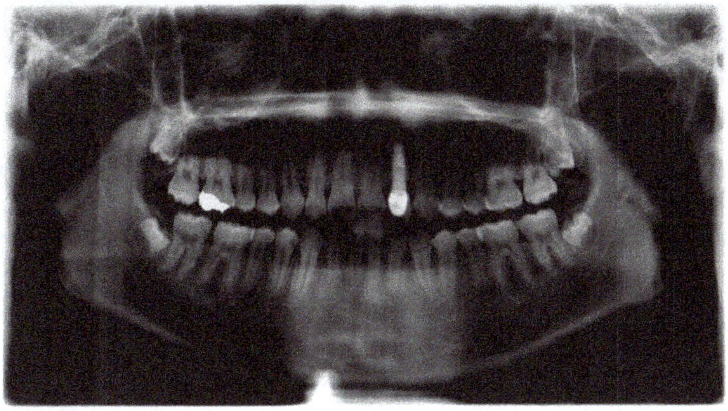

Figure 3. An orthopantomogram showing the definitive restoration.

schools [17]-[19]. General physical characteristics and dento-facial features are often reasons for social withdrawal and targets of bullying [3] [6]. The implications of bullying are extensive, and victims experience real suffering that can interfere with their social and emotional development. Studies have found links between bullying and depression, low self-esteem, contemplation of suicide, physical health problems, and poor academic performance [20]-[23].

Reservation regarding implant placement in growing patients are related to concerns over the ankylosed implant in developing dento-alveolar complex and its possible long-term sequelae. Oesterle *et al.* proposed that ankylosed implants placed in the posterior maxilla in children might become buried whereas implants in the anterior maxilla might be lost because of resorption in the infra-dental fossa and the nasal floor [13]. Cronin *et al.* warned that implants placed in the posterior mandible might become submerged in patients with rotational growth of the mandible [12]. It has been suggested implant placement should be delayed until the skeletal maturation has reached [12]-[14].

Despite the hesitation, implant placement in adolescent has the advantages of maintaining the alveolar bone and faster healing potentials [24] [25]. Ledermann *et al.* reported positive outcomes on 42 endosseous dental implants placed in 34 patients aged 9 to 18 years [25]. Brugnolo *et al.* placed single dental implants in the anterior maxilla in patients aged 11.5 to 13 years and followed up for a period of 2.5 to 4.5 years. Infra-occlusion position relative to adjacent teeth was observed and modification of the restoration was needed [26]. The authors pointed out the possible long-termimplication on the mucogingival health and the need for future corrective tissue procedures [26]. In an 8 year follow up study, Thilander *et al.* detected that infra-occlusion of maxillary anterior single implant was more severe in patients without stable incisal relationships, and suggested orthodontic alignment for stable occlusion prior to implant placement in young patients [27]. Thilander *et al.* also observed that a fixed chronological age or dental stage of fully erupted permanent teeth and skeletal maturation were not sufficient to avoid infra-occlusion of the implant-supported crown due to a slight continuous eruption of the adjacent teeth occurring in post adolescence [27].

Studies have suggested that delaying dental implant placement until the patient has reached the skeletal maturity would provide a better dental treatment outcome. However, in a retrospective study, Bernard *et al.* showed that mature adults could also exhibit vertical discrepancy after anterior restorations with osseointegrated implants to the same extent as adolescents with residual growth potential [15]. Jemt *et al.* concurred the findings and demonstrated tooth movements adjacent to single-implant restorations after more than 15 years of follow-up in adult patients. Therefore, postponing dental implant placement in young patients till skeletal maturity does not negate the possible need for future prosthetic modification or implant replacement. Furthermore, the social/psychological implication of the postponement in patients in their formative years should be explored. Clinicians must weigh the balance between the perceived ideal treatment to the need and the outcome gain of the patient. Krant suggested that the placement of implants in the anterior maxillary quadrant in young patients should only be attempted for unique treatment goals and with emphasis on the skeletal age, informed consent, and the possibility of future implant replacement [28].

With better understanding of osseointegration and improved dental implant technology, explanation and replacement of implants are no longer uncommon in the practice of implant dentistry. Treatment planning should take the patient's social psychological being into consideration and not based the decision solely on the cessation of skeletal growth. Implant treatment should be considered as a viable treatment option in young adults.

4. Conclusion

Dental implant placement can be the treatment of choice for pubescent patients if all other conventional alternatives fail to alleviate the patient's concerns both functionally and psychologically. The patient's growth pattern, individual status of the existing dentition, the functional status of mastication and phonetics, esthetic aspects, and emotional and psychological well-being are all factors that should be taken into consideration. Clinicians should consider future implant replacement rather than treatment postponement in patients who can benefit from the treatment modality.

References

[1] Cortes, M.I., Marcenes, W. and Sheiham, A. (2001) Prevalence and Correlates of Traumatic Injuries to the Permanent Teeth of School-Children Aged 9 - 14 Years in Belo Horizonte, Brazil. *Dental Traumatology*, **17**, 22-26. http://dx.doi.org/10.1034/j.1600-9657.2001.170105.x

[2] Glendor, U. (2009) Aetiology and Risk Factors Related to Traumatic Dental Injuries—A Review of the Literature. *Dental Traumatology*, **25**, 19-31. http://dx.doi.org/10.1111/j.1600-9657.2008.00694.x

[3] Hvaring, C.L., Birkeland, K. and Åstrøm, A.N. (2014) Discriminative Ability of the Generic and Condition Specific Oral Impact on Daily Performance (OIDP) among Adolescents with and without Hypodontia. *BMC Oral Health*, **14**, 57. http://dx.doi.org/10.1186/1472-6831-14-57

[4] Cortes, M.I., Marcenes, W. and Sheiham, A. (2002) Impact of Traumatic Injuries to the Permanent Teeth on the Oral Health-Related Quality of Life in 12-14-Year-Old Children. *Community Dentistry and Oral Epidemiology*, **30**, 193-198.

http://dx.doi.org/10.1034/j.1600-0528.2002.300305.x

[5] National Center for Education Statistics and Bureau of Justice Statistics. Indicators of School Crime and Safety, 2009.

[6] Shaw, W.C., Meek, S.C. and Jones, D.S. (1980) Nicknames, Teasing, Harassment and the Salience of Dental Features among School Children. *British Journal of Orthodontics*, **7**, 75-80. http://dx.doi.org/10.1179/bjo.7.2.75

[7] Seehra, J., Fleming, P.S., Newton, T. and DiBiase, A.T. (2011) Bullying in Orthodontic Patients and Its Relationship to Malocclusion, Self-Esteem and Oral Health-Related Quality of Life. *Journal of Orthodontics*, **38**, 247-56. http://dx.doi.org/10.1179/14653121141641

[8] Al-Bitar, Z.B., Al-Omari, I.K., Sonbol, H.N., Al-Ahmad, H.T. and Cunningham, S.J. (2013) Bullying among Jordanian Schoolchildren, Its Effects on School Performance, and the Contribution of General Physical and Dentofacial Features. *American Journal of Orthodontics and Dentofacial Orthopedics*, **144**, 872-878. http://dx.doi.org/10.1016/j.ajodo.2013.08.016

[9] Djemal, S., Setchell, D., King, P. and Wickens, J. (1999) Long-Term Survival Characteristics of 832 Resin-Retained Bridges and Splints Provided in a Post-Graduate Teaching Hospital between 1978 and 1993. *Journal of Oral Rehabilitation*, **26**, 302-320. http://dx.doi.org/10.1046/j.1365-2842.1999.00374.x

[10] Adell, R., Lekholm, U., Rockler, B. and Brånemark, P.I. (1981) A 15-Year Study of Osseointegrated Implants in the Treatment of the Edentulous Jaw. *International Journal of Oral Surgery*, **10**, 387-416. http://dx.doi.org/10.1016/S0300-9785(81)80077-4

[11] Buser, D., Mericske-Stern, R., Bernard, J.P., *et al.* (1997) Long-Term Evaluation of Non-Submerged ITI Implants. Part 1: 8-Year Life Table Analysis of a Prospective Multi-Center Study with 2359 Implants. *Clinical Oral Implants Research*, **8**, 161-172. http://dx.doi.org/10.1034/j.1600-0501.1997.080302.x

[12] Cronin, R.J., Oesterle, L.J. and Ranly, D.M. (1994) Mandibular Implants and the Growing Patient. *The International Journal of Oral & Maxillofacial Implants*, **9**, 55-62.

[13] Oesterle, L.J., Cronin, R.J. and Ranly, D.M. (1993) Maxillary Implants and the Growing Patient. *The International Journal of Oral & Maxillofacial Implants*, **8**, 377-387.

[14] Thilander, B., Odman, J., Grondahl, K. and Friberg B. (1994) Osseointegrated Implants in Adolescents. An Alternative in Replacing Missing Teeth? *European Journal of Orthodontics*, **16**, 84-95. http://dx.doi.org/10.1093/ejo/16.2.84

[15] Bernard, J.P., Schatz, J.P., Christou, P., Belser, U. and Kiliaridis, S. (2004) Long-Term Vertical Changes of the Anterior Maxillary Teeth Adjacent to Single Implants in Young and Mature Adults. A Retrospective Study. *Journal of Clinical Periodontology*, **31**, 1024-1028. http://dx.doi.org/10.1111/j.1600-051X.2004.00574.x

[16] Jemt, T., Ahlberg, G., Henriksson, K. and Bondevik, O. (2006) Tooth Movements Adjacent to Single-Implant Restorations after More than 15 Years of Follow-Up. *The International Journal of Prosthodontics*, **20**, 626-632.

[17] Carney, A.G. and Merrell, K.W. (2001) Perspectives on Understanding and Preventing an International Problem. *School Psychology International*, **22**, 364-382. http://dx.doi.org/10.1177/0143034301223011

[18] Spriggs, A.L., Iannotti, R.J., Nansel, T.R. and Haynie, D.L. (2007) Adolescent Bullying Involvement and Perceived Family Peer and School Relations: Commonalities and Differences across Race/Ethnicity. *Journal of Adolescent Health*, **41**, 283-293. http://dx.doi.org/10.1016/j.jadohealth.2007.04.009

[19] (2011) American Academy of Child and Adolescent Psychiatry, Bullying No. 80.

[20] Pellegrini, A.D. (1998) Bullied and Victims in School: A Review and Call for Research. *Journal of Applied Developmental Psychology*, **19**, 156-176. http://dx.doi.org/10.1016/S0193-3973(99)80034-3

[21] Analitis, F., Velderman, M.K., Ravens-Sieberer, U., Detmar, S., Erhart, M., Herdman, M., *et al.* (2009) European Kidscreen Group. Being Bullied: Associated Factors in Children and Adolescents 8 to 18 Years Old in 11 European Countries. *Pediatrics*, **123**, 569-577. http://dx.doi.org/10.1542/peds.2008-0323

[22] Kumpulainen, K. and Rasanen, E. (2000) Children Involved in Bullying at Elementary School Age: Their Psychiatric Symptoms and Deviance in Adolescence. An Epidemiological Sample. *Child Abuse & Neglect*, **24**, 1567-1577. http://dx.doi.org/10.1016/S0145-2134(00)00210-6

[23] Hawker, D.S. and Boulton, M.J. (2000) Twenty Years' Research on Peer Victimization and Psychosocial Maladjustment: A Meta-Analytic Review of Cross-Sectional Studies. *Journal of Child Psychology and Psychiatry*, **41**, 441-455. http://dx.doi.org/10.1111/1469-7610.00629

[24] Mehrali, M.C., Baraoidan, M. and Cranin, A.N. (1994) Use of Endosseous Implants in Treatment of Adolescent Trauma Patients. *The New York State Dental Journal*, **60**, 25-29.

[25] Ledermann, P.D., Hassel, T.M. and Hefti, A.F. (1993) Osseointegrated Dental Implants as Alternative Therapy to Bridge Construction or Orthodontics in Young Patients: Seven Years of Clinical Experience. *Journal of Pediatric Dentistry*, **15**, 327-332.

[26] Brugnolo, E., Mazzocco, C., Cordioli, G. and Majzoub, Z. (1996) Clinical and Radiographic Findings Following Placement of Single Tooth Implants in Young Patients—Case Reports. *International Journal of Periodontics & Restorative Dentistry*, **16**, 421-433.

[27] Thilander, B., Ödman, J. and Jemt, T. (1999) Single Implants in the Upper Incisor Region and Their Relationship to the Adjacent Teeth. An 8-Year Follow-Up Study. *Clinical Oral Implants Research*, **10**, 346-355. http://dx.doi.org/10.1034/j.1600-0501.1999.100502.x

[28] Kraut, R.A. (1996) Dental Implants for Children: Creating Smiles for Children without Teeth. *Practical Periodontics & Aesthetic Dentistry*, **8**, 909-813.

6

Impact of Rotavirus Vaccination in Severe Rotavirus Gastroenteritis Outpatient Visits at Three Pediatric Primary Care Clinics in Shibata City, Niigata Prefecture, Japan

Tomohiro Oishi[1*], Shinya Tsukano[2], Tokushi Nakano[3], Shoji Sudo[4], Hiroaki Kuwajima[5], for the Shibata RVGE Study Group

[1]Department of Pediatrics, Niigata University Medical and Dental Hospital, Niigata City, Niigata, Japan
[2]Pediatric Department, Niigata Prefectural Shibata Hospital, Shibata City, Niigata, Japan
[3]Nakano Children's Clinic, Shibata City, Niigata, Japan
[4]Sudo Pediatric Clinic, Shibata City, Niigata, Japan
[5]Pediatric Department, Kuwajima Clinic, Shibata City, Niigata, Japan
Email: *oo0612@med.niigata-u.ac.jp

Abstract

The impact of rotavirus (RV) vaccination in reducing severe rotavirus gastroenteritis (RVGE) in outpatient settings was prospectively surveyed in three pediatric clinics in Shibata City. In children younger than 3 years of age, the occurrence of severe RVGE among all acute gastroenteritis (AGE) was found to be significantly lower in three seasons after introduction of RV vaccines, compared to that in 2011, before introduction of RV vaccines. The incidence rates of severe RVGE among children younger than 3 years of age were found to be reduced by 71.2%, 47.7%, and 81.1% for 2012, 2013, and 2014, respectively, compared to that in 2011. These results suggest that the RV vaccination is effective for the prevention of severe RVGE in Japanese voluntary RV vaccination settings with estimated coverage rates of 32.5%, 40.5% and 47.1% for 2012, 2013 and 2014, respectively. It is expected that the reducing effect on severe RVGE would be persistently established by increasing the vaccine coverage rates.

Keywords

Impact of Vaccination, Rotavirus Gastroenteritis, Rotavirus Vaccine, Prospective Observation, Outpatient Settings

*Corresponding author.

1. Introduction

Rotavirus (RV) infection is the most common cause of severe diarrhea worldwide [1]. Patients with rotavirus gastroenteritis (RVGE) may develop severe dehydration, which can be life-threatening if the body fluid imbalances are not appropriately corrected. Although fatal cases are rare in Japan, it has been reported that approximately 790,000 children younger than 6 years of age visit hospitals/clinics as outpatients due to RVGE [2], and approximately 78,000 children younger than 5 years of age are hospitalized annually [3].

Currently, two oral RV vaccines, Rotarix™ (GlaxoSmithKline Biologicals, Rixensart, Belgium) and RotaTeq™ (Merck & Co., Inc., Whitehouse Station, NJ, USA), for prevention of RVGE are approved in more than 100 countries and are incorporated into national immunization programs in more than 50 countries by April 2014 [4]. In some of the countries in which these RV vaccines have been introduced, the number of hospitalizations due to RVGE has dramatically decreased by the direct and indirect effects resulting from the vaccinations [4]-[6]. Since reviewing recent evidence on efficacy and safety of RV vaccines, the WHO has recommended to use RV vaccines in all national immunization programs [7]. In Japan, Rotarix™ and RotaTeq™ have been on the market since November 2011 and July 2012, respectively. Although RV vaccination had not been adopted into the national immunization program as of 2014, an estimation of 45% uptake with a wide range of variation throughout Japan was reported in 2013 [8].

To assess the impact of the RV vaccination, an observational study design examining changes in disease burden overtime, including seasons before and after the introduction of RV vaccines, is commonly used [9]. Many of the studies reporting RV vaccine efficacy in the real world [4]-[6], indicate the impact of RV vaccination based on the data from a national database or a large insurance database. In Japan, we do not have national statistics of RV-related diseases and it is difficult to show the nationwide vaccine impact. The number of infectious gastroenteritis cases including RVGE has been collected weekly from sentinel pediatric clinics since the years before vaccine introduction, but the actual number of RVGE cases cannot be specified. For RVGE hospitalizations, the number of patients started to be collected from sentinel hospitals just after introduction of vaccines.

This study was planned to prospectively assess the impact of RV vaccines in a small city in Japan. The pragmatic design to evaluate the vaccine impact in outpatient settings using the number of severe RVGE patients as an indicator was developed by referring to some hospital-based [10]-[12] and primary practice-based [13] impact studies conducted in other countries. We previously reported the early impact by comparing the 2011 and 2012 RVGE epidemic seasons [14]. Here we report the impact observed in three RV epidemic seasons after RV vaccine introduction in 2011.

2. Method

This prospective observational study was conducted at three primary-care pediatric clinics in Shibata City, Niigata Prefecture, Japan. Shibata City is a small city with a stable population of approximately 100,000 inhabitants, and around 770 babies are born each year. In the city there are three primary-care pediatric clinics and one hospital with a pediatric ward, the Niigata Prefectural Shibata Hospital (Shibata Hospital). The three pediatric clinics serve pediatric primary medicine for people living in Shibata City and surrounding areas. The Shibata Hospital is the central facility in Kaetsu medical area, one of the seven secondary medical areas in Niigata Prefecture. We assumed that almost all children living in Shibata City would visit one of the three pediatric clinics when they have an illness such as acute gastroenteritis (AGE) and would be presented to the Shibata Hospital when they need a hospitalization care.

Children younger than 5 years of age (or 3 years of age for 2011) who visited a study site from February 2011 to May 2014 due to AGE were included. We recorded date of visit, date of birth, sex, and living area of all AGE patients with their symptoms (presence or absence of diarrhea and vomiting) and whether they required intravenous rehydration to correct dehydration. AGE was defined as occurrence of gastroenteritis symptoms for less than 14 days. Patients who required intravenous rehydration were defined as having severe AGE and were tested for fecal RV antigen. Rapid fecal rotavirus tests were performed using ImmunoCard™ ST Rotavirus (Fujirebio Inc., Tokyo, Japan) after oral informed consent was obtained from the parents/guardians of the pediatric patients. Severe AGE patients with positive RV antigen test results were defined as having severe RVGE and detailed information regarding their symptoms was collected to calculate severity score using modified Vesikari's scale [14] [15].

Clinical research records of AGE patients who lived in Shibata City were analyzed. Comparison of occurrence and incidence of RVGE before and after RV vaccine introduction was performed for only patients younger than 3 years of age during each epidemic season, because we collected the information on AGE patients younger than 3 years of age and only for epidemic months in 2011, the season before RV vaccine introduction.

A Chi-square test was used to calculate the statistical significance of differences between distributions of categorical variables, and Student's *t*-test was used to compare means of numerical variables. The incidences and 95% confidence intervals of outpatient severe RVGE, severe GE, and all acute GE were calculated based on the numbers of patients who visited the three clinics during each observation period and the number of children under 3 years of age who lived in Shibata City. These incidences were compared between 2011 and the other years using Poisson regression analysis. Microsoft Excel version 14 was used for statistical analyses.

Genotyping of rotavirus was performed when a sufficient amount of sample was obtained from a patient. Analyses were performed using reverse transcription-polymerase chain reaction at Niigata Prefectural Institute of Public Health and Environmental Sciences. All RV vaccination records in the three pediatric clinics and the Shibata Hospital were also retrospectively collected, to estimate vaccine coverage rates. The number of patients with AGE and RVGE hospitalized in the Shibata Hospital from 2008 to 2014 was retrospectively collected for reference.

This study was conducted in compliance with Ethical Guidelines for Epidemiological Research (June 17, 2002 [Partial revision: December 1, 2008] The Ministry of Education, Culture, Sports, Science and Technology; Ministry of Health, Labour and Welfare) based on the spirit of the Declaration of Helsinki - Ethical Principles for Medical Research Involving Human Subjects. Prior to conducting the study, the Ethical Review Committees of the Niigata Prefectural Shibata Hospital reviewed both ethical and scientific aspects of the study protocol (e.g., study design, population, time period, etc.) and approved the proposed study conduct.

3. Results

3.1. Number of Episodes Observed and Analyzed

In total, 3778 AGE episodes were observed in children younger than 5 years of age who lived in Shibata City at the three pediatric clinics during the study period, from February 14, 2011 to May 31, 2014. Of which, 2203 were observed during the epidemic months, from February to May. Of the total AGE episodes, 2589 occurred in children younger than 3 years of age during the extended period and 1473 during the epidemic months. The number of AGE episodes of each year is summarized in **Table 1**. We analyzed 1473 AGE episodes in children younger than 3 years of age who visited a pediatric clinic during the epidemic months.

Yearly numbers analyzed are shown in **Table 2**. Of 1473 AGE episodes, 147 (10.0%) were defined as severe AGE because intravenous rehydration was applied for them. Of 147 patients with severe AGE, 137 (93.2%) were tested for fecal RV antigen and 101 (73.7%) were confirmed as severe RVGE. For comparison of the occurrence and incidence of severe RVGE before and after RV vaccine introduction, we included 10 episodes of

Table 1. Number of AGE episodes observed.

Year	Observation period	<3 years of age	3 - 4 years of age	Total (<5 years of age)
2011	Epidemic months*	397	-	397***
	Extended period**	542	-	542***
2012	Epidemic months*	355	214	569
	Extended period**	857	407	1264
2013	Epidemic months*	398	242	640
	Extended period**	783	452	1235
2014	Epidemic months*	323	274	597
	Extended period**	407	330	737
Total	Epidemic months	1473	730	2203
	Extended period	2589	1189	3778

*Epidemic months: February 14 to May 31 for 2011, and February 1 to May 31 for 2012, 2013, 2014; **Extended period: February 14 to May 31 and October 1 to December 31 for 2011, January 1 to December 31 for 2012 and 2013, January 1 to May 31 for 2014; ***< 3 years of age.

severe AGE not tested for fecal RV antigen in addition to 101 episodes of test-confirmed severe RVGE, to avoid overestimation of the vaccine impact. Monthly numbers of AGE, severe AGE, and severe RVGE are shown in **Figure 1**. The peak month of severe RVGE was April in each year.

3.2. Changes in Occurrence of Severe RVGE

The occurrences of severe RVGE among severe AGE and all AGE, and severe AGE among all AGE are summarized in **Table 3**. The occurrences of severe RVGE among all AGE and severe AGE among all AGE in 2012,

Table 2. Number of episodes analyzed (<3 years of age, February to May).

Type of episodes	2011	2012	2013	2014	Total
AGE	397	355	398	323	1473
Severe AGE	62	31	41	13	147
Severe AGE tested for fecal RV antigen	62	28	39	8	137
Severe RVGE confirmed	52	14	29	6	101
Severe RVGE (including episodes not tested)	52	17	31	11	111

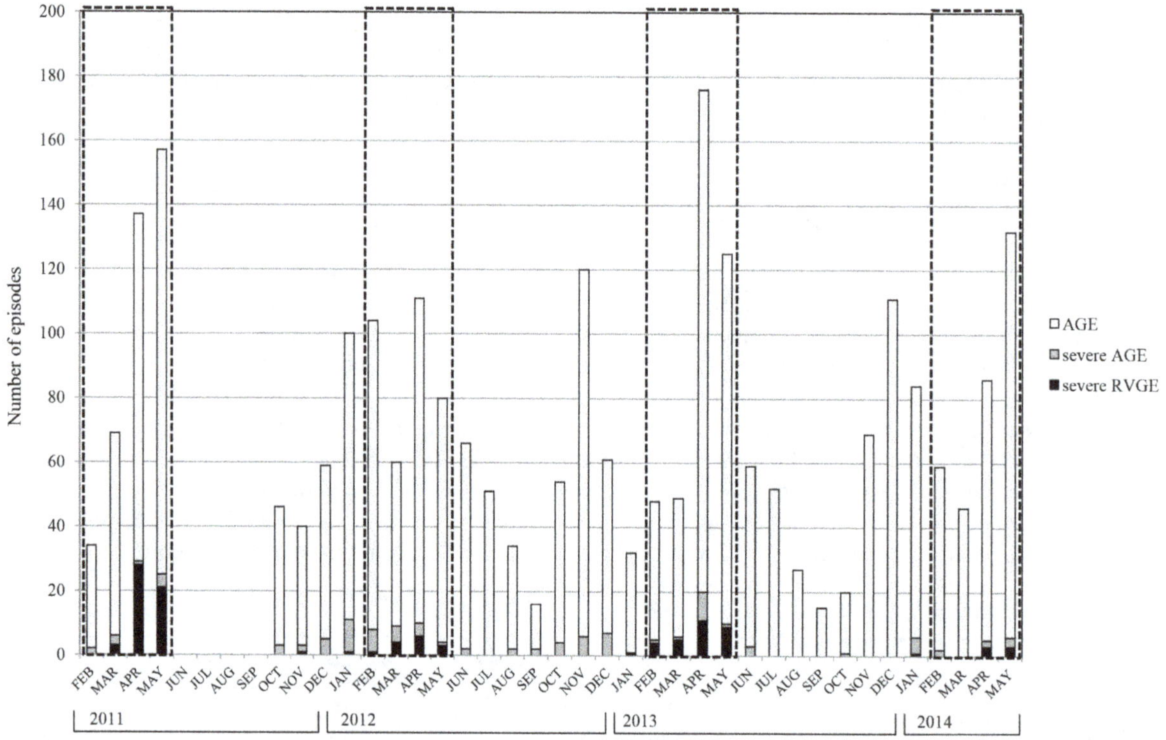

Figure 1. Monthly number of episodes of AGE, severe AGE, and severe RVGE (<3 years of age). Number of AGE (pale gray column), severe AGE (gray column) and severe RVGE (black column) episodes are indicated throughout the study periods. Severe RVGE episodes include only test confirmed episodes. Dotted squares indicate epidemic seasons. In 2011, the study was performed in only the epidemic months from February to May and the months from October to December. The peak month of severe RVGE was April in each year.

Table 3. Occurrence of severe RVGE or severe AGE among all AGE or severe AGE patients.

Occurrence of	2011	2012	2013	2014
Severe RVGE/all AGE	13.1% (52/397)	4.8%** (17/355)	7.8%* (31/398)	3.4%** (11/323)
Severe RVGE/severe AGE	83.9% (52/62)	54.8%** (17/31)	75.6% (31/41)	84.6% (11/13)
Severe AGE/all AGE	15.6% (62/397)	8.7%** (31/355)	10.3%* (41/398)	4.0%** (13/323)

*$p < 0.05$; **$p < 0.01$

2013, and 2014, seasons after RV vaccine introduction, were lower than in 2011, the season before RV vaccine introduction. The occurrences of severe RVGE among severe AGE were similar in each year except for 2012, indicating that the majority of severe GE episodes that require intravenous rehydration in outpatient settings are possibly attributable to rotavirus during RV epidemic months.

3.3. Changes in Incidence of Severe RVGE

The incidence rates of severe RVGE were significantly reduced, by 71.2%, 47.7%, and 81.1% for 2012, 2013, and 2014, respectively, compared to that in 2011, the season before RV vaccine introduction (**Table 4**). Similar reductions were observed in the incidence rates of severe AGE. Reduction in the incidence rates of AGE were seen in 2012 (21.3%) and 2014 (27.4%), but not in 2013.

3.4. Profiles of Patients with Severe RVGE

The descriptions of children with severe RVGE are shown in **Table 5**. The peak months of age were 12 to 23

Table 4. Incidence rates of severe RVGE, severe AGE, and AGE among children younger than 3 years of age.

/1000 person-years (95% CI)	2011	2012	2013	2014
Severe RVGE	77.1 (57.6 - 99.5)	22.2 (12.9 - 33.9)**	40.3 (27.4 - 55.7)**	14.6 (7.3 - 24.4)**
% reduction	-	71.2% (50.3 - 83.4%)	47.7% (18.4 - 66.5%)	81.1% (63.8 - 90.1%)
Severe AGE	92.0 (70.5 - 116.2)	40.5 (27.5 - 55.9)**	53.3 (38.3 - 70.9)**	17.2 (9.2 - 27.8)**
% reduction	-	56.0% (32.3 - 71.4%)	42.1% (13.9 - 60.9%)	81.3% (66.0 - 89.7%)
AGE	588.8 (532.3 - 648.1)	463.4 (416.4 - 512.8)**	517.8 (468.2 - 569.9)	427.7 (382.3 - 475.6)**
% reduction	-	21.3% (9.2 - 31.8%)	12.1% (−1.1 - 23.5%)	27.4% (15.9 - 37.3%)

**$p < 0.01$ vs 2011; Number of children younger than 3 years of age in population as of March 31; 2011: 2300; 2012: 2311; 2013: 2338; 2014: 2297. Observation period: 2011: 107 days (Feb 14 to May 31); 2012: 121 days (Feb 1 to May 31); 2013: 120 days (Feb 1 to May 31); 2014: 120 days (Feb 1 to May 31).

Table 5. Profile of severe RVGE patients.

		2011	2012	2013	2014
Total number	52	17	31	11	
Sex	Male	27	9	16	5
	Female	25	8	15	6
Age in months	0 to 5	2	1	0	0
	6 to11	7	3	0	1
	12 to 23	24	6	18	2
	24 to 35	19	7	13	8
Months	February	0	1	4	1
	March	3	5	5	0
	April	28	8	13	5
	May	21	3	9	5
Vaccinated	-	0	1	2	
				Rotarix^{TM} 1	Rotarix^{TM} 1
					RotaTeq^{TM} 1
Severity Score	11-point Vesikari Scale	6.04 (1.88)	7.00 (1.90)	5.77 (2.37)	7.00 (2.12)
Mean (SD)	20-point Vesikari Scale	-	12.00 (2.90)	11.68 (2.10)	10.20 (1.64)
	Number evaluated	52	11	22	5

months in 2011 and 2013 and 24 to 35 months in 2012 and 2014. The peak month of epidemic season was April. Yearly variation was not detected in the mean severity score calculated using 11-point and 20-point Vesikari's scales [14]. There were 3 severe RVGE episodes observed in children who had received RV vaccine before the onsets: 1 in 2013 and 2 in 2014 (**Table 6**). All 3 episodes were observed more than one year after vaccination.

3.5. Genotypes of Rotaviruses

Genotypes of rotaviruses in feces collected from the study site and Shibata Hospital are summarized in **Table 7**. The majority genotype was G3P [8] in 2011, G1P [8] and G9P [8] in 2012, G1P [8] in 2013, and G9P [8] in 2014. Epidemic viruses might change year by year.

3.6. Estimated Vaccine Coverage Rate

In Shibata City, voluntary RV vaccination started from the end of November 2011. Vaccination costs should have been paid by parents or guardians of infants. From the number of patients who were vaccinated with at least one dose of Rotarix™ or RotaTeq™ at the three pediatric clinics and the Shibata Hospital during the study period, vaccine coverage rate in the birth cohort was estimated as 32.5%, 40.5%, and 47.1% as of the end of May in 2012, 2013, and 2014.

3.7. Changes in RVGE Hospitalization

The number of children younger than 3 years of age who lived in Shibata City and hospitalized in the Shibata Hospital due to RVGE and AGE was retrospectively collected for reference of long-term trends. **Figure 2** indicates numbers of hospitalizations due to RVGE and non-RV GE by year. The proportion of RVGE among AGE was 26.9% in the period after RV vaccine introduction (from January 2012 to May 2014), significantly lower ($p = 0.018$) compared with 44.7% in the period before (from January 2008 to December 2011). Although year-to-year variation was seen in numbers of hospitalizations due to RVGE and AGE, the proportion of RVGE among AGE reduced after RV vaccine introduction.

Table 6. Profiles of severe RVGE patients with vaccination history.

	No. 1	**No. 2**	**No. 3**
Date of diagnosis	2013/2/28	2014/4/28	2014/5/12
Age in months	17	25	15
Sex	Male	Female	Male
Vaccinated with	Rotarix™	Rotarix™	RotaTeq™
Vaccinated in	2012/1; 2012/2	2012/6; 2012/8	2013/4; 2013/5; 2013/6
Severity Score			
20-point Vesikari Scale	11	Not available	11
10-point Vesikari Scale	6	Not available	9

Table 7. Genotypes of rotaviruses detected during the study period.

	2011		**2012**		**2013**		**2014**	
	n	(%)	*n*	(%)	*n*	(%)	*n*	(%)
G1P [8]	1	5.9	18	45	39	88.6	0	0
G2P [4]	1	5.9	1	2.5	5	11.4	1	16.7
G3P [8]	14	82.4	1	2.5	0	0	0	0
G9P [8]	1	5.9	20	50.0	0	0	5	83.3
Total	17		40		44		6	

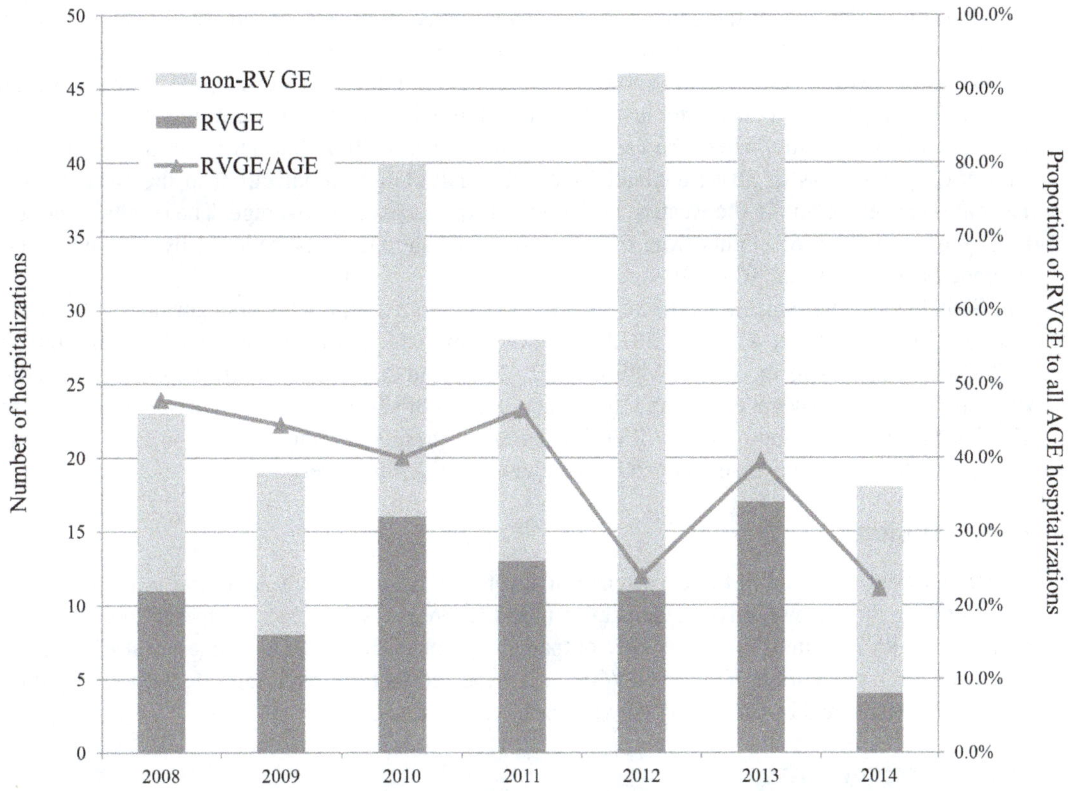

Figure 2. Numbers of RVGE and non-RV GE hospitalizations (children younger than 3 years of age). Numbers of hospitalizations among children younger than 3 years of age who lived in Shibata City are indicated in dark gray column (due to RVGE) and pale gray column (due to non-RV GE) by year. The proportion of RVGE among AGE reduced after the introduction of RV vaccines compared with the years before. All patients hospitalized due to AGE had RV tests to determine the cause of AGE.

4. Discussion

Consistent reduction in the occurrence and incidence rates of severe RVGE in children less than 3 years of age observed in three seasons after RV vaccine introduction may be explained by the vaccine impact. As in many other studies [4]-[6], the results suggest indirect benefits for older children, in addition to the children who were targeted for vaccination. Patel MM *et al.* described that indirect benefits were noted in the first or the second year after vaccine introduction, while only infants were eligible to receive vaccination, potentially implicating infants as the primary transmitters of infection [6].

In spite of consistent reduction after RV vaccine introduction, relative increases in the incidence rates of AGE, severe AGE, and severe RVGE were seen in 2013, the second season after vaccine introduction. Biennial epidemic peaks after RV vaccine introduction were also observed in some other studies [6] [16]. The biennial pattern was explained by accumulation of unimmunized susceptible children during seasons with low rotavirus activity and the higher number of susceptible children to facilitate transmission during a subsequent season [6] [16].

The occurrence of severe RVGE among severe AGE decreased in 2012 but did not in 2013 and 2014. We consider that a substantial proportion of AGE patients less than 3 years old who require intravenous rehydration therapy are RVGE patients during epidemic months in outpatient settings. The reduction of occurrence in 2012 might be influenced by AGE epidemic of other pathogens such as noro virus.

A major limitation of this study was that we had only one season of observation data as a reference. However, although there was year-to-year variation in numbers of severe RVGE and severe AGE after RV vaccine introduction, consistent reduction in the occurrence and incidence rates of severe RVGE was observed in the three seasons after RV vaccine introduction. It may be reasonable to consider that the reduction is due to RV vaccine impact.

Another limitation is that the study was conducted under circumstances in which the vaccine coverage rates were not sufficiently high. There are some studies reporting vaccine impact under relatively low vaccine coverage rates [11] [13] [17]-[20]. Zeller reported 35% reduction in the RV-positive rate among hospitalized patients aged less than 5 years at a university hospital in Belgium when the vaccine coverage rate was estimated as 65% [11]. A study in Germany, where the vaccine was introduced in 2006 but not incorporated into the national immunization program as of 2012, evaluated the rates of RVGE hospitalization in the eastern region with high vaccination coverage and in the western region with low vaccination coverage. The results suggested the rates of RVGE hospitalization of infants from 6 to 11 months of age would be reduced by 42% when the vaccination coverage rates increase to 50% [19].

In Shibata City, the incidence rates of severe RVGE among outpatients younger than 3 years of age were reduced by 71.2% in 2012, 47.7% in 2013, and 81.1% in 2014. Estimated vaccine coverage rates were 32.5%, 40.5%, and 47.1% as of the end of May in 2012, 2013, and 2014. There were no direct associations observed between the vaccine coverage rates and the reduction rates of severe RVGE. We assume that the vaccine may be effective for the prevention of severe RVGE even under these moderate vaccination rates in Japan, and that the year-to-year variation may be explained by the biennial epidemic pattern.

5. Conclusion

Reductions were observed in the occurrence of severe RVGE among all AGE and in the incidence rates of severe RVGE in three consecutive seasons after introduction of RV vaccine, compared to that in 2011, before introduction of RV vaccines in primary care outpatient settings. These results suggest that RV vaccination may be effective for the prevention of severe RVGE. It is expected that the reducing effect on severe RVGE would be persistently established by increasing the vaccine coverage rates.

Acknowledgements

This study was supported in part by a research grant from the Investigator-Initiated Studies Program of GlaxoSmithKline Biologicals and Japan Vaccine Co., Ltd.

We would like to thank Dr. Tsutomu Tamura at Niigata Prefectural Institute of Public Health and Environmental Sciences for his cooperation in genotyping of rotavirus. We would also like to thank Satoshi Osaga and Hiromi Sugawara at MC&P Co., Ltd. for their assistance in statistical analyses and medical writing.

References

[1] Tate, J.E., Burton, A.H., Boschi-Pinto, C., Steele, A.D., Duque, J. and Parashar, U.D., the WHO-coordinated Global Rotavirus Surveillance Network (2011) 2008 Estimate of Worldwide Rotavirus-Associated Mortalityin Children Younger than 5 Years before the Introduction of Universal Rotavirus Vaccination Programmes: A Systematic Review and Meta-Analysis. *The Lancet Infectious Diseases*, **12**, 136-141. http://dx.doi.org/DOI:10.1016/S1473-3099(11)70253-5

[2] Yokoo, M., Arisawa, K. and Nakagomi, O. (2004) Estimation of Annual Incidence, Age-Specific Incidence Rate, and Cumulative Risk of Rotavirus Gastroenteritis among Children in Japan. *Japanese Journal of Infectious Diseases*, **57**, 166-171.

[3] Nakagomi, T., Nakagomi, O., Takahashi, Y., Enoki, M., Suzuki, T. and Kilgore, P.E. (2005) Incidence and Burden of Rotavirus Gastroenteritis in Japan, as Estimated from a Prospective Sentinel Hospital Study. *The Journal of Infectious Diseases*, **192**, S106-S110. http://dx.doi.org/10.1086/431503

[4] Yen, C., Tate, J.E., Hyde, T.B., Cortese, M.M., Lopman, B.A., Jiang, B., Glass, R.I. and Parashar, U.D. (2014) Rotavirus Vaccines—Current Status and Future Considerations. *Human Vaccine & Immunotherapeutics*, **10**, 1-13. http://dx.doi.org/10.4161/hv.28857

[5] Patel, M.M., Glass, R., Desai, R., Tate, J.E. and Parashar, U.D. (2012) Fulfilling the Promise of Rotavirus Vaccines: How Far Have We Come Since Licensure? *The Lancet Infectious Diseases*, **12**, 561-570. http://dx.doi.org/10.1016/S1473-3099(12)70029-4

[6] Patel, M.M., Steele, D., Gentsch, J.R., Wecker, J., Glass, R.I. and Parashar, U.D. (2011) Real-World Impact of Rotavirus Vaccination. *Pediatric Infectious Disease Journal*, **30**, S1-S5. http://dx.doi.org/10.1097/INF.0b013e3181fefa1f

[7] World Health Organization (2013) Rotavirus Vaccines WHO Position Paper—January 2013. *Weekly Epidemiological record*, **88**, 49-64.

[8] Committee for National Immunization Policy (2013) Interim Report of rotavirus Vaccination Working Group (in Japanese).
http://www.mhlw.go.jp/file/05-Shingikai-10601000-Daijinkanboukouseikagakuka-Kouseikagakuka/0000029637.pdf

[9] Weinberg, G.A. and Szilagyi, P.G. (2010) Vaccine Epidemiology: Efficacy, Effectiveness, and the Translational Research Roadmap. *The Journal of Infectious Diseases*, **201**, 1607-1610. http://dx.doi.org/10.1086/652404

[10] Clark, H.F., Lawley, D., Mallette, L.A., Dinubile, M.J. and Hodinka, R.L. (2009) Decline in Cases of Rotavirus Gastroenteritis Presenting to The Children's Hospital of Philadelphia after Introduction of a Pentavalent Rotavirus Vaccine. *Clinical and Vaccine Immunology*, **16**, 382-386. http://dx.doi.org/10.1128/CVI.00382-08

[11] Zeller, M., Rahman, M., Heylen, E., De Coster, S., De Vos, S., Arijs, I., Novo, L., Verstappen, N., Van Ranst, M. and Matthijnssens, J. (2010) Rotavirus Incidence and Genotype Distribution before and after National Rotavirus Vaccine Introduction in Belgium. *Vaccine*, **28**, 7507-7513. http://dx.doi.org/10.1016/j.vaccine.2010.09.004

[12] Rae, M., Strens, D., Vergison, A., Verghote, M. and Standaert, B. (2011) Reduction in Pediatric Rotavirus-Related Hospitalizations after Universal Rotavirus Vaccination in Belgium. *The Pediatric Infectious Disease Journal*, **30**, e120-e125. http://dx.doi.org/10.1097/INF.0b013e318214b811

[13] Bégué, R.E. and Perrin, K. (2010) Reduction in Gastroenteritis with the Use of Pentavalent Rotavirus Vaccine in a Primary Practice. *Pediatrics*, **126**, e40-e45. http://dx.doi.org/10.1542/peds.2009-2069

[14] Oishi, T., Taguchi, T., Nakano, T., Sudo, S. and Kuwajima, H. (2014) The Occurrence of Severe Rotavirus Gastroenteritis in Children under 3 Years of Age before and after the Introduction of Rotavirus Vaccine: A Prospective Observational Study in Three Pediatric Clinics in Shibata City, Niigata Prefecture, Japan. *Japanese Journal of Infectious Diseases*, **67**, 304-306. http://dx.doi.org/10.7883/yoken.67.304

[15] Ruuska, T. and Vesikari, T. (1990) Rotavirus Disease in Finnish Children: Use of Numerical Scores for Clinical Severity of Diarrhoeal Episodes. *Scandinavian Journal of Infectious Diseases*, **22**, 259-267.
http://dx.doi.org/10.3109/00365549009027046

[16] Tate, J.E., Haynes, A., Payne, D.C., Cortese, M.M., Lopman, B.A., Patel, M.M. and Parashar, U.D. (2013) Trends in National Rotavirus Activity before and after Introduction of Rotavirus Vaccine into the National Immunization Program in the United States, 2000 to 2012. *The Pediatric Infectious Disease Journal*, **32**, 741-744.
http://dx.doi.org/10.1097/INF.0b013e31828d639c

[17] Curns, A.T., Steiner, C.A., Barrett, M., Hunter, K., Wilson, E. and Parashar, U.D. (2011) Reduction in Acute Gastroenteritis Hospitalizations among US Children after Introduction of Rotavirus Vaccine: Analysis of Hospital Discharge Data from 18 US States. *The Journal of Infectious Diseases*, **201**, 1617-1624. http://dx.doi.org/10.1086/652403

[18] Gil-Prieto, R., Gonzalez-Escaladaa, A., Alvaro-Mecaa, A., Garcia-Garciaa, L., San-Martinb, M., González-Lópezb, A. and Gil-de-Miguela, A. (2013) Impact of Non-Routine Vaccination on Hospitalizations for Diarrhoea and Rotavirus Infections in Spain. *Vaccine*, **31**, 5000-5004. http://dx.doi.org/10.1016/j.vaccine.2013.05.109

[19] Dudareva-Vizule, S., Koch, J., an der Heiden, M., Oberle, D., Keller-Stanislawski, B. and Wichmann, O. (2012) Impact of Rotavirus Vaccination in Regions with Low and Moderate Vaccine Uptake in Germany. *Human Vaccine & Immunotherapy*, **8**, 1407-1415. http://dx.doi.org/10.4161/hv.21593

[20] Steyer, A., Sagadin, M., Kolenc, M. and Poljšak-Prijatelj, M. (2014) Molecular Characterization of Rotavirus Strains from Pre- and Post-Vaccination Periods in a Country with Low Vaccination Coverage: The Case of Slovenia. *Infection, Genetics and Evolution*, in press. http://dx.doi.org/10.1016/j.meegid.2014.06.021

7

Focused Assessment with Sonography in Trauma (FAST) Scans Are Not Sufficiently Sensitive to Rule out Significant Injury in Pediatric Trauma Patients

Clare Skerritt, Saira Haque, Erica Makin

Department of Pediatric Surgery, The Royal London Hospital, London, UK
Email: erica.makin@ntlworld.com

Abstract

Aim: To assess the sensitivity and specificity of FAST scans in pediatric trauma in a dedicated pediatric trauma centre. Method: A 3-year (2008-2011) analysis of prospectively collected data looking at the results of FAST scans compared to Computed Tomography (CT) or laparotomy findings. Results: There were 482 pediatric trauma calls of which 166 patients had suspected intra-abdominal injury. 163 patients underwent CT scans of which 89 (55%) had FAST scans prior to CT. 3 patients had FAST scans without CT; 1 patient went straight to theatre (positive FAST) and 2 patients died in the department before any further imaging. The sensitivity of FAST scans to detect abdominal injury is 23% and the specificity is 97%. The injuries missed on FAST scan were: liver lacerations (n = 3), splenic lacerations (n = 5), 1 combined liver and kidney injury and 1 combined splenic injury and small bowel perforation. Conclusions: FAST scans in trauma have a low sensitivity in pediatric patients with the possibility of missing significant intra-abdominal injury. They do not obviate the need for CT scan when clinical suspicion is high.

Keywords

Blunt Trauma, Ultrasound, FAST

1. Introduction

The clinical use of Focused Assessment with Sonography in Trauma (FAST) scans has gained increasing acceptance in the management of adult trauma patients and is used in up to 96% of adult trauma centers in the

United States. However, its adoption into pediatric trauma centers is considerably less at 15% [1].

Debate still continues as to their accuracy in assessing pediatric trauma patients. Some centers favor formal ultrasound instead of FAST scans. Retzlaff *et al.* showed that ultrasound was effective in managing 97% of pediatric patients who had suffered intra-abdominal injuries as a result of blunt abdominal trauma and that CT only influenced decision making in 1 out of their 35 patients [2].

Our hospital is a level-one trauma center and FAST scans are performed routinely in adults, the results of which are relied upon to guide management. The same emergency department (ED) trauma team also covers pediatric trauma calls and performs FAST scans in pediatric patients. There has been continued debate between ED staff and the pediatric surgeons as to the reliability of these scans to influence management in pediatric patients. During the study period due to concerns about their sensitivity in children, we had a low threshold for CT scanning all haemodynamically stable children with a significant mechanism of injury.

The aim of the study is to determine the sensitivity and specificity of FAST scans in assessing pediatric trauma patients to establish if they can be a reliable alternative to CT scanning and thus reduce radiation exposure [3]-[5] which may lead to an increased lifetime risk of malignancy.

2. Materials and Methods

Data were analyzed from a prospectively maintained database of all pediatric trauma patients over a 3-year period from May 2008 to May 2011. FAST scans were performed by either an emergency department physician (minimum of level-1 in ultrasound training accredited by the College of Emergency Medicine) or a Radiologist (Specialist Trainee year 1 and above). FAST scans were used following blunt trauma and the scan was limited to 4 views (left and right upper abdominal quadrants, pelvic and pericardial) looking for the presence of free fluid. It did not assess the integrity of solid intra-abdominal organs. The result was recorded as positive if any free fluid was identified. No attempt was made to quantify the volume of free fluid. There were some shifts when trained FAST practitioners did not staff the department and therefore not all trauma patients received FAST scans.

Patients who were haemodynamically stable and had either a mechanism of injury that could have caused intra-abdominal injury or abdominal tenderness then underwent CT scans with intravenous contrast. The departmental protocol aims to scan haemodynamically stable patients within 10 minutes of arrival and there was minimal delay between the FAST and CT scan. All CT scans demonstrating an intra-abdominal injury have been secondarily reviewed by a Consultant Pediatric Radiologist with respect to grading of solid organ injuries in alignment with the American Association for the Surgery of Trauma (AAST) classification, together with an assessment of the degree of free fluid within the abdominal cavity.

Patients were excluded from the study if no FAST was performed or if no further imaging/CT scans were available for comparison. We did not use clinical follow-up alone as definitive evidence of no intra-abdominal injury. CT scan or findings at laparotomy were considered the gold standard for comparison of FAST scan findings.

Statistical analysis was performed using Graphpad Prism V 5.0 to determine sensitivity, specificity, positive and negative predictive values of FAST scans in detecting intra-abdominal injury following blunt trauma.

3. Results

There were 482 pediatric trauma calls secondary to blunt trauma over a three year period. 166 patients had suspected intra-abdominal injuries, of these 163 patients had CT scans. 89 (55%) received FAST scans prior to the CT. 3 further patients had FAST scans. 1 patient went straight to theatre due to haemodynamic instability (positive FAST) and underwent a splenectomy, 2 patients were pronouced dead on arrival in the emergency department prior to any further imaging.

The median age at time of injury was 10.2 years (range 0.5 - 16.3 yrs). 70 patients were male (76%) and the median Injury Severity Score (ISS) was 11 (range 0 - 75) of which 46% had an ISS >15 indicating severe trauma. The median time from injury to arrival in the emergency department resuscitation room was 59 minutes (range 7 - 418 minutes).

The commonest mechanism of injury was road traffic accidents (n = 66) and reflecting our hospital's inner city setting the majority of patients (75%) had been pedestrians hit by vehicles rather than passengers. The second commonest mechanism of injury was falls from height. (n = 22) (**Table 1**).

Table 1. Mechanism of Injuries.

Mechanism of Injury	Number of Patients	Median Age (yrs) [Range]	Median Injury Severity Score [Range]
All	92	10.2 [0.5 - 16.3]	11 [0 - 75]
Road traffic accidents			
Pedestrian vs. car	49	10.0 [0.5 - 16.3]	11 [0 - 50]
Passenger	11	11.0 [2.8 - 14.3]	10 [2 - 29]
Cyclist	2	11.5 [7.8 - 15.2]	3 [1 - 5]
Motorbike	4	14.1 [11.3 - 15.9]	8.5 [4 - 15]
Fall from height	22	10.4 [1.4 - 16.3]	10 [0 - 75]
*Miscellaneous	4	6.3 [3.0 - 11.8]	27 [2 - 45]

Miscellaneous = hit by metal bar from loader, trapped by electric gates, unknown = 2.

Seven patients had a positive FAST scan (6 road traffic accidents (RTA) and 1 fall from a height). Of these, 5 had significant injuries (ISS > 15). Two patients were declared dead on arrival in the emergency department without surgery (a 5 yrs old boy who was knocked down by a lorry and an 18 mth old boy who had fallen from a 4th floor). These patients were excluded from the analysis of sensitivity of FAST scans. A 3 yrs old boy who was hit by a car required an emergency splenectomy. 2 patients sustained solid organ injuries, one liver injury (AAST grade 3) and one splenic laceration (AAST grade 2), both were successfully managed conservatively. However there were 2 patients with positive FAST scans in whom CT findings were negative.

There were 10 patients (RTA n = 7, fall n = 3) in whom FAST scans were reported as negative when in fact significant injuries were then discovered on CT scans. The missed injuries included 3 liver lacerations, 1 combined liver and right kidney laceration (**Figure 1**), 5 splenic injuries and 1 combined splenic injury and small bowel perforation. All injuries were managed conservatively apart from one patient who required a laparotomy to repair a jejunal perforation (**Table 2**).

Overall mortality was 3.3% (n = 3). Two were declared dead on arrival and have already been described. One further patient died within 24 hours of admission following a massive head injury having been a passenger in an RTA.

For the 90 patients that had a FAST scan followed by either a CT scan or laparotomy the sensitivity to detect intra-abdominal injury was 23%, specificity 97% with a positive predictive value of 60% and a negative predictive value of 88% (**Table 3**).

4. Discussion

Our study indicates that FAST scans in children have a sensitivity of 23% and are not sensitive enough to exclude significant intra-abdominal injury. Preliminary studies in children have suggested that ultrasound scans could reduce the use of CT scans in pediatric trauma patients [6] [7]. These studies involved either a full abdominal ultrasound or included assessment of parenchymal integrity of the solid intra-abdominal organs. Richards *et al.* [8] reported the largest study of ultrasound in pediatric trauma patients. A comparison was made between ultrasound findings and CT/laparotomy in 744 patients. When ultrasound was used to look for free fluid alone the sensitivity to detect intra-abdominal injury was 56%. This improved marginally to 68% when solid organ parenchyma was also examined. FAST scans in our hospital are restricted to looking for free fluid only. This enables the scan to be performed quickly and negates the need to have extensive radiology training. It could be argued that dedicated medical sonographers or radiologists would obtain more accurate results. However, Mutagabani *et al.* reported a similar sensitivity to our study of 30% when all the FAST scans in their study were performed by pediatric radiologists [9].

An explanation for the low sensitivity of FAST in children is that not all intra-abdominal injuries in children are associated with free intra-peritoneal fluid. Taylor and Sivit found that 37% of intra-abdominal injuries detected by CT were not associated with free fluid [10]. Our study supports this finding since 5 out of the 10 intra-abdominal injuries missed on FAST scan had no or trace free fluid detected on CT scan. There is no litera-

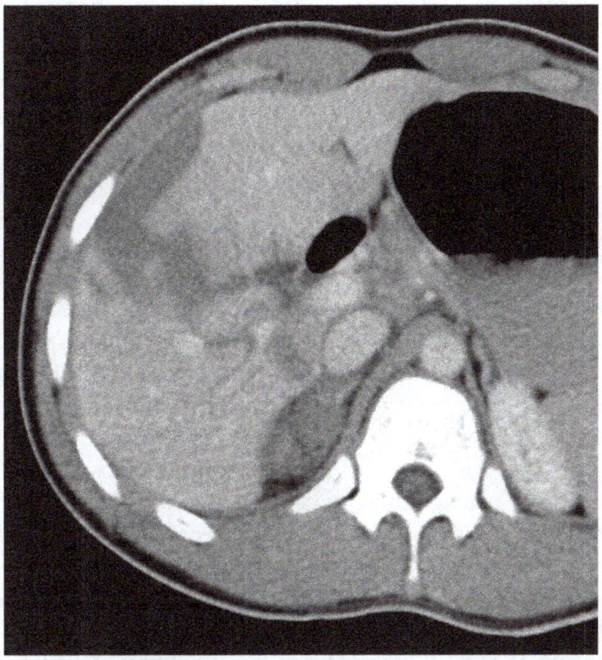

Figure 1. Grade IV liver laceration missed on FAST scan: 9 cm liver laceration affecting segment V and VIII, traversing the portal vein.

Table 2. Demographics and injuries sustained when FAST was negative.

Patient No	Sex	Age (yrs)	Mechanism Injury	Injury Severity Score	Injury	AAST Grade	Free Fluid on CT	Treatment
1	M	12.4	RTA	34	Liver trauma	3	Small	Conservative
2	M	13.9	Fall	10	Liver trauma	4	Trace	Conservative
					R Renal trauma	3		
3	F	15	RTA	43	Liver trauma	3	Trace	Conservative
4	M	11.8	RTA	45	Liver trauma	2	Trace	Conservative
5	M	9.8	RTA	41	Splenic trauma	2	Trace	Conservative
6	M	13	Fall	21	Splenic trauma	3	Nil	Conservative
7	M	6	Fall	4	Splenic trauma	4	Moderate	Conservative
8	M	7.6	RTA	27	Splenic trauma	2	Small	Conservative
9	M	6.8	RTA	21	Splenic trauma	2	Small	Conservative
10	F	4.3	RTA	9	Splenic trauma Jejunal perforation	1	Small	Laparotomy, oversewing jejunum

Abbreviations: M = male, F = female, RTA = Road Traffic Accident, AAST = American Association Surgery of Trauma. Definitions free fluid on CT: Trace = Fluid seen on one 5 mm CT section, Small = Fluid seen on 2 - 3 consecutive 5 mm CT sections, Moderate = Fluid seen on 4 - 5 consecutive 5 mm CT sections, Marked = Fluid seen on >6 consecutive 5 mm sections.

Table 3. Sensitivity and Specificity of FAST scans in pediatric trauma.

	CT Positive/Laparotomy	CT Negative
FAST positive	3	2
FAST negative	10	75

Sensitivity = 23% (95% CI 5% to 54%), Specificity = 97% (95% CI 90% to 99%). PPV = 60% (95% CI 15% to 93%), NPV = 88% (95% CI 79% to 94%).

ture available to suggest how much free fluid needs to be present within the peritoneal cavity of children before it is detectable with ultrasound. A blinded study in adults where fluid for diagnostic peritoneal lavage was infused into patients whilst they were continually scanned with ultrasound over Morison's pouch found that the average volume infused was 400 mls before it was detected [11]. This study is unlikely to be repeated in children however it is possible that injuries are missed due to lower volumes of fluid in the peritoneal cavity in children.There is evidence that FAST scans in children become more accurate in hypotensive patients who have suffered large bleeds [12].

We chose to only look at those patients who had FAST scans followed by CT scan or laparotomy. Those studies [2] [6] [13] [14] supporting the use of FAST scans tend to use clinical follow-up as evidence of no intra-abdominal injury which may well account for their apparent better sensitivity. In adults observation may well be an adequate control, however particularly in young children symptoms and signs may not always manifest until too late. Some authors argue that missed injuries may not be clinically significant and knowledge of the injury does not necessarily influence management. However, in our series two grade IV liver and splenic injuries were missed (**Figure 1**). These patients were successfully managed conservatively, but knowledge of the extent of solid organ injuries and reassurance of no active bleeding (absent contrast blush on CT) [15] is necessary to support the decision to manage these patients conservatively, preferably on a high dependency unit where any clinical deterioration could be immediately detected. In addition quantification of the extent of injury at the time of trauma provides guidance for planning follow-up imaging to assess for significant sequelae of solid organ injuries such as biliary leaks, urinomas and pseudoaneurysms (both hepatic and splenic) [16].

There have been several papers reporting the sensitivity of FAST scans can be improved when combined with other tests [17] [18]. Suthers *et al.* [17] reported that the sensitivity of FAST reaches 100% when considered jointly with the physical examination of the patient performed by the surgeon attending the trauma call. We would argue that in a multiply injured child with a depressed level of consciousness a physical examination will not provide adequate information for decision making and in fact a CT scan becomes vital to ensure no occult injuries are missed.

Within adult practice some authors are beginning to question the role of FAST scans in haemodynamically stable patients [19] [20]. Natarajan *et al.* [20] looked at over 2000 patients who had undergone FAST scans for blunt trauma and found that in the haemodynamically stable patients there 60 patients with true positive FAST scans and 87 patients with false negative FAST scans. Sensitivity was only 41% and amongst the false negative FAST scans over a third of patients underwent emergency laparotomy for their injuries. Due to the low sensitivity of FAST scans, a haemodynamically stable patient with a negative scan will still require a CT to avoid missing injuries and a positive FAST scan will also need a confirmatory CT to provide a better understanding of the injuries to guide management. Therefore the authors concluded that FAST scans should be restricted to those patients who are haemodynamically unstable. A recent meta-analysis of FAST scans in children supported this approach [21]. When only the most methodologically sound papers were included in analysis, FAST scan sensitivity was 66% (56% - 75%) and specificity 95% (93% - 97%) for detecting intra-abdominal trauma.

We recognize that our study has limitations. It was performed retrospectively and not all blunt abdominal trauma patients had FAST scans. However it reflects real-life use of FAST scans in the busiest trauma center in the UK. We conducted the study to inform the ongoing debate between emergency department physicians and pediatric surgeons in our hospital regarding how FAST scans can be used to influence management. Scaife *et al.* [22] conducted a prospective study of the use of FAST scans performed by pediatric trauma surgeons and found very similar results to our study. Interestingly, once the findings were analyzed and reported to staff the use rate decreased from 70% to 30% of potential intra-abdominal injury trauma cases. There may be a select group of patients who are haemodynamically unstable at presentation in whom FAST scans may help to determine which body cavity to open first, specifically if there is evidence of cardiac tamponade. However our study does not support the routine use of FAST scans in assessing pediatric trauma patients for the presence of intra-abdominal injury.

5. Conclusion

In conclusion, FAST scans are not sensitive enough to rule out significant intra-abdominal injuries in pediatric trauma patients. We would advocate that all haemodynamically stable patients undergo a CT scan when there is a moderate probability of intra-abdominal injury determined by the mechanism of injury.

Conflicts of Interest

None.

References

[1] Scaife, E.R., Fenton, S.J., Hansen, K.W. and Metzger, R.R. (2009) Use of Focused Abdominal Sonography for Trauma at Pediatric and Adult Trauma Centers: A Survey. *Journal of Pediatric Surgery*, **44**, 1746-1749. http://dx.doi.org/10.1016/j.jpedsurg.2009.01.018

[2] Retzlaff, T., Hirsch, W., Till, H. and Rolle, U. (2010) Is Sonography Reliable for the Diagnosis of Pediatric Blunt Abdominal Trauma? *Journal of Pediatric Surgery*, **45**, 912-915. http://dx.doi.org/1016/j.jpedsurg.2010.02.020

[3] Rice, H.E., Frush, D.P., Farmer, D., Waldhausen, J.H. and APSA Education Committee (2007) Review of Radiation Risks from Computed Tomography: Essentials for the Pediatric Surgeon. *Journal of Pediatric Surgery*, **42**, 603-607. http://dx.doi.org/10.1016/j.jpedsurg.2006.12.009

[4] Fenton, S.J., Hansen, K.W., Meyers, R.L., Vargo, D.J., White, K.S., Firth, S.D. and Scaife, E.R. (2004) CT Scan and the Pediatric Trauma Patient—Are We Overdoing It? *Journal of Pediatric Surgery*, **39**, 1877-1881. http://dx.doi.org/j.jpedsurg.2004.08.007

[5] Brenner, D.J. (2002) Estimating Cancer Risks from Pediatric CT: Going from the Qualitative to the Quantitive. *Pediatric Radiology*, **32**, 228-231. http://dx.doi.org/10.1007/s00247-002-0671-1

[6] Akgur, F.M., Aktug, T., Olguner, M., Kovanlikaya, A. and Hakgüder, G. (1997) Prospective Study Investigating Routine Usage of Ultrasonography as the Initial Diagnostic Modality for the Evaluation of Children Sustaining Blunt Abdominal Trauma. *Journal of Trauma*, **42**, 626-628.http://dx.doi.org/10.1097/00005373-199704000-00007

[7] Katz, S., Lazar, L., Rathaus, V. and Erez, I. (1996) Can Ultrasonography Replace Computed Tomography in the Initial Assessment of Children with Blunt Abdominal Trauma? *Journal of Pediatric Surgery*, **31**, 649-651. http://dx.doi.org/10.1016/S0022-3468(96)90666-1

[8] Richards, J.R., Knopf, N.A., Wang, L. and McGahan, J.P. (2002) Blunt Abdominal Trauma in Children: Evaluation with Emergency Ultrasound. *Radiology*, **222**, 749-754.http://dx.doi.org/10.1148/radiol.2223010838

[9] Mutabagani, K.H., Coley, B.D., Zumberge, N., McCarthy, D.W., Besner, G.E., Caniano, D.A. and Cooney D.R. (1999) Preliminary Experience with Focused Abdominal Sonography for Trauma (FAST) in Children: Is It Useful? *Journal of Pediatric Surgery*, **34**, 48-54. http://dx.doi.org/10.1016/S0022-3468(99)90227-0

[10] Taylor, G.A. and Sivit, C.J. (1995) Post Traumatic Fluid: Is It A Reliable Indicator of Intra-Abdominal Injury in Children? *Journal of Pediatric Surgery*, **30**, 1644-1648. http://dx.doi.org/10.1016/0022-3468(95)90442-5

[11] Branney, S.W., Wolfe, R.E., Moore, E.E., Albert, N.P., Heinig, M., Mestek, M. and Eule, J. (1995) Quantitative Sensitivity of Ultrasound in Detecting Free Intraperitoneal Fluid. *Journal of Trauma*, **39**, 375-380. http://dx.doi.org/10.1097/00005373-199508000-00032

[12] Holmes, J.F., Brant, W.E., Bond, W.F., Sokolove, P.E. and Kuppermann, N. (2001) Emergency Department Ultrasonography in the Evaluation of Hypotensive and Normotensive Children with Blunt Abdominal Trauma. *Journal of Pediatric Surgery*, **36**, 968-973. http://dx.doi.org/10.1053/jpsu.2001.24719

[13] Soudack, M., Epelman, M., Maor, R., Hayari, L., Shoshani, G., Heyman-Reiss, A., Michaelson, M. and Gaitini, D. (2004) Experience with Focused Abdominal Sonography for Trauma (FAST) in 313 Pediatric Patients. *Journal of Clinical Ultrasound*, **32**, 53-61.http://dx.doi.org/10.1002/jcu.10232

[14] Patel, J.C. and Tepas III, J.J. (1999) The Efficacy of Focused Abdominal Sonography for Trauma (FAST) as a Screening Tool in the Assessment of Injured Children. *Journal of Pediatric Surgery*, **34**, 44-47. http://dx.doi.org/10.1016/S0022-3468(99)90226-9

[15] Van der Vlies, C.H., Saltzherr, T.P., Wilde, J.C.H., van Delden, O.M., de Haan, R.J. and Goslings, J.C. (2010) The Failure Rate of Nonoperative Management in Children with Splenic or Liver Injury with Contrast Blush on Computed Tomography: A Systematic Review. *Journal of Pediatric Surgery*, **45**, 1044-1049. http://dx.doi.org/10.1016/j.jpedsurg.2010.01.002

[16] Safavi, A., Beaudry, P., Jamieson, D. and Murphy, J.J. (2011) Traumatic Pseudoaneurysms of the Liver and Spleen in Children: Is Routine Screening Warranted? *Journal of Pediatric Surgery*, **46**, 938-941. http://dx.doi.org/10.1016/j.jpedsurg.2011.02.035

[17] Suthers, S.E., Albrecht, R., Foley, D., Mantor, P.C., Puffinbarger, N.K., Jones, S.K. and Tuggle, D.W. (2004) Surgeon-Directed Ultrasound for Trauma Is a Predictor of Intra-Abdominal Injury in Children. *American Surgeon*, **70**, 164-167.

[18] Sola, J.E., Cheung, M.C., Yang, R., Koslow, S., Lanuti, E., Seaver, C., Neville, H.L. and Schulman, C.I. (2009) Pediatric FAST and Elevated Liver Transaminases: An Effective Screening Tool in Blunt Abdominal Trauma. *Journal of Surgical Research*, **157**, 103-107. http://dx.doi.org/10.1016/j.jss.2009.03.058

[19] Miller, M.T., Pasquale, M.D., Bromberg, W.J., Wasser, T.E. and Cox, J. (2003) Not So FAST. *Journal of Trauma*, **54**, 52-60. http://dx.doi.org/10.1097/00005373-200301000-00007

[20] Natarajan, B., Gupta, P.K., Cemaj, S., Sorensen, M., Hatzoudis, G.I. and Forse, R.A. (2010) FAST Scan: Is It Worth Doing in Hemodynamically Stable Blunt Trauma Patients? *Surgery*, **148**, 695-701. http://dx.doi.org/10.1016/j.surg.2010.07.032

[21] Holmes, J.F., Gladman, A. and Chang, C.H. (2007) Performance of Abdominal Ultrasonography in Pediatric Blunt Trauma Patients: A Meta-Analysis. *Journal of Pediatric Surgery*, **42**, 1588-1594. http://dx.doi.org/10.1016/j.jpedsurg.2007.04.023

[22] Scaife, E.R., Rollins, M.D., Barnhart, D.C., Downey, E.C., Black, R.E., Meyers, R.L., Stevens, M.H., Gordon, S., Prince, J.S., Battaglia, D., Fenton, S.J., Plumb, J. and Metzger, R.R. (2013) The Role of Focused Abdominal Sonography for Trauma (FAST) in Pediatric Trauma Evaluation. *Journal of Pediatric Surgery*, **48**, 1377-1383. http://dx.doi.org/10.1016/j.jpedsurg.2013.03.038

8

The Use of Trans-Esophageal Electrophysiology Study to Identify a High Risk Asymptomatic Wolff Parkinson White Syndrome Patient

Manoj Gupta[1,2], Walter Hoyt[3], Christopher S. Snyder[1,2*]

[1]Division of Pediatric Cardiology, Department of Pediatrics, Rainbow Babies and Children's Hospital, Cleveland, OH, USA
[2]School of Medicine, Case Western Reserve University, Cleveland, OH, USA
[3]Division of Pediatric Cardiology, Department of Pediatrics, School of Medicine, University of Virginia, Charlottesville, VA, USA
Email: *Christopher.Snyder@UHhospitals.org

Abstract

Patients with a Wolff-Parkinson-White (WPW) pattern on their ECG can experience symptoms such as syncope, palpitations, supraventricular tachycardia, and atrial fibrillation, or they can be asymptomatic (aWPW). All patients with WPW, regardless of the presence or absence of symptoms, are at risk of sudden death. Therefore, it is recommended that younger patients with WPW undergo studies to determine their risk. We report a previously asymptomatic WPW patient identified as high risk for sudden death due to rapid conduction down her accessory pathway during atrial fibrillation induced during a trans-esophageal electrophysiology study.

Keywords

Wolff-Parkinson-White Syndrome, Risk Assessment

1. Background

Approximately 0.15% of the general population is affected with Wolff-Parkinson-White (WPW) syndrome [1]. The presence of symptoms, such as syncope, palpitations, supraventricular tachycardia, atrial fibrillation (A fib)

*Corresponding author.

or sudden death (SCD) in addition to the ECG findings of a short PR interval and the presence of a delta wave meets the criteria initially spelled out by Drs. Wolff, Parkinson and White for the diagnosis of WPW [2]. Many patients with aWPW pattern on their ECG do not manifest symptoms and are subsequently referred to as either asymptomatic ventricular pre-excitation or asymptomatic Wolff-Parkinson-White (aWPW) [3]-[4]. The exact number of patients with aWPW remains unknown, but it is accepted to be approximately 50% of all WPW patients [3]-[4].

Regardless of symptomatology, all patients with WPW are capable of rapid conduction down their accessory pathway (AP) during atrial fibrillation (A fib) which can lead to ventricular fibrillation and SCD [5]-[7]. Although the overall incidence of SCD in WPW patients is low, estimated at approximately 4.5 per 1000 patient-years, the catastrophic nature of this manifestation suggests an important role for risk stratification and treatment for those who are at risk [8]. A number of methods are currently available to risk assessment of WPW patients, ranging from non-invasive studies such as exercise stress testing (EST) to invasive studies including trans-esophageal or trans-venous electrophysiology studies [9] [10].

We report on a previously asymptomatic WPW patient identified as high risk for SCD due to rapid conduction down her accessory pathway during A fib, shortest pre-excited RR interval of 172 msec, induced during a transesophageal electrophysiology study.

2. Case Report

A previously healthy 16-year-old female was referred for evaluation of chest pain. Her history and physical examination were unremarkable, but her ECG revealed WPW (**Figure 1**). Because she was asymptomatic, the decision was made to risk assessing her proceeding from non-invasive (EST) to invasive (transvenous electrophysiology study) testing.

During her exercise stress test, the accessory pathway persisted to the peak heart rate of 205 bpm. Due to the fact that her ECG did not normalize (loss of pre-excitation), her risk could not be determined. She subsequently underwent a minimally invasive transesophageal electrophysiology study (TEEPS).

The TEEPS was performed under general mask anesthesia using a single, 5 French trans-esophageal electrophysiology catheter (TAPCATH 205® bipolar pacing and recording catheter). The catheter was passed via the naso-esophageal route and placed in her mid esophagus where atrial tracings were noted. After atrial pacing was confirmed, atrial burst pacing was performed to a cycle length of 200 milliseconds until A fib was induced (**Figure 2**)

Her shortest preexcited R-R interval during A fib measured 172 msec, placing her at high risk for SCD. Due to this risk, her TEEPS was converted to a transvenous electrophysiology study where her AP was located and successfully ablated (**Figure 3**).

3. Discussion

In symptomatic patients with WPW, current practice dictates that these patients benefit from a transvenous electrophysiology study because the accessory pathway can be both risk-assessed and ablated during the same procedure. Currently, no guidelines exist for the management of aWPW patients.

A previous Italian study [11] which followed 184 asymptomatic children with WPW pattern on their ECG,

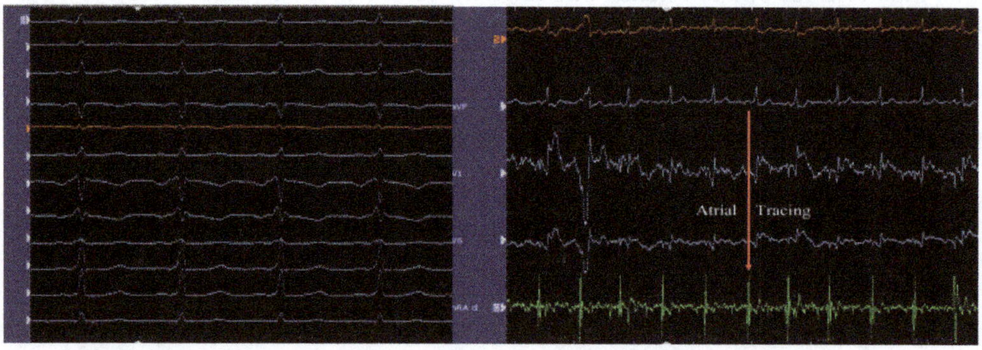

(a) (b)

Figure 1. (a): WPW pattern. (b): Atrial tracing.

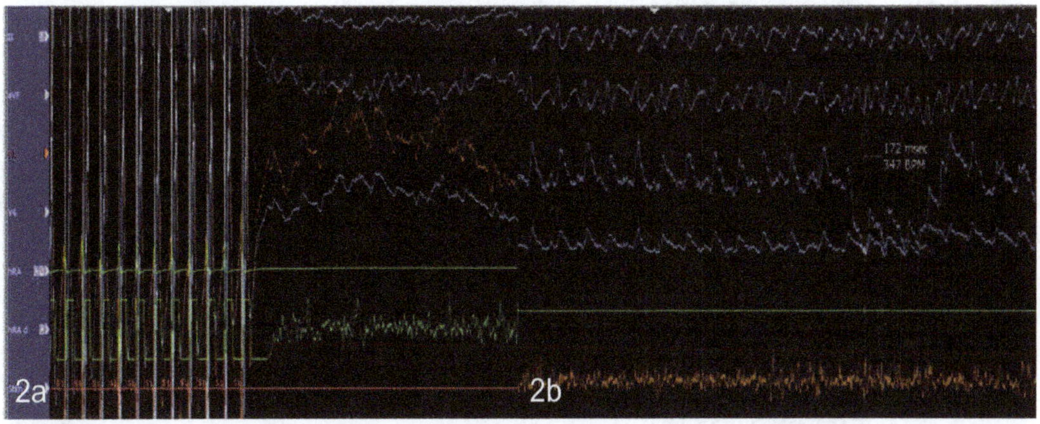

Figure 2. Induction of A fib during atrial burst pacing.

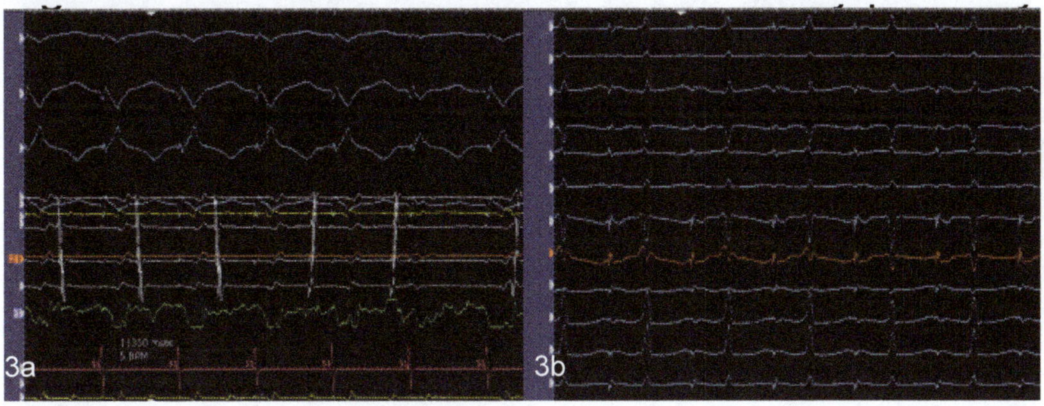

Figure 3. Localization & ablation of accessory pathway.

found 19 patients during 60 months follow-up who developed potentially life threatening arrhythmias and three of these patients died secondary to these tachyarrhythmias.

In an effort to risk assessing patients with aWPW, our institution developed an algorithm for risk stratification which progresses from least to most invasive testing [12] (**Table 1** and **Figure 4**).

4. Asymptomatic WPW Algorithm

This decision tree commences with a non-invasive EST. During this test, the physician monitors the patients ECG for either normalization of the QRS or loss of preexcitation. If the patient does not lose preexcitation during the EST, then their risk cannot be determined. While EST is easily performed in the office on the same day of evaluation, the disadvantage is that the EST provides successful risk assessment in only 8% of all aWPW patients [13] [14].

If the EST fails to risk assessing a patient, then the next step in our algorithm is to perform a transesophageal electrophysiology study; as this test is minimally invasive, requires no intravenous access, only limited anesthesia, and saving patient from invasive transvenous electrophysiology study. During TEEPS, if A fib is successfully induced and the shortest pre-excited RR interval is equal to or greater than 250 millliseconds then there is no risk of SCD and no further testing is required. If A fib is not inducible or the shortest pre-excited RR interal during A Fib is less than 250 milliseconds, then the next step in the algorithm is to perform a transvenous electrophysiology study [12].

In our patient, we were able to induce A fib with TEEPS where her shortest RR interval was 172 milliseconds, placing her at high risk for sudden cardiac death. Due to her risk, the TEEPS was converted to a transvenous electrophysiology study at which time the accessory pathway was localized and successfully ablated. On her follow up visits, she is asymptomatic from a cardiovascular standpoint with no evidence of preexcitation on her ECG.

Table 1. Risk factors and grading.

Risk factors\Grading	Low risk	Intermediate risk	High risk
SPERRI	>250 ms	220 - 250 ms	<220 ms
Intermittent pre-excitation	Yes	-	-
Multiple accessory pathway	-	-	Yes
Disappearance of AP on EST	Yes	-	-

SPERRI: Shortest pre-excited R-R interval; AP: Accessory pathway; EST: Exercise stress test.

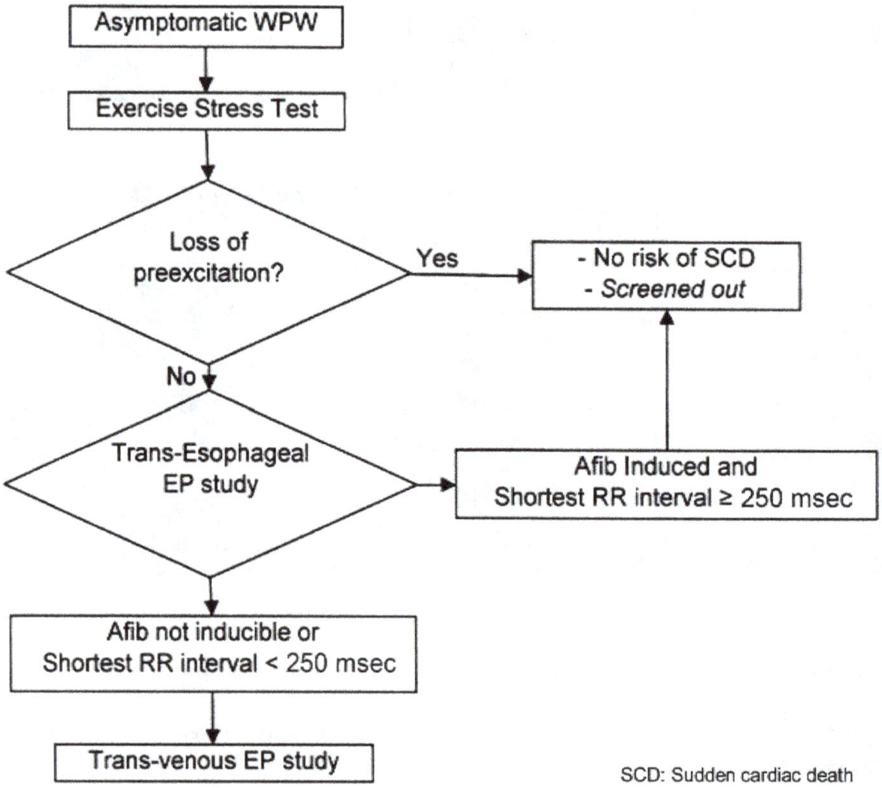

Figure 4. Risk stratification algorithm.

5. Conclusion

This report describes the identification of a previously asymptomatic patient with Wolff-Parkinson-White as one who has high risk for sudden cardiac death. This documentation of her risk was performed using the minimally invasive transesophageal procedure. Performance of this procedure on previously asymptomatic patients with Wolff-Parkinson-White syndrome can be very helpful in determining their risk for sudden cardiac death.

References

[1] Munger, T.M., Packer, D.L., Hammil, S.C., Feldman, B.J., Bailey, K.R., Ballard, D.J., Holmes Jr., D.R. and Gersh, B.J. (1993) A Population Study of the Natural History of Wolff-Parkinson-White Syndrome in Olmsted County, Minnesota, 1953-1989. *Circulation*, **87**, 866-873 http://dx.doi.org/10.1161/01.CIR.87.3.866

[2] Perry, J. (1998) Supraventricular Tachycardia. In: Garson Jr., A., Bricker, J.T., Fisher, D.J. and Neish, S.R., Eds., *Science and Practice of Pediatric Cardiology*, Williams & Wilkins, Baltimore, 2059-2101.

[3] Wellens, H.J., Rodriguez, L.M., Timmermans, C. and Smeets, J.L. (1997) The Asymptomatic Patient with Wolff-Parkinson-White Electrocardiogram. *PACE*, **20**, 2082-2086. http://dx.doi.org/10.1111/j.1540-8159.1997.tb03633.x

[4] Goudevenos, J.A., Katsouras, C.S., Graekas, G., *et al.* (2000) Ventricular Preexcitation in the General Population: A Study on the Mode of Presentation and Clinical Course. *Heart*, **83**, 29-34. http://dx.doi.org/10.1136/heart.83.1.29

[5] Pietersen, A.H., Andersen, E.D. and Sandoe, E. (1992) Atrial Fibrillation in the Wolff-Parkinson-White Syndrome. *The American Journal of Cardiology*, **70**, 38A-43A. http://dx.doi.org/10.1016/0002-9149(92)91076-G

[6] Klein, G.J., Bashore, T.M., Sellers, T.D., Pritchett, E.L., Smith, W.M. and Gallagher, J.J. (1979) Ventricular Fibrillation in the Wolff-Parkinson-White Syndrome. *The New England Journal of Medicine*, **301**, 1080-1085. http://dx.doi.org/10.1056/NEJM197911153012003

[7] Bromberg, B.I., Lindsay, B., Cain, M. and Cox, J. (1996) Impact of Clinical History and Electrophysiologic Characterization of Accessory Pathways on Management Strategies to Reduce Sudden Death among Children With Wolff-Parkinson-White Syndrome. *Journal of the American College of Cardiology*, **27**, 690-695. http://dx.doi.org/10.1016/0735-1097(95)00519-6

[8] PACES/HRS(2012) Expert Consensus Statement on the Management of the Asymptomatic Young Patient with a Wolff-Parkinson-White (WPW, Ventricular Preexcitation) Electrocardiographic Pattern. *Heart Rhythm*, **9**, 1006-1024 http://dx.doi.org/10.1016/j.hrthm.2012.03.050

[9] Gaita, F., Giusteto, C., Riccardi, R., Mangiardi, L. and Brusca, A. (1989) Stress and Pharmacologic Tests as Methods to Identify Patients with Wolff-Parkinson-White Syndrome at Risk of Sudden Death. *The American Journal of Cardiology*, **64**, 487-490. http://dx.doi.org/10.1016/0002-9149(89)90426-8

[10] Sharma, A., Yee, R., Guiraudon, G. and Klein, G. (1987) Sensitivity and Specificity of Invasive and Non-invasive Testing for Risk of Sudden Death in Wolff-Parkinson-White Syndrome. *Journal of the American College of Cardiology*, **10**, 373-381 http://dx.doi.org/10.1016/S0735-1097(87)80021-9

[11] Santinelli, V., *et al.* (2009) The Natural History of Asymptomatic Ventricular Pre-Excitation: A Long-Term Prospective Follow-Up Study of 184 Asymptomatic Children. *Journal of the American College of Cardiology*, **53**, 275-280. http://dx.doi.org/10.1016/j.jacc.2008.09.037

[12] Pappone, C., Santinelli, V., Rosanio, S., Vicedomini, G., Nardi, S., Pappone, A., Tortoriello, V., Manguso, F., Mazzone, P., Gulletta, S., Oreto, G. and Alfieri O. (2003) Usefulness of Invasive Electrophysiologic Testing to Stratify the Risk of Arrhythmic Events in Asymptomatic Patients with Wolff-Parkinson-White Pattern: Results from a Large Prospective Long-Term Follow-Up Study. *Journal of the American College of Cardiology*, **41**, 239-244. http://dx.doi.org/10.1016/S0735-1097(02)02706-7

[13] Bricker, J.T., Co-Burn, J., Garson Jr., A., Gillete, P.C., McVey, P., Malinda, T. and McNamara, D. (1984) Exercise Testing in Children with Wolff-Parkinson-White Syndrome. *The American Journal of Cardiology*, **55**, 1001-1004. http://dx.doi.org/10.1016/0002-9149(85)90734-9

[14] Moltedo, J.M., Iyer, R.V., Forman, H., Fahey, J., Rosenthal, G. and Snyder, C.S. (2006) Is Exercise Stress Testing a Cost-Saving Strategy for Risk Assessment of Pediatric Wolff-Parkinson-White Syndrome Patients? *The Ochsner Journal*, **6**, 64-67.

9

Segmental Pigmentation Disorder with Congenital Heterochromia Iridis

Carmen Madrigal Díez[1*], Sara Rodríguez Prado[2], José Héctor Fernández Llaca[3]

[1]Primary Paediatric Health Care, Centro de Salud Bezana, Servicio Cántabro de Salud, Spain
[2]Department of Opthalmology, Hospital de Sierrallana, Torrelavega, Cantabria, Spain
[3]Department of Dermatology, Hospital Universitario Marqués de Valdecilla, Santander, Cantabria, Spain
Email: [*]c.madrigaldiez@yahoo.es

Abstract

We report the case of a 10-year-old girl with congenital complete heterochromia iridis and segmental pigmentation disorder in its hyperpigmented form. We have found no publication that mentions the combination of these 2 disorders.

Keywords

Congenital Heterochromia Iridis, Segmental Pigmentation Disorder, Café-au-Lait Macules

1. Case Report

During a routine checkup, a 10-year-old girl had noticeably different colors in her irises and had large hyperpigmented spots on her skin. According to her mother, both irises were blue during the child's first month of life; however, in the following months, the left iris remained blue while the right darkened until reaching its definitive brown color by 10 months of age. During her second year of life, two spots appeared on the child's back that were darker brown than her normal skin, which progressively spread towards the front. During the summer when the child was 10 years of age, her family noticed a spot on the left side of her face with a similar color to that on her chest. This new spot had not been detected before. During the autumn, the spot progressively faded until it almost disappeared. The girl's development has been normal, with no clinical suspicion of endocrine, sensory or neurological disorders or other significant manifestations. There is no similar medical history in the girl's family.

The physical examination confirmed the presence of two large café-au-lait spots, with irregular coloration and edges. The spots extended from the lumbosacral region towards both sides of the trunk through the flanks

[*]Corresponding author.

(**Figure 1**) until reaching the spot on the right side of the midline of the abdomen, where it ended neatly and without going past the line (**Figure 2**). The lateral edges of both spots were more irregular. In the paravertebral region, the intensity of the pigmentation progressively diminished until it was almost imperceptible. In the right intercostal area of the chest, the girl had another isolated spot of the same color as the previous ones although smaller. On the left side of the face, there was another hyperpigmented spot, with an irregular border that extended over the forehead, the periorbital region and the cheek. On the forehead, the border between the normal skin and the hyperpigmented skin was well defined and showed a tendency to respect the midline, although it slightly exceeded it in the upper area (**Figure 3**). In the periorbital area and cheek, the borderline was diffuse, and the pigmentation faded until disappearing (**Figure 4**). We also observed complete heterochromia iridis, with the right iris going brown and the left remaining blue (**Figure 3**). A thorough ophthalmologic examination ruled out the presence of any underlying refractive problem or ocular disease. The girl's physical and psychological development was normal, and there were no other associated organ disorders or signs of advanced puberty.

The results of an extensive laboratory study were normal and included serum calcium and phosphate levels (10.02 and 4.19 mg/dl, respectively) and 24-hour phosphaturia (950 ml daily and 864 mg/dl). The hormone levels of prolactin, TS4, T4, LH, FSH and estradiol were also normal for a prepubescent girl. There were no apparent skeletal disorders (including the head) in the radiological examination. The patient's bone age (10 years) matched her chronological age. The girl and her family rejected the possibility of performing skin biopsies.

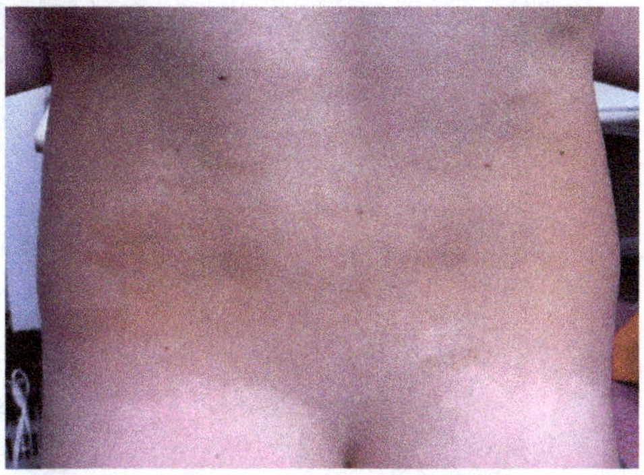

Figure 1. Two lumbosacral bilateral café-au-lait macules, with irregular edges. Their color fades out as they approach the dorsal midline.

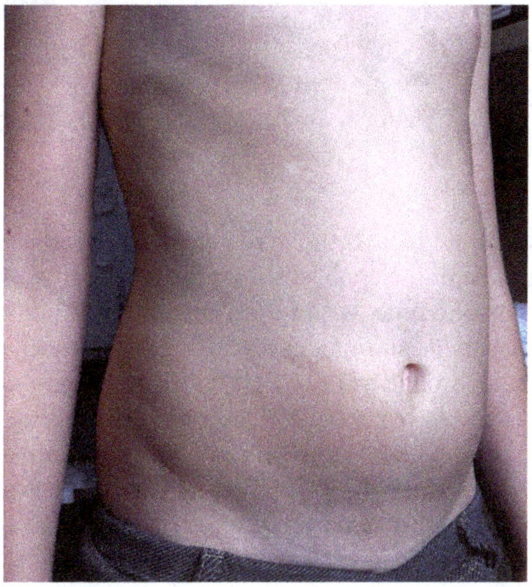

Figure 2. On the right side, the macule stops with a clean edge at the ventral midline without going over it. In the intercostal region, another less extensive macule can be observed.

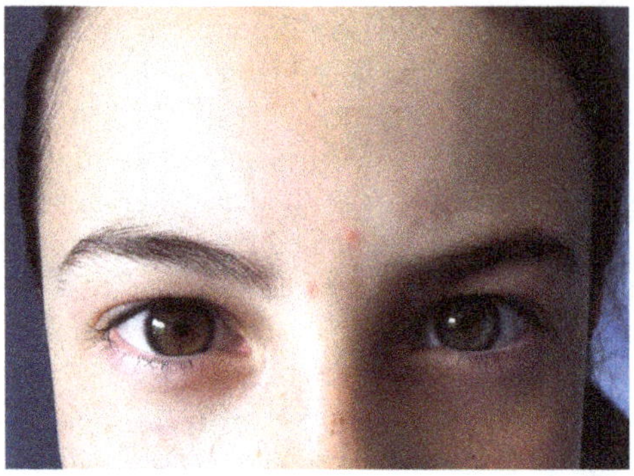

Figure 3. Café-au-lait facial macule. In the front left region, the macule slightly surpasses the midline; its edge is clearly delimited from the unaffected skin. Complete heterochromia iridis, with a darker right iris.

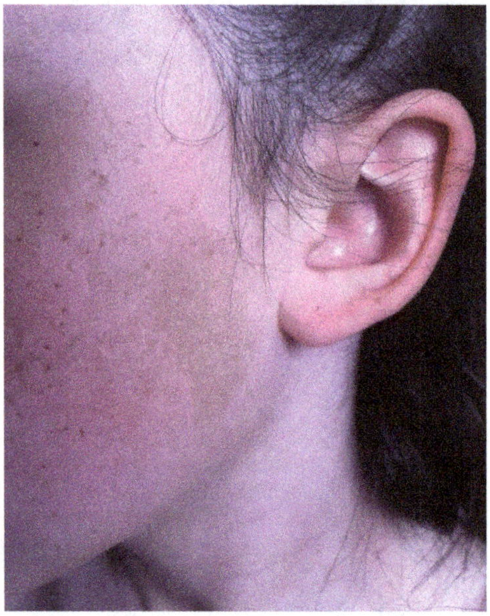

Figure 4. On the cheek, the edge is more blurred.

2. Discussion

Eye and skin color are two of the most distinctive personal appearance traits. The two have a common process that creates them: the migration of melanoblasts from the neural crest to their destination points, their maturation to melanocytes and the metabolic process of formation and distribution of melanin. However, while skin melanocytes release melanosomes to the surrounding cells, the uveal melanocytes do not release them [1].

Complete congenital heterochromia iridis (CCHI) and the café-au-lait macules (CALM) are two pigmentation disorders of the eyes and skin. At birth, neither the migration or maturation processes of the iris melanocytes have been completed. Therefore, CCHI is not typically observed until after the first months of life [1]. The same occurs with CALM, which can go unnoticed for the first few years, especially in children with pale skin [2].

CCHI can present as an isolated disorder or associated with other organ disorders. With an incidence lower than 1/200.000, isolated CCHI is included by the Genetic and Rare Diseases Information Center (GARD) within the rare diseases group. Other times, CCHI is included in diseases or syndromes that, along with other symptoms, include heterochromia iridis due to hypochromia (Hirschsprung's disease, congenital Horner's syndrome, Waardenburg syndrome and hypomelanosis of Ito) or to hyperchromia of the affected iris (oculodermal melanocytosis or nevus of Ota (ODM) and Sturge-Weber syndrome).

Our patient is a carrier of complete heterochromia iridis, which, as occurs with CCHI, was already apparent in the first months of life, with no apparent associated sign that would lead to the suspicion that the patient had Hirschsprung's disease, Horner's syndrome, Waardenburg syndrome, Sturge-Weber syndrome or hypomelanosis of Ito.

In our patient, the simultaneous onset of CCHI with diffuse macular edges, observed at prepubescence in skin areas innervated by the first two branches of the trigeminal nerve, with diffuse edges and with seasonal variations in intensity, could suggest an ODM. However, the skin macula was soft brown and on the left side of the face, while the brown iris was in the right eye. In contrast, facial macula in ODM tends to be grey-blue, and the dark iris is on the same side as the skin macula [2] [3].

In CALM, there is an increase in the melanin contained in the basal melanocytes and keratinocytes, with no increase in the quantity of melanocytes [3] [4]. CALM are more common than CCHI, especially when they are few, small, isolated, symmetrical and well-defined, which occurs in more than 10% of healthy children. In such cases, CALM represents a personal characteristic, with no pathological meaning. CALM are significantly rarer when they increase in number and size, with asymmetric forms and irregular edges [2] [4].

The characteristics of our patient's macules are similar to those of segmental pigmentation disorder (SegPD), a condition described by Metzker [5] and in subsequent reviews by Hogeling [6]. The name was employed to refer to a subgroup of patients with large hypopigmented or hyperpigmented skin macules, which had well-defined borders in the body's midline, especially the ventral. These macules do not usually spread beyond the midline, although they occasionally overlap by a few centimeters [6], and have more diffuse lateral edges. Of the patterns described by Happle [7] as a reflection of mosaic skin pigmentation, the archetype that most resembles the form and distribution of our patient's macules is type 2 checkerboard. However, it is not always possible to fit all SegPDs in this classification [8], which likely would extend with the incorporation of an additional archetype [9]. The histological findings in cases of SegPD with hyperpigmentation in which skin biopsies were performed have been similar to those found with classic CALM [4] [5]. Therefore, the current criteria for the diagnosis of SegPD are mainly clinical [6] [8] [10]. The risk that SegPD is associated with other systemic disorders is low; however, in cases with highly extensive spots, a more thorough study that rules out their presence is recommended [6] [10].

In the forms with hyperpigmentation, the differential diagnosis should be established with McCune-Albright syndrome (MAS), giant and isolated CALMs, neurofibromatosis (NF), speckled lentiginous nevus and nevoid hyperpigmentation [2] [9].

Although they do not always match these characteristics, CALMs of MAS are typically described as large, unilateral macules, with irregular and asymmetrical edges ("coast of Maine" pattern), not exceeding the midline, following the broad band pattern of Blaschko's lines and are accentuated with exposure to the sun [2] [11]. These macules are usually the first observed manifestation of MAS. They should therefore not be underestimated, and their observation should lead to the necessary tests to rule out the presence of fibrous dysplasia and/or undetected hyperfunctioning endocrinopathies, which, when present, are detectable before 10 years of age in the vast majority of cases [9] [11]. For our patient, the normal results from the endocrine and radiological tests allowed us to reasonably rule out MAS.

The large isolated CALMs preserve the morphological peculiarities of classic CALMs, without the lateral blurring seen with our patient and with no relation to the midline [4] [6].

CALMs of NF usually present the "coast of California" pattern; their abundance in the axilla and groin originate the Crowe sign. The neurofibromas usually appear later, during adolescence. Lisch nodules, which can change the color of the iris, are present in both eyes, usually appear during late childhood and are more abundant in the lower hemisphere [1]. Segmental NF is a variant of NF caused by a postzygotic mosaicism and only presents in a body segment in which the characteristic manifestations of NF appear [1] [8]. For our patient, the CALMs did not correspond to the coast of California pattern. The heterochromia was present at birth, and she did not have Crowe's sign or Lisch nodules.

Speckled lentiginous nevus can present demarcation in the body midline, but the characteristic darker specks that stand out over the flat brown macula are very obvious at 10 years of age [6].

Nevoid hyperpigmentation follows the pattern of narrow Blaschko lines, which is very different from that of our case.

Although not a rare clinical condition, the SegPD described by Metzker is still not well defined. This lack of definition is due in part to the considerable diversity in terminology with which the condition is reported and to the lack of clarity in terms of its clinical characteristics and potential associations, which makes it more difficult to study and characterize [6] [8]. Therefore, it is advisable to report the characteristics of SegPD observed during clinical practice [8].

We have presented a case of a girl with SegPD, who was also a carrier of CCHI but with no other associated anomaly. Both CCHI and SegPD are the results of a disorder in the biological process responsible for melanin pigmentation in the iris and skin, respectively. Although skin pigmentation disorders associated with ocular disorders have been reported, we have found no reports that refer to the simultaneous onset of SegPD and CCHI in one individual. There has been a reported case of an 11-year-old girl with a large facial CALM associated with CCHI, who also had a large hemangioma in one of the buttocks [12]. The report does not explicitly reference the possibility of the condition being a SegPD, and the skin lesion was considered a large segmental CALM.

Due to its incidence, which is estimated at approximately 0.35% [6] [7], SegPD cannot be considered a rare disease; however, the very low incidence of CCHI means that the probability of the two conditions casually coinciding is very low ($<1/57 \times 10^6$). Reports of other cases in which the two disorders coincided would suggest some type of correlation between them.

Conflict of Interest

The authors declare no conflict of interest.

References

[1] Rennie, I.G. (2012) Don't It Make My Blue Eyes Brown: Heterochromia and Other Abnormalities of the Iris. *Eye*, **26**, 29-50. http://dx.doi.org/10.1038/eye.2011.228

[2] Shah, K.N. (2010) The Diagnostic and Clinical Significance of Café-au-Lait Macules. *Pediatric Clinics of North America*, **57**, 1131-1153. http://dx.doi.org/10.1016/j.pcl.2010.07.002

[3] Sinha, S., Cohen, P.J. and Schwartz (2008) Nevus of Ota in Children. *Cutis*, **82**, 25-29.

[4] Landau, M. and Krafchik, B.R. (1999) The Diagnostic Value of Café-au-Lait Macules. *Journal of the American Academy of Dermatology*, **40**, 877-890. http://dx.doi.org/10.1016/S0190-9622(99)70075-7

[5] Metzker, A., Morag, C. and Weitz, R. (1983) Segmental Pigmentation Disorder. *Acta Dermato-Venereologica*, **63**, 167-169.

[6] Hogelin, M. and Frieden, I.J. (2010) Segmental Pigmentation Disorder. *British Journal of Dermatology*, **162**, 1337-1341. http://dx.doi.org/10.1111/j.1365-2133.2010.09702.x

[7] Happle, R. (1993) Mosaicism Human Skin Understanding the Patterns and Mechanism. *JAMA Dermatology*, **129**, 1460-1470. http://dx.doi.org/10.1001/archderm.1993.01680320094012

[8] Orion, E., Matz, H. and Wolf, R. (2003) Café au lait Has a Hue of Its Own. *Dermatology Online Journal*, **9**, **8**.

[9] Happle, R. and Bittar, M. (2006) Patrones del mosaicismo en la piel humana: Comprendiendo aspectos actuales y futuros. *Dermatol Pediatr Lat*, **4**, 171-181.

[10] Treta, J. (2010) Patterned Pigmentation in Children. *Pediatric Clinics of North America*, **57**, 1121-1129. http://dx.doi.org/10.1016/j.pcl.2010.07.007

[11] Collins, M.T., Cantante, R.F. and Eugster, E. (2012) McCune-Albright Syndrome and the Extraskeletal Manifestations of Fibrous Dysplasia. *Orphanet Journal of Rare Diseases*, **7**, S4. http://www.ojrd.com/content/7/S1/S4

[12] Quilan, K. and Shwayder, T. (2005) Café au lait Macule Associated with Heterochromia Iridis. *Pediatric Dermatology*, **22**, 177-178. http://dx.doi.org/10.1111/j.1525-1470.2005.22220.x

10

Lipodystrophy among Children Infected with Human Immunodeficiency Virus and on Antiretroviral Treatment in Ouagadougou

Caroline Yonaba[1], Aïssata Ouedraogo[2*], Sylvie Armelle Pingwende Ouédraogo[2], Bourama Ouattara[2], Angel Kalmogho[1], Fla Koueta[2], Diarra Yé[2], Ludovic Kam[1]

[1]Department of Pediatric, Yalgado Ouedraogo University Teaching Hospital, Ouagadougou, Burkina Faso
[2]Department of Pediatric, Charles de Gaulle Pediatric University Teaching Hospital, Ouagadougou, Burkina Faso
Email: [*]sita_kab@yahoo.fr

Abstract

Management of Human Immunodeficiency Virus infection remains a major challenge in many sub-Saharan African countries. Antiretroviral drugs which have reduced significantly the mortality rate of this pandemic disease are a source of side effects. Among these side effects, adult lipodystrophy has already been described by several authors. The aim of this study is to determine the prevalence of lipodystrophy and associate factors in children on antiretroviral therapy, managed at Charles De Gaulle Children University Hospital and Yalgado Ouedrago University Hospital in Ouagadougou, Burkina Faso. This is a cross-sectional study conducted from June 2013 to January 2014. We included children aged 2 to 15 years who had been on antiretroviral treatment for at least six months with no severe acute malnutrition (wasting). Lipodystrophy was diagnosed clinically after assessment of morphological changes. Overall, 323 children complying with the inclusion criteria were examined. The average duration of antiretroviral therapy was 5.3 years. Forty five children had lipodystrophy, *i.e.* 13.9% prevalence rate. One hundred and twenty seven different lipodystrophic lesions were noted, hence 82.7% lipoatrophy and 17.3% lipohypertrophy. The most common presentations were: face (32%), lower limbs (26%) and upper limbs (15.7%). Factors associated with lipoatrophy were: age above 10 years ($P = 0.004$); male gender ($P = 0.0004$); antiretroviral treatment duration of more than 60 months ($P < 0.001$) and treatment with stavudine ($P = 0.01$). Our study showed that lipodystrophy is not exceptional in children on antiretroviral therapy in Ouagadougou. However, more researches on lipid profiles of these children are necessary to prevent other common complications related to fat accumulation.

[*]Corresponding author.

Keywords

HIV, Children, Lipodystrophy, Burkina-Faso

1. Introduction

Lipodystrophy is a condition characterized by morphological changes due to a disorder in the distribution of fat in Human immune deficient virus (HIV) infected people treated with antiretroviral therapy. It remains a major issue because of the psychosocial stigma [1] and the atherogenic risk [2]-[4].

A prevalence rate of 20% to 80% has been reported [5] [6]. Several authors have shown that lipid disorders due to the long term antiretroviral use, notably hypertriglyceridemia and dyslipidemia [6]-[9].

Dollfus *et al.* in France in 2001 found 13 cases of lipodystrophy in 39 children under antiretroviral therapy. These children were aged 5 to13 years [10].

Piloya *et al.* in Uganda found in a study including 364 HIV-infected children and under antiretroviral treatment, 27% of lipodystrophy and 34% of hyperlipidemia [11].

The European group found through a study including 477 children in 30 pediatric clinics, 26% of lipodystrophy among which 8.8% of lipohypertrophy, 7.55% of lipoatrophy and 9.64% for the mixed form [12].

Nucleoside inhibitors of the reverse transcriptase are the most responsible of lipodystrophy [2] [13]. In 2013, less toxic regimens were not widely available for children in Burkina Faso [14]. Our aim is to describe lipodystrophy cases and to determine associated factors in children on antiretroviral therapy in two hospitals of Ouagadougou.

2. Materials and Method

This is a descriptive and analytical cross-sectional study. We included HIV-infected children on antiretroviral therapy managed as outpatients at Charles De Gaulle University Hospital (CHUP CDG) and Yalgado Ouedraogo University Hospital (CHUYO). The two hospitals together manage a population of 891 HIV infected children and among them 606 were on antiretroviral therapy.

Children who were on antiretroviral therapy for at least 6 months and aged between 2 and 15 years were included. A parent's or tutor's consent was required for all children to participate in the study. We excluded children who had severe malnutrition or other chronic diseases (carditis, kidney failure, tuberculosis, etc.).

Data on clinical symptoms were collected on each medical visit. Weight and height were assessed in order to check for any morphological changes. We paid special attention to fat loss areas (lipoatrophy), notably arms (thinning and decrease in the upper arm circumference), legs (thinning with abnormal visualization of veins), face (widening of cheeks or the temporal region) and buttocks (flattening). Areas of lipohypertrophy or fat accumulation were investigated on the abdomen (increase of the volume with an enlargement of waist size), chest, breast, pelvis, and neck (buffalo hump). Blood pressure assessment at rest completed the examination.

Each child's blood tests of less than 3 months were registered. Blood samples were taken on an empty stomach and then analyzed in each hospital's laboratory. Lipids measurement included only total cholesterol and tryglyceridemia. Antiretroviral treatments at admission and at the time of the survey were registered.

In our study, were analyzed antiretroviral (ARV) regimens those including the start of antiretroviral therapy, zidovudine (AZT), stavudine (D4T) or protease inhibitors (IP). Protease inhibitor available in both hospitals for the monitoring of children was ritonavir-boosted lopinavir (lopi/rt).

Data were entered and processed with Epi Info software, version 3.5.1, SPSS Version 17, Word and Excel 2007. Chi^2 statistical test was used to compare variables. Statistical gaps were significant when $P < 0.05$.

Factor analysis consisted in comparing (using Chi^2 test) the frequency of some of the characteristics between the group of children with lipodystrophies and those without. These characteristics included age, gender, treatment regimen at admission, the length of the treatment and the WHO clinical level at admission. The same characteristics (except clinical level) were compared for lipoatrophy.

3. Results

3.1. Population Description

Overall 323 children who met the inclusion criteria were examined. The average age was 9.9 years and 167 of them (51.7%) were above 10 year-old. Male represented 50.2%.

Children were HIV1 infected in 98.8% cases (N = 319) and HIV2 in 1.2% cases (N = 4).

At the initiation of antiretroviral therapy, TCD4 lymphocytes count was available for 135 children, among them 38.5% had severe immune deficiency (TCD4 lymphocytes rate <200 cells/mm³).

Body mass index (BMI) was calculated in 289 children aged above five years and nine of them (3.1%) were obese (BMI > 30).

One hundred and sixty four (164) children had reached puberty and among them 111 (67%) were above Tanner stage 2.

Six children (2.1%) out of 282 who had their blood pressure checked, were found to have high blood pressure.

The average duration of antiretroviral therapy was 55.9 months ± 15 months with extremes of 7 and 121 months.

All the patients were on Highly Active Antiretroviral Therapy (HAART). First line treatments included the association of "zidovudine-lamivudine-nevirapine" or "stavudine-lamivudine-nevirapine" respectively in 34.7% and 30.7% of our patients.

Other characteristics of children on antiretroviral treatment are listed in **Table 1**.

At the time of the survey, among 152 children who had their blood tests available, hyperglycemia (>7.1 mmol/l) was noted in 3 children (2%); total hypercholestérolemia (>4.5 mmol/l) in 9 children (6%) and hypertrigly-ceridemia (>1.55 mmol/l) in 12 children (7.9%).

Lipodystrophy was found in 45 (13.9%) children out of 323 examined, among them 29 (62.2%) were male.

3.2. Types and Locations of Lipodystrophy

Among 45 children who had lipodystrophy, 10.8% had lipoatrophy, 1.9% had mixed type and 1.2% had lipohypertrophy.

Several locations of lipodystrophy were noticed. Some of the children presented more than one location. On the whole, 127 lesions were found in 45 children, including 82.7% of lipoatrophy and 17.3% of lipohypertrophy.

Table 2 summarizes the distribution of lipodystrophy per type and location.

The face and limbs (upper and lower) were the most common locations both for lipodystrophy and lipoatrophy.

Table 1. General characteristics of 323 children on antiretroviral therapy.

Characteristics	Number (n)	Percentage (%)
Age (years)		
≤10	156	48.3
>10	167	51.7
WHO Clinical stage*		
Stage 1	3	0.9
Stage 2	61	18.9
Stage 3	234	72.5
Stage 4	25	7.7
Social status		
Orphan**	210	65.0
Non orphan	113	35.0
Treatment duration		
≤60 mois	189	58.5
>60 mois	134	41.5
Initial Treatment regimen		
AZT+	178	55.2
D4T+	139	43.0
Other regimens	6	1.8

*WHO 2013 Classification, **orphan of one or two parents. (AZT+) = regimen containing zidovudine (AZT), (D4T+) = regimen containing stavudine (D4T).

Table 2. Distribution of lipodystrophy per type of location.

Locations	Lipoatrophy	Lipohypertrophy	Number (n)	Percentage (%)
Face	41	0	41	32.2
Lower limbs	33	0	33	26.0
Upper limbs	20	0	20	15.7
Buttocks	10	2	12	9.4
Abdomen	0	10	10	7.9
Breast	0	5	5	4.0
Brain area	1	2	3	2.4
Pubis	0	3	3	2.4

3.3. ART Regimens of Children Presenting with Lipodystrophy

Among the children presenting with lipodystrophy, 35 (77.8%) started their treatment with D4T and 9 (20%) with AZT. At the time of the survey, AZT was used in 34 (75.6%) patients, D4T in four (8.9%) patients and protease inhibitors in 12 (26.7%).

3.4. Associated Factors

We studied on one hand, the association between lipodystrophy and some of the clinical and therapeutic factors, and on the other hand, the association between lipoatrophy and the same factors listed above. Results are shown on **Table 3** and **Table 4**.

The frequency of lipoatrophy was significantly higher in patients whom antiretroviral treatment duration was more than 60 months and those whose treatment included stavudine.

4. Discussion

Patients' mean age was 9.9 years. This was also the case for Piloya in Uganda, Dollfus in France and Vigano in Italy, who recorded a mean age of 9.8 years; 9.1 years and 9.78 years in their studies respectively [10] [11] [15].

Inefficient programs for the prevention of mother-to-child transmission of HIV (PMTCT) may explain our results. The extension of the PMTCT program started in 2006 in Burkina Faso. Therefore, the majority of children born before 2006 did not benefit from this program; this accounts for the predominance of above 10 year-old patients in our study.

The first line treatment used in our study is that recommended in Burkina Faso [14].

AZT and D4T have long been the basis of the first line antiretroviral treatment in most developing countries. The process of switching D4T to AZT was done in keeping with D4T switching plan recommended by World Health Organization (WHO) in 2010 [16].

To reduce the occurrence of new cases of lipodystrophy this process must be accelerated in our hospitals.

Lipodystrophy prevalence rate (13.9%) was fairly high in our study.

The European Group of Pediatric lipodystrophy had reported a prevalence rate of 26% in France, including 7.5% for lipoatrophy, 8.8% for lipohypertrophy and 9.6% for the mixed syndrome in a prospective study covering 477 HIV infected children [12].

Piloya in Uganda found a prevalence rate of 27% of lipodystrophy in 364 HIV infected children [11]. However, Kinabo *et al.* in Tanzania reported lipodystrophy prevalence rate of 30%, including 19% for lipoatrophy, 3.8% for lipohypertrophy and 7.1% for mixed forms in a cross-sectional study on 210 HIV infected children and adolescents aged 1 to 18 years [17].

The prevalence of lipodystrophy therefore varies from one study to another. In all these three researches mentioned above, study design included adolescents aged 18 years in whom the risk of occurrence of lipodystrophy is higher than that of under 15 years [5] [10] [11]. Other diagnostic methods are more accurate and should be used whenever possible; skin fold measurement or muscles Dexa-scan and body fat assessment [18] [19].

In our series, several locations of lipodystrophy were found including 32% in the face, 26% on the lower limbs. Our results are similar to those of Joly in France who found 49% and 48% of locations on the face and lower limbs [13].

Table 3. Factors associated with lipodystrophy.

Associated factors	Number	Lipodystrophy		Odds ratio	P
		Yes N (%)	No N (%)	(IC)	
Age (years)					
≤10	156	15 (9.6)	141 (90.4)	1	
>10	167	30 (18)	137 (82)	0.5 (0.3 - 1)	0.005
Sex					
Female	161	17 (10.6)	144 (89.4)	1	
Male	162	28 (17.3)	134 (82.7)	1 (0.9 - 1.1))	0.042
Clinical stage					
1	2	1 (50)	1 (50)	1	
2	62	3 (4.8)	59 (95.2)	7.5 (5.2 - 9.4)	0.5
3	233	39 (16.7)	194 (83.3)	0.3 (0.2 - 0.8)	0.001
4	26	2 (7.7)	24 (92.3)	2.4 (0.9 - 5.5)	0.06
Treatment duration ARV					
≤60	189	12 (6.3)	177 (93.7)	1	
>60	134	33 (24.6)	101 (75.4)	0.4 (0.2 - 0.7)	<0.001
Initial treatment regimen					
AZT−	145	36 (24.8)	109 (75.2)	1	
AZT+	178	9 (5)	169 (95)	6.3 (0.2 - 8.2)	0.41
D4T−	184	10 (5.4)	174 (94.6)	1	
D4T+	139	35 (25.2)	104 (74.8)	0.2 (0.1 - 0.3)	<0.001
Lopi/rt−	271	33 (12.2)	238 (87.8)	1	
Lopi/rt+	52	12 (23)	40 (77)	0.4 (0.2 - 0.6)	0.06

(AZT−) = Treatment regimen not containing zidovudine; (AZT+) = Treatment regimen containing zidovudine; (D4T−) = Treatment regimen not containing zidovudine; (D4T+) = Treatment regimen containing stavudine; (Lopi/rt−) = Treatment regimen not containing lopinavir/ritonavir; (Lopi/rt+) = Treatment regimen containing lopinavir/ritonavir.

Table 4. Factors associated with the presence of lipoatrophy.

Associated factors	Number	Lipodystrophy		Odds ratio	P
		Yes N (%)	No N (%)	(CI)	
Age (years)					
≤10	156	11 (7)	145 (93)	1	
>10	167	24 (14.4)	143 (85.6)	0.5 (0.3 - 1)	0.004
Sex					
Female	161	8 (5)	153 (95)	1	
Male	162	27 (16.7)	135 (83.3)	0.3 (0.2 - 0.6)	0.0004
Treatment duration (month)					
≤60	189	8 (4.2)	181 (95.8)	1	
>60	134	27 (2)	107 (98)	0.2 (0.1 - 0.3)	<0.001
Initial treatment					
AZT−	145	30 (2)	115 (98)	1	
AZT+	178	5 (2.8)	173 (97.2)	8.6 (5.8 - 9.8)	0.49
D4T−	184	6 (3.3)	178 (96.7)	1	
D4T+	139	29 (2)	110 (98)	0.1 (0.09 - 0.2)	0.01

On the contrary, the European Group of Pediatric Lipodystrophy found that the trunk was the most affected area in 66% of cases, followed by the lower limbs, the face, the upper limbs, the buttocks in 40%; 39%; 37% and 22% of cases respectively [12].

The development of lipodystrophy and especially lipoatrophy may be a source of stigma. Likewise, patients who link lipodystrophy to antiretroviral do not usually adhere to that treatment [12].

Lipoatrophy treatment is not well codified which makes it difficult for patients to get appropriate care. In adults, medical treatment with statines or plastic surgery has provided contradictory results [6] [20]. In our working context, psychological support remains the sole accessible solution. At the time of the survey, the national plan to switch D4T to other less toxic regimens was still underway.

In univariate and multivariate analysis, age above 10 years was significantly associated with lipodystrophy (P = 0.005). This result is similar to that found by other authors [10] [12] [17]. Morphological changes therefore increase with age.

Contrary to our study, Aurpibul in Thailand had noticed that lipodystrophy was more common in girls than boys, 61% and 39% of cases respectively [5]. Actually, there are seemed to be gender-based physiological differences in the occurrence of lipodystrophy. At puberty, estrogen and progesterone hormones contribute to fat accumulation in girls whereas in boys, testosterone, an anabolic hormone, maintains little fat accumulation. Thus, lipohypertrophy should normally be expected to be more common in girls than boys. However this was not the case in our study, the frequency of lipoatrophy among boys (16.7%) was higher than that of girls (5%) (P = 0.004).

We found no connection between hypercholesterolemia, hypertriglyceridemia, hyperglycemia and the presence of lipodystrophy in children. We think that these biological disturbances were transient and not associated with metabolic syndrome.

Lipodystrophy was found in all antiretroviral therapy regimens in our series. AZT and D4T of Nucleoside Reverse Transcriptase Inhibitors class (NRTIs), historically linked to lipodystrophy, and were used in 20% and 77.8% of our patients with lipodystrophy. Our results are very similar to those of Dollfus *et al.* who found that D4T was used in 92% of patients presenting lipodystrophy compared to 42% for AZT [10].

We found that D4T was significantly associated with the presence of lipodystrophy (P < 0.001) and especially lipoatrophy (P = 0.01). Our results are similar to those of Viard in France who, in a randomized trial on D4T and risk of lipoatrophy, found 3.6 times higher the risk of developing lipoatrophy when using D4T than AZT [13].

NRTIs particularly thymidinic derivatives (D4T and AZT), have a direct impact on mitochondria. They decrease the mitochondrial DNA and the respiratory chain proteins and increase the production of reactive oxygen. D4T and AZT induce lipolysis and, under certain circumstances, an apoptosis of adipocytes. These molecules interfere with adipocyte differentiation and contribute to activate the production of pro-inflammatory cytokines; while the other NRTIs do not change the rate of the mitochondrial DNA significantly [2].

Proteases inhibitors used in ARV regimen were found in 26.7% of patients presenting with lipodystrophy, this rate is lower than that found by Dollfus *et al.* of 79% [10]. In statistical analysis, there was no link between an exposure to PIs and the development of lipodystrophy (P = 0.06). However, some authors found a statistically significant link between exposure to PIs and the occurrence of lipodystrophy [17]. Indeed, protease inhibitors are associated with an alteration of the adipocyt differentiation, an oxidative stress and the production of pro-inflammatory cytokines.

5. Limits for This Study Were

- The method used to diagnosis lipodystrophy (morphological change) might have under estimated the disorder.
- The study was conducted in two hospitals of Ouagadougou and might not represent the profile of all HIV infected children on antiretroviral therapy in Burkina Faso.

6. Conclusion

We found a high prevalence rate of lipodystrophy in HIV-infected children on antiretroviral treatment. Age older than 10 years, WHO clinical stage 3, and long-term exposure to antiretroviral treatment especially D4T were factors most associated with lipoatrophy. Our results highlight the need to make available less toxic antiretroviral drugs for pediatric population. We'll have to try and make health professionals aware of screening for lipodystrophy. More researches on larger cohort in our setting are necessary to determine other metabolic disorders and associated factors in HIV-infected children treated with antiretroviral.

References

[1] Mutimura, E., Stewart, A. and Crowther, N.J. (2007) Assessment of Quality of Life in HAART-Treated HIV-Positive Subjects with Body Fat Redistribution in Rwanda. *AIDS Research and Therapy*, **4**, 19. http://dx.doi.org/10.1186/1742-6405-4-19

[2] Capeau, J., Caron, M., Vigouroux, C., Carvera, P., Kim, M., Maachi, M., *et al.* (2006) Les lipodystrophy secondaires aux traitements ARV de l'infection par le VIH. *Médecine Sciences*, **22**, 531-536. http://dx.doi.org/10.1051/medsci/2006225531

[3] Mercier, S., Gueye, N.F.N., Cournil, A., Fontbonne, A., Copin, N., Ndiaye, I., *et al.* (2009) Lipodystrophy and Metabolic Desorders in HIV-1-Infected Adults on 4- to 9-Year Antiretroviral Therapy in Senegal: A Case Control Study. *Journal of Acquired Immune Deficiency Syndromes*, **51**, 224-230. http://dx.doi.org/10.1097/QAI.0b013e31819c16f4

[4] Thiébaut, R., Daucourt, V., Mercié, P., Ekouévi, D.K., Malvy, D., Morlat, P., *et al.* (2000) Lipodystrophy, Metabolic Disorders, and Human Immunodeficiency Virus Infection: Aquitaine Cohort. *Clinical Infectious Diseases*, **31**, 1482-1487. http://dx.doi.org/10.1086/317477

[5] Aurpibul, L., Puthanakit, T., Lee, B., Mangtaburks, A., Sirisanthana, T. and Sirisanthana, V. (2007) Lipodystrophy and Metabolic Changes in HIV-Infected Children on Non-Nucleoside Reverse Transcriptase Inhibitor-Based Antiretroviral Therapy. *Antiviral Therapy*, **12**, 1247-1254.

[6] Capeau, J. and Valantin, M.-A. (2011) Syndrome lipodystrophique au cours du traitement antirétroviral in HIV; édition doin. 525-540.

[7] Chironi, G., Simon, A. and Vittecoq, D. (2004) Le risque cardiovasculaire au cours des traitements ARV, effets indésirables et alternatives thérapeutiques. *Médecine Thérapeutique*, **10**, 120-128.

[8] Lapphra, K., Vanprapar, N., Phongsmart, W., *et al.* (2005) Dyslipidemia and Lipodystrophy in HIV-Infected Thai Children on Highly Active Antiretroviral Therapy (HAART). *Journal of the Medical Association of Thailand*, **88**, 956-965.

[9] Hammond, E. and Noland, D. (2007) Adipose Tissue Inflammation and Altered Adipokine and Cytokine Production. *Antiretroviral Therapy-Associated Lipodystrophy*, **2**, 274-281.

[10] Dollfus, C., Jaquet, D., Levine, M., Ortoga-Rodriguez, E., Faye, A., Polak, M., *et al.* (2000) Clinical and Metabolic Presentation of the Lipodystrophic Syndrome in HIV-Infected Children. *AIDS*, **14**, 2123-2128. http://dx.doi.org/10.1097/00002030-200009290-00008

[11] Piloya, T., Bakeera-Kitaka, S., Kekitiinwa, A. and Kamya, M.R. (2012) Lipodystrophy among HIV-Infected Children and Adolescents on Highly Active Antiretroviral Therapy in Uganda: A Cross Sectional Study. *Journal of International AIDS Society*, **15**, 17427. http://dx.doi.org/10.7448/IAS.15.2.17427

[12] European Paediatric Lipodystrophy Group (2004) Antiretroviral Therapy, Fat Redistribution and Hyperlipidaemia in HIV-Infected Children in Europe. *AIDS*, **18**, 1443-1435. http://dx.doi.org/10.1097/01.aids.0000131334.38172.01

[13] Joly, V., Flandre, P., Meiffredy, V., Leturgue, N., Harel, M., Aboulker, J.P., *et al.* (2002) Increased Risk of Lipoatrophy under Stavudine in HIV-1-Infected Patients: Results of a Substudy from a Comparative Trial. *AIDS*, **16**, 2447-2454. http://dx.doi.org/10.1097/00002030-200212060-00010

[14] Ministère de la santé du Burkina Faso (2009) Comité ministériel de lutte contre le VIH/SIDA au Burkina Faso, normes et protocoles de prise en charge médicale des personnes vivant avec le VIH au Burkina Faso. 200 p.

[15] Vigano, A., Mora, S., Testolin, C., Beccio, S., Schneider, L., Bricalli, D., *et al.* (2003) Increased Lipodystrophy Is Associated with Increased Exposure to HAART in HIV-Infected Children. *Journal of AIDS*, **32**, 482-489. http://dx.doi.org/10.1097/00126334-200304150-00003

[16] WHO (2014) Antiretroviral Therapy for HIV Infection in Infants and Children. http://www.who.int/hiv/pub/paediatric/infants2010/en/

[17] Kinabo, G.D., Sprengers, M., Msuya, L.J., Shayo, A.M., Van Asten, H., Dolmans, W.M., *et al.* (2012) Prevalence of Lipodystrophy in HIV-Infected Children in Tanzania on Highly Active Antiretroviral Therapy. *The Pediatric Infectious Disease Journal*, **32**, 39-44.

[18] Hartman, K., Verweel, G., Groot, R. and Hartwig, N.G. (2006) Detection of Lipoatrophy in Human Immunodeficiency Virus-1-Infected Children Treated with HAART. *The Pediatric Infectious Disease Journal*, **25**, 427-431. http://dx.doi.org/10.1097/01.inf.0000215003.32256.aa

[19] Padilla, S., Gallego, J.A., Masia, M. and Gutierrez, F. (2004) Single-Slice Computed Tomography and Antropometric Skinfold Analysis for Evaluation of Facial Lipoatrophy in HIV-Infected Patients. *Clinical Infectious Diseases*, **39**,

1848-1851. http://dx.doi.org/10.1086/426072

[20] Levan, P., Nguyen, T.H., Lallemand, F., Mazetier, L., Mimoun, M., Rozenbaum, W., *et al.* (2002) Correction of Facial Lipoatrophy, in HIV-Infected Patients on HAART by Injection of Autologous Fatty Tissue. *AIDS*, **16**, 1985-1987. http://dx.doi.org/10.1097/00002030-200209270-00026

11

The Influence of Pain: Quality of Life after *Pectus excavatum* Correction

Wietse P. Zuidema[1,2*], Alida F. W. van der Steeg[2,3], Jan W. A. Oosterhuis[1], Christien Sleeboom[2], Stefan M. van der Heide[4], Elly S. M. de Lange-de Klerk[5], Hugo A. Heij[2]

[1]Department of Surgery, VU University Medical Center, Amsterdam, The Netherlands
[2]Pediatric Surgical Center of Amsterdam, Emma Children's Hospital AMC and VU University Medical Center, Amsterdam, The Netherlands
[3]Center of Research on Psychology in Somatic Diseases (CoRPS), Tilburg University, Tilburg, The Netherlands
[4]Department of Cardio-Thoracic Surgery, Radboud University Medical Center, Nijmegen, The Netherlands
[5]Department of Epidemiology and Biostatistics, VU University Medical Center, Amsterdam, The Netherlands
Email: [*]w.zuidema@vumc.nl

Abstract

Introduction: The main indication for surgery of thoracic wall deformities (TWD) is psychological due to cosmetic complaints. The assumption is that appearances have a negative effect on self-esteem and quality of life (QoL). Correction should result in improvement. Methods: Prospective trial. QoL was assessed using the CHQ and the WHOQOL-bref. Measurements were taken before surgery (T1) and 6 weeks thereafter (T2). Results: Forty-two patients were included. WHOQOL-bref showed differences between pre-operative and six weeks past surgery on facet body image ($p = 0.003$). Self-esteem (CHQ) did not show a significant improvement at T2. Concerning the scores on the single step questionnaire (SSQ), 33 patients were "very" to "extremely satisfied" with appearance and increased self-esteem ($p < 0.001$). Concerning the domain "pain and physical complaints", CHQ did show a significant change ($p < 0.001$) with more complaints at T2. Conclusion: Six weeks after surgical correction of a TWD satisfaction with the "new" chest is good; pain seems to be a problem with possible negative influence on self-esteem.

Keywords

Pain, Quality of Life (Qol), Pectus, Chest Wall Deformity

[*]Corresponding author.

1. Introduction

The most important anterior chest wall deformity is the *Pectus excavatum* (PE). It predominantly affects males. The incidence of PE is about 1 in 400 [1]. The most important complaint is cosmesis although a substantial part of the patients also complains of physical impairments, especially shortness of breath during exercise.

The NUSS procedure and the Ravitch procedure are used for correction of PE. Both procedures have been reported to give good cosmetic results [2]. In addition, studies reporting physical improvement after correction of PE are increasing in number [3] [4].

Both physical and cosmetic issues may lead to a decreased quality of life (QoL) and body image, especially in adolescents who are vulnerable to peer pressure [5]. Quality of life is defined by the World health Organization as "an individual's perception of his/her position in life in context of the culture and value systems in which he/she lives and in relation to his/her goals, expectations, standards and concerns" [6]. Thus, QoL refers to satisfaction with functioning in a wide range of areas.

Since the primary goal of surgical correction of a *Pectus excavatum* is improvement of cosmesis and thus body image and QoL, it is important to assess the factors that may negatively influence QoL.

A major concern in the early post-operative phase after pectus correction is pain [7]. In the literature this problem is recognized, however most studies only focus on pain management in the first days after surgery and describe methods to alleviate the pain immediately post-operatively [7]-[9]. The severity of post-operative pain is influenced by anxiety, with more anxious individuals reporting higher pain-scores [10]-[12]. So far, however, no studies have looked into the relation between anxiety and post-operative pain or assessed the influence of post-operative pain on QoL after *Pectus excavatum* correction.

The present study has a longitudinal, prospective set-up and aims to evaluate the early changes in QoL after surgical *Pectus excavatum* correction and assess the influence of pain on QoL.

We hypothesized that severe post-operative pain would negatively influence QoL scores in both adolescents and young adults.

2. Methods

2.1. Patients

Since October 2011 all consecutive patients who were referred to our outpatient clinic with a PE were asked to participate in this study. Patients younger than 12 years of age were not eligible for correction at our institution and therefore did not participate.

Patients or parents with insufficient knowledge of the Dutch language in reading or writing were excluded. Patients with Marfan's syndrome or other associated connective tissue diseases were allowed to participate.

All patients over the age of sixteen gave informed consent.

Patients under the age of sixteen gave informed consent as did their parents.

The medical ethics committee approved the study.

2.2. Surgery

In patients with a PE the Nuss procedure was performed [13]. Surgery was performed by one of 6 surgeons. Post-operative pain management was preferably done with patient controlled epidural analgesia. Patients who refused an epidural or patients who did not experience sufficient pain relief with epidural analgesia received patient controlled intravenous analgesia using morphine and occasionally ketamin.

On the third day post-operative it was tried to decrease the epidural or intravenous analgesia and switch to oral pain medication (e.g. paracetamol in combination with an NSAID). With this medication patients were usually discharged and were advised to diminish the dosage at home, based on the pain they experienced.

2.3. Questionnaires

Patients were divided into 3 groups based upon age, being younger than 16 years, 16 - 18 years and older than 18 years of age. Questionnaires used differed per age group. Socio-demographic characteristics of the three age groups are shown in **Table 1**.

Measurement moments were pre-operatively and 6 weeks post-operative.

Quality of life was assessed using the Dutch version of the Child Health Questionnaire (CHQ-87) in patients

Table 1. Socio-demographic characteristics in the three age groups.

Socio-demographic characteristics	<16 years	16 < x < 18 years	>18 years
Mean age	14.6 years	16.9 years	20.6 years
Gender (male/female)	21/2	7/3	8/1
Education level	low 7, middle 9, high 7	Low 3, middle 4, high 3	Low 3, middle 3, high 3
Average family size	4.1	4.0	2.7

A higher score on education represents a more demanding school type. Average family size represents the number of currently together living family members which can include one or both parents.

younger than 16 and between 16 and 18 years of age and with the short version of the World Health Organization Quality of Life assessment instrument (WHOQL-bref) in patients between 16 and 18 years and older than 18 years of age.

The CHQ-87 is a generic QoL assessment tool that has good reliability and validity [14]. This questionnaire covers the physical, emotional and social well-being of children. Items are scored using a four to six point Likert scale and converted to a 0 to 100 point continuum, with higher scores indicating a better QoL. Norm values of the Dutch population are available and allow for comparison with "healthy" children [15].

The WHOQOL-bref is the short version of the WHOQOL-100 [16]. It consists of questions assessing QoL in four domains being physical health, psychological health, social relationships and environment and a general evaluative facet (overall quality of life and general health). For the purpose of our study two facets of the WHOQOL-100 have been added to the WHOQOL-bref being the facet pain and discomfort and the facet body image. Items are scored on a four point Likert scale. Higher scores indicate a better QoL.

Anxiety was assessed using the short versions of the State and Trait Anxiety Inventory [17] [18]. Trait anxiety concerns differences in individuals in the disposition to respond to stressful situations with varying levels of anxiety.

State anxiety refers to the momentarily experienced feeling of apprehension and tension. Items are scored on a four point Likert scale, these scores are added up and then dichotomized in high or not-high, with cut-off scores derived from the manual. The short versions have good reliability and validity [19].

In order to measure the satisfaction with surgery and the post-operative appearance of the thorax the single step questionnaire was used [4]. This assessment tool uses 16 questions to assess satisfaction. Scores are added and a score above 41, with a maximum score of 84 is considered to be a satisfactory outcome. This questionnaire was only completed post-operatively at T2. The concept of the questionnaire is that one measurement moment gives information concerning pre-operative and post-operative satisfaction.

Pain in rest and during activity post-operatively was measured using a 100 mm Visual Analogue Scale [20].

2.4. Statistical Analysis

Data analyses were conducted using IBM SPSS 20 software (SPSS Inc. Chicago, IL, USA). Descriptive statistics for variables of interest in this study are presented as percentage; means and SDs. Comparison between scores at measurement moment T1 and T2 for the enlisted variables from the study group were calculated using the paired Student T-test. The cut off point for significance was set at $p < 0.05$.

3. Results

Between October 2011 and July 2013 42 patients were included, 36 males and 6 females. All patients underwent a Nuss procedure because of a PE. The mean age was 16.4 years (SD 3.02) with 23 patients under the age of 16 years, 10 patients between 16 and 18 years and 9 patients being older than 18 years of age.

Scores on the WHOQOL-bref showed only a significant differences between pre-operative and six weeks past surgery on facet body image ($p = 0.003$). Scores on the CHQ showed a significant increase in bodily pain and discomfort after 6 weeks ($p < 0.001$; see **Table 2**).

State anxiety was significantly diminished after 6 weeks compared with the pre-operative scores ($p = 0.009$).

Concerning the scores on the single step questionnaire (SSQ) 33 out of 42 patients were very to extremely satisfied with the overall post-operative appearance. Scores on post-operative self-esteem were significantly higher

Table 2. Comparison between scores on WHOQOL, CHQ, and STAI for T1 and T2.

Measurement moment	T1	T2	p-value
WHOQOL			
Facet pain	9.9 (2.3)	9.4 (2.5)	0.53
Facet body image	12.1 (3.7)	16.5 (3.0)	0.003
Overall Quality of life	7.8 (1.2)	8.0 (1.6)	0.54
CHQ			
Mental health	73.4 (16.1)	78.0 (17.4)	0.11
Self-esteem	73.2 (15.2)	75.7 (14.7)	0.26
Bodily pain and discomfort	74.5 (19.6)	51.3 (21.7)	0.001
General health	79.7 (18.2)	76.5 (20.1)	0.42
STAI			
State anxiety	11.3 (3.7)	9.6 (3.2)	0.009

Scores are represented in means (SD). Concerning scores: a higher score represents improvement, with the exception of pain measured with CHQ (higher score represents less pain) and scores on state anxiety (lower score, less anxiety).

compared with scores pre-operatively (8.1 (SD 1.4) on a score of 1 - 10 and 5.5 (SD 1.8) respectively; $p < 0.001$). However, only 27 patients (64.3%) replied with yes on the question "going back, would you have the operation again". Eleven patients were unsure and 4 patients said no.

Pain during hospital stay was severe to very severe in 30 patients, and pain at six weeks was still present in 32 of the patients with 5 still needing painkillers.

VAS-scores in rest at six weeks were 2.7 (2.3) and in activity 3.4 (2.3) (with scores ranging from 0 to 10).

4. Discussion

The primary goal of pectus correction is improvement of self-esteem body image and quality of life. However, certain surgery related factors may negatively influence the aforementioned outcome.

In this study it was found that even though the large majority of patients are very satisfied with the result of the surgery about a third would not have the surgery again. The only other factor that significantly changed between pre- and post-operative measurement moments is pain. Six weeks post-surgery almost two third of the patients still experience pain and 12% still need painkillers.

Considering the fact that other studies have shown a positive relationship between surgical correction of a thoracic wall deformity and improvement of body image and QoL [2] [3], the assumption is that 6 weeks after surgery pain is of such a large influence it hampers the improvement of QoL.

Factors that influence postoperative pain are age, anticipatory anxiety and total analgesics administered [12].

During the first informative outpatient consult concerning surgical correction of the pectus pain is mentioned extensively and patients are informed about the (possible) severity and the necessity of epidural analgesia post-operative in combination with oral pain medication.

The questions used in the current study did not inquire into the correctness of the information provided and whether or not the experienced pain fitted the expectations. This will be included in future questionnaires.

The relationship between pain and anxiety is known, especially in the early postoperative phase. Both the anxiety of patients and the anxiety of their parents have a negative influence on the level of pain, e.g. the higher the level of anxiety the higher the pain score [10] [11] [21].

Anxiety can be divided in momentarily experienced anxiety (state anxiety) and the personality characteristic anxiety e.g. the proneness to respond with anxiety to certain stressful situations (trait anxiety). Concerning trait anxiety 7 out of the 42 patients scored high on the questionnaire, implying that they are likely to respond with higher anxiety levels in certain situations. The levels of state anxiety however showed high scores for 15 out of the 42 patients pre-operatively and decreased to 2 out of 42 post-operatively. Because of the relatively small numbers included so far a significant relationship found between total score trait anxiety and pain in rest at six weeks post-operatively ($p < 0.001$), should be interpreted with caution.

Factors that may influence pain intensity are pain education [22] [23] and coping instructions [24]. Both studies show that being prepared and being able to cope does not necessarily reduce the experienced pain [22] but does prevent negative feelings concerning the pain and the medical care.

Limitations of this study are the relative small sample size, which makes it necessary to interpret the results with caution. Also the fact that the forty-two surgical procedures were carried out by 6 different surgeons, may have let to small variation in technique and hereby to possible variation in post-operative pain level.

5. Conclusions and Future Directions

Six weeks after surgical correction of a TWD satisfaction with the "new" chest is good; pain seems to be a problem with possible negative influence on self-esteem.

Future studies concerning pain after surgical correction of thoracic wall defects should include interventional studies using coping strategies and anxiety-reducing psychosocial interventions.

In addition, longer follow-up is necessary in the current study to see whether the equilibrium between pain and QoL shifts in favor of QoL.

References

[1] Shamberger, R.C. (1996) Congenital Chest Wall Deformities. *Current Problems in Surgery*, **33**, 469-552. http://dx.doi.org/10.1016/S0011-3840(96)80005-0

[2] Lam, M.W.C., Klassen, A.F., Montgomery, C.J., LeBlanc, J.G., Skarsgard, E.D. (2008) Quality-of-Life Outcomes after Surgical Correction of *Pectus excavatum*: A Comparison of the Ravitch and Nuss procedures. *Journal of Pediatric Surgery*, **43**, 819-825. http://dx.doi.org/10.1016/j.jpedsurg.2007.12.020

[3] Kelly, R.E., Cash, T.F., Shamberger, R.C., *et al.* (2008) Surgical Repair of *Pectus excavatum* Markedly Improves Body Image and Perceived Ability for Physical Activity: Multicenter Study. *Pediatrics*, **122**, 1218-1222. http://dx.doi.org/10.1542/peds.2007-2723

[4] Krasopoulos, G., Dusmet, M., Ladas, G. and Goldstraw, P. (2006) Nuss Procedure Improves the Quality of Life in Young Male Adults with *Pectus excavatum* Deformity. *European Journal Cardio-Thoracic Surgery*, **29**, 1-5. http://dx.doi.org/10.1016/j.ejcts.2005.09.018

[5] Steinmann, C., Krille, S., Mueller, A., Weber, P., Reingruber, B. and Martin, A. (2011) *Pectus excavatum* and Pectus Carinatum Patients Suffer from Lower Quality of Life and Impaired Body Image: A Control Group Comparison of Psychological Characteristics Prior to Surgical Correction. *European Journal Cardio-Thoracic Surgery*, **40**, 1138-1145.

[6] WHOQOL Group (1994) Development of the WHOQOL: Rationale and Current Status. *International Journal of Mental Health*, **23**, 24-56.

[7] Densmore, J.C., Peterson, D.B., Stahvic, L.L., *et al.* (2010) Initial Surgical and Pain Management Outcomes after Nuss Procedure. *Journal of Pediatric Surgery*, **45**, 1767-1771.

[8] Futagawa, K., Suwa, I., Okuda, T., Kamamoto, H., Sugiura, J., Kajikawa, R. and Koga, Y. (2006) Anesthetic Management for the Minimally Invasive Nuss Procedure in 21 Patients with *Pectus excavatum*. *Journal of Anesthesia*, **20**, 48-50. http://dx.doi.org/10.1007/s00540-005-0367-4

[9] Soliman, I.E., Apuya, J.S., Fertal, K.M., Simpson, P.M. and Tobias, J.D. (2009) Intravenous versus Epidural Analgesia after Surgical Repair of *Pectus excavatum*. *American Journal of Therapeutics*, **16**, 398-403. http://dx.doi.org/10.1097/MJT.0b013e318187de3e

[10] LaMontagne, L.L., Hepworth, J.T. and Salisbury, M.H. (2001) Anxiety and Post-Operative Pain in Children Who Undergo Major Orthopedic Surgery. *Applied Nursing Research*, **14**, 119-124. http://dx.doi.org/10.1053/apnr.2001.24410

[11] Palermo, T.M., Drotar, D.D. and Lambert, S. (1998) Psychosocial Predictors of Children's Postoperative Pain. *Clinical Nursing Research*, **7**, 275-291. http://dx.doi.org/10.1177/105477389800700305

[12] Palermo, T.M. and Drotar, D. (1996) Prediction of Children's Postoperative Pain: The Role of Presurgical Expectations and Anticipatory Emotions. *Journal of Pediatric Psychology*, **21**, 683-698.

[13] Nuss, D., Kelly Jr., R.E., Croitoru, D.P. and Katz, M.E. (1998) A 10-Year Review of a Minimally Invasive Technique for the Correction of *Pectus excavatum*. *Journal of Pediatric Surgery*, **33**, 545-552. http://dx.doi.org/10.1016/S0022-3468(98)90314-1

[14] Landgraf, J.M., Abetz, L. and Ware, J.A. (1996) The CHQ User Manual. The Health Institute, New England Medical Center, Boston.

[15] Raat, H., Landgraf, J.M., Bonsel, G.J., Gemke, R.J. and Essink-Bot, M.L. (2002) Reliability and Validity of the Child Health Questionnaire-Child Form (CHQ-CF87) in a Dutch Adolescent Population. *Quality of Life Research*, **11**, 575-581. http://dx.doi.org/10.1023/A:1016393311799

[16] WHOQOL Group (1998) Development of the World Health Organization WHOQOL-BREF Quality of Life Assessment. *Psychological Medicine*, **28**, 551-558. http://dx.doi.org/10.1017/S0033291798006667

[17] Spielberger, C.D., Gorsuch, R.L. and Lushene, R.E. (1970) The State-Trait Anxiety Inventory Manual. Consulting Psychologists Press, Palo Alto.

[18] Van der Ploeg, H.M., Defares, P.B. and Spielberger, C.D. (1980) ZBV. A Dutch-Language Adaptation of the Spielberger State-Trait Anxiety Inventory. Swets & Zeitlinger, Lisse.

[19] Van der Bij, A.K., de Weerd, S., Cikot, R.J.L.M., Steegers, E.A.P. and Braspenning, J.C.C. (2003) Validation of the Dutch Short Form of the State Scale of the Spielberger State-Trait-Anxiety Inventory: Considerations for Usage in Screening Outcomes. *Journal of Community Genetics*, **6**, 84-87. http://dx.doi.org/10.1159/000073003

[20] Huskisson, E. (1974) Measurement of Pain. *The Lancet*, **304**, 1127-1131. http://dx.doi.org/10.1016/S0140-6736(74)90884-8

[21] Kain, Z.N., Mayes, L.C., O'Connor, T.Z. and Cicchetti, D.V. (1996) Preoperative Anxiety in Children. Predictors and Outcomes. *Archives of Pediatrics and Adolescent Medicine*, **150**, 1238-1245. http://dx.doi.org/10.1001/archpedi.1996.02170370016002

[22] Crandall, M., Lammers, C., Senders, C., Braun, J.V. and Savedra, M. (2008) Children's Pre-Operative Tonsillectomy Pain Education: Clinical Outcomes. *International Journal of Pediatric Otorhinolaryngology*, **72**, 1523-1533. http://dx.doi.org/10.1016/j.ijporl.2008.07.004

[23] Sjöling, M., Nordahl, G., Olofsson, N. and Asplund, K. (2003) The Impact of Preoperative Information on State Anxiety, Postoperative Pain and Satisfaction with Pain Management. *Patient Education and Counseling*, **51**, 169-176. http://dx.doi.org/10.1016/S0738-3991(02)00191-X

[24] LaMontagne, L.L., Hepworth, J.T., Salisbury, M.S. and Cohen, F. (2003) Effects of Coping Instruction in Reducing Young Adolescents' Pain after Major Spinal Surgery. *Orthopaedic Nursing*, **22**, 398-403. http://dx.doi.org/10.1097/00006416-200311000-00005

12

Evaluation of a Pediatric Mock Code Educational Training Program at a Large, Tertiary Care Pediatric Hospital

Ayelet Rimon[1,2*], Amit Hess[1,2*], Dennis Scolnik[3], Oren Tavor[1,2], Shirley Friedman[2,4], Miguel Glatstein[1,2#]

[1]Pediatric Emergency Medicine, Dana-Dwek Children's Hospital, Tel-Aviv, Israel
[2]Sackler School of Medicine, Tel Aviv University, Tel-Aviv, Israel
[3]Divisions of Pediatric Emergency Medicine and Clinical Pharmacology and Toxicology, Department of Pediatrics, The Hospital for Sick Children, University of Toronto, Toronto, Canada
[4]Pediatric Intensive Care, Dana-Dwek Children's Hospital, Tel-Aviv, Israel
Email: [#]Nopasara73@hotmail.com

Abstract

Background: Management of the acutely ill children represents one of the more complex clinical skills required of pediatric physicians. Our goal was to develop and evaluate a multidisciplinary pediatric mock code training program for the pediatric residents in our institution. Methods: We performed a before and after evaluation of pediatric residents. The residents were educated by attending five mock code scenarios, followed by debriefing. Before and after the five sessions, the residents completed a self-assessment questionnaire. Results: Residents reported a significant improvement in their comfort in all aspects of managing pediatric resuscitations, with notable improvement seen in running a resuscitation requiring airway management, managing fluid resuscitation and performing endotracheal intubation. The most prominent change was demonstrated in the comfort level of the overall management of a pediatric resuscitation. Conclusion: The pediatric mock code educational training program improved residents' self-reported knowledge and comfort level in managing pediatric emergency situations.

Keywords

Education, Mock Code, Pediatric Residents, Emergency Medicine

[*]The authors have the equal contribution.
[#]Corresponding author.

1. Background

Management of acutely ill children represents one of the more complex clinical skills required of physicians, especially in the pediatric emergency department where severe medical conditions, behavioral crises, and accidental/intentional injuries are commonly encountered [1] [2]. The ability of the physician to competently and effectively manage these varied medical conditions depends both on their total caseload and the frequency of exposure to these types of injuries and situations [3]. Although pediatric residents are expected to acquire this set of skills during their training since they are often the primary care givers during resuscitations, their degree of confidence and knowledge levels in managing these situations remains unclear [4]. Critical decisions regarding very ill children presenting to the emergency department often have to be taken by pediatric residents before the arrival of the sub-specialties such as anesthesia, general surgery and pediatric critical care. Teaching interventions have been designed to address residents' needs in these areas. PALS is also evidence based and a standard of care, although skills retention beyond 6 months decreases. Although the Pediatric Advanced Life Support (PALS) course has been shown to be an effective teaching program, it has several limitations including extensive facility and faculty requirements, high cost and limited availability [5]. PALS is also evidence based and a standard of care, although skills retention beyond 6 months decreases. Mock code training is an effective training tool for pediatric acute care providers who have limited exposure to critically ill patients [6] [7], and pediatric "mock codes" have been utilized to increase the emergency preparedness of inpatient medical units for several decades [8]. Repetitive pediatric simulation of this type provides learners with a discrete opportunity to apply their knowledge [9]. These practice drills have been shown to both increase practitioners' confidence and decrease anxiety during actual resuscitations [2]. Data obtained from medical trainees can also be used to design future skill-based educational initiatives [5].

The objective of this educational study was to improve medical caregivers' skills in pediatric resuscitation at our institution. The low fidelity simulation training was administered in the actual emergency department in order to provide pediatric residents with as real an experience as possible and to facilitate their transition into becoming a part of the pediatric emergency team. We hypothesized that weekly training, comprised of multiple mock code scenarios, for two months would increase pediatric residents' reported levels of knowledge and comfort in leading a real code.

2. Methods

Over a period of two months (from April 1, 2014 to May 31, 2014), all junior and senior residents in the pediatric residency program of our institution were invited voluntary to attend weekly mock code teaching and debriefing sessions. Prior to beginning the course of mock code educational sessions, residents completed a self-assessment questionnaire (pre). Questions regarding their comfort in dealing with emergency situations and confidence in performing specific life-saving skills were addressed, using a five-point Likert scale ranging from 1 = "strongly disagree" to 5 = "strongly agree" for each item (see **Appendix 1**). Once the training was completed each resident completed the same self-assessment questionnaire (post) to measure changes resulting from the intervention. Data was also recorded regarding the number of occasions each resident had participated in emergency interventions or resuscitations before starting the training program.

The intention of each mock code scenario was to provide specific opportunities for the residents to care for seriously ill pediatric patients. Participants were exposed to situations that required immediate attention to the "ABCs" (airway, breathing and circulation) of pediatric resuscitation using a traditional plastic mannequin (Laerdal Medical Corporation, USA). The transition from basic to advanced life support techniques was inherent in each mock code scenario. We hoped to bring all residents to a self-assessed knowledge and skill level of at least "average" (2.5/5) in each skill assessed and also aimed to eliminate responses indicating the lowest levels of confidence (strongly disagree or disagree with having good resuscitation knowledge and skills). In order to create a realistic simulation, nurses were included in the mock code training and the training took place in the resuscitation room of the emergency department. The necessary equipment was present, but had been not set up or connected before the start of the scenario.

The 15 - 20 minute scenarios were designed and facilitated by emergency medicine physicians, and were followed by a 20 minute debriefing session. They were designed to be realistic and practical; life-threatening situations encompassing the wide range of childhood illnesses and injuries that practitioners may well have to address were specifically chosen. There were five different scenarios, all involving management of airway, breathing and circulation, due to different emergencies. Practical skills such as endotracheal intubation and obtaining intra-osseous access were incorporated in most scenarios.

Each of the five mock code scenarios was designed to encourage the development of a particular skill set: 1) **Drowning**: to familiarize residents with management priorities when dealing with drowning patients, recognize and treat hypothermia and its complications and also to consider potential associated problems like intoxication, head and cervical injury; 2) **septic shock—meningococcemia**: to enhance recognition of fever and petechiae as a medical emergency, to understand that systolic blood pressure can be preserved until late in the course of shock in children and to become cognizant that early and aggressive fluid resuscitation and vasopressor therapy are lifesaving; 3) **altered mental status—ketoacidosis**: to recognize and manage patients with altered mental status, identify the presenting signs and symptoms of diabetic ketoacidosis (DKA), to treat DKA and manage increased intracranial pressure associated with DKA; 4) **apnea—bronchiolitis**: to identify respiratory distress and impending respiratory failure, acutely manage apnea and respiratory failure, and to be aware of the association between apnea and bronchiolitis; 5) **cardiac arrest**: to rapidly start protocolized management of cardiac arrest and to acquire an initial approach to cardiac emergencies.

All codes were assessed for patient management and team function by an observing pediatric emergency medicine attending physician. At the completion of each scenario, the participating residents took part in a debriefing session with the attending physician, which pointed out the strengths and weaknesses of the team.

Statistical Analysis: In addition to using descriptive statistics to describe findings data from the pre and post self assessment questionnaire responses were compared using the Wilcoxon Signed Rank Test.

3. Results

Forty four pediatric residents participated in the pediatric mock code educational initiative, and completed both a pre and a post questionnaire. The group consisted of 33 (75%) female residents, 11 males, ages 28 - 35 years. Six residents were unable to enter the training, as a result of leave of absence or rotations in a unit which refused nonattendance. Information regarding the characteristics of the participating residents is summarized in **Table 1**. The majority of the residents were junior, within the first two years of a five year residency. Twenty seven residents (61%) had completed PALS training before the beginning of the training program. Previous experience in real resuscitations was variable: 36% of residents had no resuscitation experience, and 86% had been directly involved in five or less pediatric resuscitations.

Responses for all questions were calculated and reported as median scores before and after the mock code training (**Table 2**). Before the intervention the only skill the residents were comfortable performing was bag-mask-ventilation, with a median score of four (agree with the phrase "I am comfortable performing bag-mask-ventilation"). Low scores were found on assessments of theoretical knowledge of airway management

Table 1. Demographic information of residents participating in the pediatric mock code educational initiative.

Characteristics of the 44 participants	n (%)
Resident year of training	
First (junior)	12 (27%)
Second (junior)	14 (32%)
Third (senior)	5 (11%)
Fourth (senior)	7 (16%)
Fifth (senior)	6 (14%)
Completed PICU rotation	12 (27%)
Completed PALS training	27 (61%)
Actual resuscitation experience (number of cases)	
None	16 (36%)
1 - 2	14 (32%)
3 - 5	8 (18%)
6 - 10	6 (14%)

Table 2. Summary of resident responses to the pre- and post-intervention questionnaire.

Question	Pre-intervention (median, range)	Post-intervention (median, range)	p value
I have good knowledge on how to manage a resuscitation requiring airway management	2.5, 5	4, 5	<0.001
I feel comfortable running a resuscitation requiring airway management	2, 5	3, 5	<0.001
I have good knowledge on how to manage a resuscitation of shock requiring fluid resuscitation	3, 5	4, 5	<0.001
I feel comfortable running a resuscitation of shock requiring fluid resuscitation	3, 5	4, 5	<0.001
I am comfortable performing bag-mask-ventilation	4, 5	4.5, 5	<0.001
I am comfortable performing endotracheal intubation	2, 5	4, 5	<0.001
I feel comfortable managing a pediatric resuscitation	2, 5	3.5, 5	<0.001

Table 3. Numbers of students scoring in lowest 2 categories pre- and post-mock code training.

Question	Bottom 1 + 2 score pre-intervention, *n*	Bottom 1 + 2 score post-intervention, *n*	Observed change
I have good knowledge on how to manage a resuscitation requiring airway management	22	5	17
I feel comfortable running a resuscitation requiring airway management	33	5	28
I have good knowledge on how to manage a resuscitation of shock requiring fluid resuscitation	15	0	15
I feel comfortable running a resuscitation of shock requiring fluid resuscitation	20	0	20
I am comfortable performing bag-mask-ventilation	7	0	7
I am comfortable performing endotracheal intubation	29	9	20
I feel comfortable managing a pediatric resuscitation	33	2	31

during resuscitation and fluid management in shock.

Numbers of residents who assessed themselves as being in the weakest categories of knowledge and resuscitation skills pre- and post-mock code training are displayed in **Table 3**. The biggest change by the end of the program was in overall comfort level in the management of a pediatric resuscitation, with a decrease from 33 physicians in the bottom scores (1 or 2/5) pre-intervention (75%) to two physicians (5%) post-intervention. Notable improvement was also seen in running a resuscitation requiring airway management, fluid resuscitation for shock and performing endotracheal intubation. A small group of seven residents (16%) reported having a low comfort level in bag-mask ventilation pre-intervention, in comparison to none in the post-intervention assessment.

4. Discussion

Pediatric residents are frequently the first responders in emergency situations in the emergency department even though they may have only modest experience as members of a pediatric resuscitation team and despite reporting low self-assessments of knowledge and skills of resuscitation. The "pre" results of our study clearly confirm the need for resuscitation training in the curriculum of residents. We have shown that a two-month simulation program involving five resuscitation scenarios can improve their self-assessment of knowledge and resuscitation skills.

The ability to lead resuscitation is one of the goals of training a pediatric resident. Traditionally, residents training in pediatrics gain much of their experience in resuscitation through exposure to real cases, with the only mandatory training being PALS. Despite the fact that our institution does not have the capability of high fidelity simulation, we demonstrated the after two months of intensive low fidelity weekly mock codes we were able to improve residents' knowledge and comfort level in managing emergency situations.

In a cross sectional study of pediatric residents Friedman *et al.* [8] showed that one year after starting a mock code program, residents attended more mock codes and reported more comfort with knowledge in codes. A second one year study also showed that mock codes improved resident confidence and self-assessment of their resuscitation skills [10]. Our study demonstrated an increase in residents' comfort managing pediatric resuscitations and performing procedural skills after an intensive two month training program.

This study has several limitations. Firstly, given that the study was initiated due to an urgent need to train our residents, they served as their own control group through pre-post mock-code training. Secondly, the evaluation tool was resident self-assessment regarding knowledge and skills rather than a measure of real-life performance. Thirdly, previous studies have shown that participants in advanced life support courses have significant deterioration of their skills and knowledge over time [11] [12] and the sustainability of the observed improvements was not measured in our study. However, it may be reasonable to presume that residents' improvements will be reinforced by the real-life situations they deal with as they mature into fully-fledged pediatricians.

5. Conclusion

Our study stresses the need for mock code training in the curriculum of pediatric residents. It suggests a method whereby knowledge and skills can be developed and enhanced through the use of five common clinical scenarios, delivered on a weekly basis over two months, using low fidelity mock code training.

References

[1] Mikrogianakis, A., Osmond, M.H., Nuth, J.E., Shephard, A., Gaboury, I. and Jabbour, M. (2008) Evaluation of a Multidisciplinary Pediatric Mock Trauma Code Educational Initiative: A Pilot Study. *The Journal of Trauma*, **64**, 761-767.

[2] Toback, S.L., Fiedor, M., Kilpela, B. and Reis, E.C. (2006) Impact of a Pediatric Primary Care Office-Based Mock Code Program on Physician and Staff Confidence to Perform Life-Saving Skills. *Pediatric Emergency Care*, **22**, 415-422. http://dx.doi.org/10.1097/01.pec.0000221342.11626.12

[3] Cappelle, C. and Paul, R.I. (1996) Educating Residents: The Effects of a Mock Code Program. *Resuscitation*, **31**, 107-111. http://dx.doi.org/10.1016/0300-9572(95)00919-1

[4] Tofil, N.M., Lee White, M., Manzella, B., McGill, D. and Zinkan, L. (2009) Initiation of a Pediatric Mock Code Program at a Children's Hospital. *Medical Teacher*, **31**, e241-e247. http://dx.doi.org/10.1080/01421590802637974

[5] Popp, J., Yochum, L., Spinella, P.C., Donahue, S. and Finck, C. (2012) Simulation Training for Surgical Residents in Pediatric Trauma Scenarios. *Connecticut Medicine*, **76**, 159-162.

[6] Weinberg, E.R., Auerbach, M.A. and Shah, N.B. (2009) The Use of Simulation for Pediatric Training and Assessment. *Current Opinion in Pediatrics*, **21**, 282-287. http://dx.doi.org/10.1097/MOP.0b013e32832b32dc

[7] Ralston, M.E., Day, L.T., Slusher, T.M., Musa, N.L. and Doss, H.S. (2013) Global Paediatric Advanced Life Support: Improving Child Survival in Limited-Resource Settings. *Lancet*, **381**, 256-265. http://dx.doi.org/10.1016/S0140-6736(12)61191-X

[8] Friedman, D., Zaveri, P. and O'Connell, K. (2010) Pediatric Mock Code Curriculum: Improving Resident Resuscitations. *Pediatric Emergency Care*, **26**, 490-494. http://dx.doi.org/10.1097/PEC.0b013e3181e5bf34

[9] Auerbach, M., Kessler, D. and Foltin, J.C. (2011) Repetitive Pediatric Simulation Resuscitation Training. *Pediatric Emergency Care*, **27**, 29-31. http://dx.doi.org/10.1097/PEC.0b013e3182043f3b

[10] Trainor, J.L. and Krug, S.E. (2000) The Training of Pediatric Residents in the Care of Acutely Ill and Injured Children. *Archives of Pediatrics and Adolescent Medicine*, **154**, 1154-1159.

[11] Gass, D.A. and Curry, L. (1983) Physicians' and Nurses' Retention of Knowledge and Skill after Training in Cardiopulmonary Resuscitation. *Canadian Medical Association Journal*, **128**, 550-551.

[12] Andreatta, P., Saxton, E., Thompson, M. and Annich, G. (2011) Simulation-Based Mock Codes Significantly Correlate with Improved Pediatric Patient Cardiopulmonary Arrest Survival Rates. *Pediatric Critical Care Medicine*, **12**, 33-38. http://dx.doi.org/10.1097/PCC.0b013e3181e89270

Appendix 1

Self-Assessment Questionnaire

Gender Male/Female
Year of residency 1 2 3 4 5
Have you completed a rotation in the PICU? Yes/No
Have you completed a PALS course in the past 2 years? Yes/No
How many pediatric resuscitations have you taken part in? 0/1 - 2/3 - 5/6 - 9/10 or more

Rate You Level of Agreement with the Following Sentences

	Strongly disagree	disagree	neutral	agree	strongly agree
I have good knowledge on how to manage a resuscitation requiring airway management	1	2	3	4	5
I feel comfortable running a resuscitation requiring airway management	1	2	3	4	5
I have good knowledge on how to manage a resuscitation requiring fluid resuscitation	1	2	3	4	5
I feel comfortable running a resuscitation of shock requiring fluid resuscitation	1	2	3	4	5
I am comfortable performing bag-mask ventilation	1	2	3	4	5
I am comfortable performing endotracheal intubation	1	2	3	4	5
I feel comfortable managing a pediatric resuscitation	1	2	3	4	5

13

The Incidence of Respiratory Distress Syndrome among Preterm Infants Admitted to Neonatal Intensive Care Unit: A Retrospective Study

Maryam Saboute[1], Mandana Kashaki[1], Arash Bordbar[1], Nasrin Khalessi[2*], Zahra Farahani[3]

[1]Department of Pediatrics, Akbarabadi Hospital, Iran University of Medical Sciences, Tehran, Iran
[2]Department of Pediatrics, Ali Asghar Hospital, Iran University of Medical Sciences, Tehran, Iran
[3]Maternal Fetal and Neonatal Research Center, Tehran University of Medical Sciences, Tehran, Iran
Email: *nasrinkhalessi@yahoo.com

Abstract

Background: Respiratory distress syndrome (RDS) or hyaline membrane disease (HMD) is the most common cause of neonatal morbidity and mortality in preterm infants. We aimed to determine the frequency of RDS among 3 groups of preterm infants and the value of some related factors. Methods: A cross-sectional, descriptive analytical investigation was carried out in the NICU ward of Akbarabadi Hospital (Tehran-Iran) during spring 2011. Newborns' data were collected and assessed by using their hospital medical records. Seventy-three preterm infants with gestational age < 34 weeks were hospitalized in the NICU. All participants were divided into 3 groups: extremely preterm (<28 weeks), very preterm (28 to <32 weeks) and moderate preterm (32 to 34 weeks). Frequency of RDS and some related factors were compared among 3 groups. Results: RDS was observed in 65.6% of all participants; however frequency of RDS was not different between three groups. An inversely correlation was found between gestational age and mortality rate (p = 0.05). In regard to Betamethasone administration prior to birth, this interval was significantly longer in alive neonates in comparison to infants who died (p < 0.05). Conclusion: RDS was frequent in preterm neonates with gestational age < 32 weeks. Time of Betamethasone administration prior to birth can significantly influence on neonatal mortality rate.

Keywords

Respiratory Distress Syndrome, Neonatal Intensive Care Unit, Preterm Infant, Mortality Rate

*Corresponding author.

1. Introduction

Respiratory distress syndrome (RDS) or hyaline membrane disease (HMD) is a main cause of morbidity and mortality in the early neonatal period. Related to the degree of prematurity, it occurs in 7% - 50% of neonates. It is also responsible for 30% - 40% of newborns' hospital admission. The significant cause of RDS is deficiency of alveolar surfactants due to immaturity of Type II pneumocyte, resulting low compliance of lungs, alveolar surface tension, decreased gas exchange and a demand for high ventilatory pressures. The clinical manifestation of RDS includes apnea, cyanosis, grunting, inspiratory stridor, nasal flaring, poor feeding, tachypnea, retractions in the intercostals, subcostal, or suprasternal spaces. These signs and symptoms are present at birth or shortly afterwards with getting worse over the first 48 - 72 hours of infant's life [1]-[5].

Before 1960 oxygen therapy was the only treatment for infants born with RDS. Continuous positive airway pressure (CPAP) was designed in the early 1970's and antenatal corticosteroids were introduced in 1972. After 1990 Surfactant treatment, new ventilators and developed ventilation techniques were the last treatments which dramatically improved the outcomes of infants with RDS [6].

Preterm labor is the most common problem (7% to 10% of deliveries) lead to the neonatal death in the second half of pregnancy and RDS is the most common cause of neonatal morbidity and mortality in preterm infants [7] [8]. Many studies confirmed an inverse relationship between RDS and gestational age [9] [10]. In contrary much progress in perinatal care, respiratory disrtress syndrome still remains a major neonatal problem [11]. In the present study we aimed to determine the incidence of RDS between 3 groups of preterm infants (extremely, very and moderate) then we assessed the value of some related factors.

2. Method and Material

A cross sectional, descriptive analytical investigation was performed at the NICU ward of Akbarabadi Hospital; a tertiary referral center and also one of the teaching hospitals affiliated to Iran University of Medical Sciences (Tehran-Iran) during spring 2011.

Infants with gestational age ≤ 34 weeks who admitted to the NICU for at least a day due to RDS from April 1, 2011 to June 31, 2011 entered the study. Exclusion criteria were missing data, congenital malformation and RDS accompanied by other complications. The charts of all infants were studied by using their hospital medical records and newborns' data were collected. The basic information including sex, weight, height, head and chest circumference, history of RDS, treatment (mechanical ventilation), prevention (betamethasone administration prior birth), complications (mortality) and some para clinical data (cranial ultrasound finding) were gathered and recorded in some check lists. RDS diagnosis had been established based on clinical symptoms and chest X-ray findings. To determine the association between RDS and mother's preeclampsia, simultaneously we assessed maternal obstetric medical records. All preterm subjects were divided into 3 groups based on WHO identification [12]; extremely preterm (<28 weeks), very preterm (28 to <32 weeks) and moderate preterm (32 to 34 weeks). Finally we compared frequency of RDS among 3 groups and evaluated correlations between some related factors, as well. The software package SPSS version 19 was used to perform the statistical analysis. The Student's T test, Chi Square and Mann-Whitney analysis were applied where applicable. With the proposed sample size of 78, the study had a power of 80%. The level of significant was considered $p < 0.05$.

Patients' data were considered secret and as no intervention was carried out in our study, we did not ask for patients consent. Ethics approval for the study was obtained from the institutional review board of Iran University of Medical Sciences.

3. Result

Of 78 NICU admitted preterm neonates (≤34 weeks), 5 newborns were excluded due to missing data, severe cardiac congenital anomalies, RDS accompanied by sepsis and meconium aspiration syndrome. The target population consisted of 73 preterm neonates of three groups (extremely preterm, very preterm and moderate preterm). Mothers of 7 neonates (9.58%) had preeclampsia. Cranial ultrasound had been performed for 24 cases. All demographic data are shown in **Table 1**.

A positive relationship was seen between anthropometric measurements and gestational age. Of all participants, 42 cases (65.6%) with mean birth weight 1464.7619 ± 478.05622 gram suffered from RDS. Although no significant correlations were seen among 3 groups' gestational age and RDS ($p = 0.207$), this syndrome was

Table 1. Demographic characteristics of all participants.

Variables	n (%)
Type of delivery	
C/S	40 (54.5)
NVD	33 (45.5)
Sex	
Male	45 (61.9)
Female	28 (38.1)
Weight	
<1000	12 (16.4)
1000 - 1500	38 (52.5)
>1500	22 (30.1)
G/age	
<28 week	13 (17.8)
28 - 32 week	38 (52.1)
32 - 34 week	22 (30.1)
Mechanical ventilation	
No	48 (56.9)
Yes	25 (43.1)
Mother's preeclamsia	7 (9.58)
Cranial ultrasound	
Normal	24
Abnormal	2

Table 2. Comparison of factors between 3 groups.

Age	Weight Mean ± SD gr	HC Mean ± SD Cm	CC Mean ± SD Cm	Length Mean ± SD Cm	RDS n (%)	Mortality n (%)	Duration of hospitalization Mean ± SD (days)
<28 week	1020 ± 238.88	25.77 ± 1.69	22.27 ± 2.41	36.54 ± 2.54	$\frac{8}{13}$ (61)	$\frac{10}{13}$ (76)	27 ± 20.99
28 - 32 week	1421.57 ± 257.5	28.10 ± 10.71	24.75 ± 2.25	40.49 ± 3.65	$\frac{24}{38}$ (63)	$\frac{13}{38}$ (34)	13.71 ± 11.86
32 - 34 week	2049.09 ± 326.25	30.97 ± 1.16	27.9 ± 1.70	46.52 ± 2.66	$\frac{10}{22}$ (45)	$\frac{3}{22}$ (13)	13.33 ± 8.30
P value	0.00*	0.00*	0.00*	0.00*	0.207	0.05*	0.122

HC: head circumference, CC: Chest circumference.

more frequent in two groups with gestational age < 32 weeks than neonates with gestational age 32 - 34 weeks (61% - 63% vs. 45%). An inversely significant correlation was observed between gestational age and mortality rate ($p = 0.05$, $r = 0.01$); 76.9% of extremely preterm neonates died in neonatal period. No relationship was found between RDS and sex or birth weight of neonates ($p = 0.317$, 0.065). Neonatal mortality did not differ among 2 genders (male; 56.5%, female 43.5%, p value = 0.137), as well. Although extremely preterm neonates had longer hospitalization period in compare to those in other groups, this difference was not significant (p value = 0.122) (**Table 2**). In regard to single dose Betamethasone administration in admission time prior to child birth, there was no statistically significant difference between healthy neonates and cases with RDS (17.56 ± 30.57 vs. 22.44 ± 41.17 hours; p value = 0.676). On the other hand interval between corticosteroids administration and birth was significantly longer in alive neonates in compare to infants who died (27.92 ± 46.42, 9.35 ± 11.98 hours, $p = 0.048$). No correlation was also found between time of Betametasone administration and need for mechanical ventilation (p value = 0.286). The correlation between preeclampsia and RDS was not statistically significant ($p = 0.38$). Mann-Whitney Test also showed no association between abnormal brain finding via ultrasound examination and gestational age (p value = 0.067).

4. Discussion

As the majority of RDS cases occur in preterm infants, obstetric and neonatal strategies are needed to prevent premature delivery and its related morbidity and mortality [1]. In the present study we have reviewed the incidence of respiratory distress in preterm infants. Based on our results 65.6% of population study had history of RDS which is higher than that were reported by previous studies. Zhang pointed to 50% as the incidence of RDS in preterm infants born before 30 weeks of gestation [4]. Khattab also reported Respiratory distress syndrome in 30% - 40% as the cause of admission in the neonatal period [3]. RDS was also shown in 23% of neonates admitted to the NICU with gestational age > 28 wks by Arit *et al.* [13]. Caner *et al.* indicated the incidence of RDS in 40.6% of 613 premature infants who admitted to the neonatal intensive care unit [14]. The reasons for these differences in the epidemiology may relate to differences in the categorized gestational age of participant.

No significant correlations were observed between 3 groups' gestational age and frequency of RDS that may due to our small sample size. RDS was more frequent in neonates with gestational age < 28 and 28 - 32 weeks by 61% - 3% and in newborns 32 - 34 weeks by 45%. This finding showed that all preterm infants with gestational age ≤ 34 weeks are at approximately equal risk for RDS.

Results showed an inversely correlation between gestational age and mortality rate. In compatible to our results Arit demonstrated much of the mortality rate in neonates with low gestational age and low birth weight [13]. Fidanovski also detected higher risk of mortality in infants with lower birth weight and shorter gestational age in 126 premature infants hospitalized at Pediatric Intensive Care Unit [15].

According to the findings a longer term interval between corticosteroids administration and birth (27.92 ± 46.42 hours) significantly reduced mortality rate ($p < 0.05$). In consistent to our results, Morris *et al.* showed that antenatal corticosteroids prior to premature delivery have had a crucial impact on neonatal mortality. They reported the greatest benefit in neonates born between 1 and 7 days after receiving corticosteroids [1].

Several studies assessed the incidence of RDS in preterm infants but our study suggests that respiratory distress from any cause may occur in more than half of preterm infants with gestational age ≤ 34 weeks. More over this report provides evidences that RDS may relate other important factors like neonate's weight, apgar score, mode of delivery. However we suggest this topic should be considered in future studies. On the other hand this study had some limitations. The number of our sample size was too small. We did not consider some other factors like apgar score, surfactant replacement therapy, number of antenatal corticosteroids doses administered prior to birth. Several relevant clinical data were not available in the neonates' hospital records that certainly affected on our results.

5. Conclusion

RDS was frequent in preterm neonates with gestational age < 32 weeks. Time of Betamethasone administration prior to birth can significantly influence on neonatal mortality rate. Focus on predicting RDS and risk factors have the potential effects on RDS incidence.

Conflict of Interest

The authors declare that there is no conflict of interests.

References

[1] Morris, I. and Adappa, R. (2012) Minimizing the Risk of Respiratory Distress Syndrome. *Paediatrics and Child Health*, **22**, 513-517. http://dx.doi.org/10.1016/j.paed.2012.08.012

[2] Edwards, M.O., Sarah, J. and Kotecha, S.K. (2013) Respiratory Distress of the Term Newborn Infant. *Paediatric Respiratory Reviews*, **14**, 29-37. http://dx.doi.org/10.1016/j.prrv.2012.02.002

[3] Khattab, A. (2015) Tei index in Neonatal Respiratory Distress and Perinatal Asphyxia. *The Egyptian Heart Journal*, **67**, 243-248. http://dx.doi.org/10.1016/j.ehj.2013.12.084

[4] Zhang, L., Cao, H., Zhao, S., Yuan, L., Han, D., Jiang, H. and EI, A.L. (2015) Effect of Exogenous Pulmonary Surfactants on Mortality Rate in Neonatal Respiratory Distress Syndrome: A Network Meta-Analysis of Randomized Con-

trolled Trials. *Pulmonary Pharmacology & Therapeutics*. In Press, Accepted Manuscript, Available Online 18 August 2015.

[5] Varvarigou, A.A., Thomas, I., Rodi, M., Economou, L., Mantagos, S. and Mouzaki, A. (2015) Respiratory Distress Syndrome (RDS) in Premature Infants Is Underscored by the Magnitude of Th1 Cytokine Polarization. *Cytokine*, **58**, 355-360. http://dx.doi.org/10.1016/j.cyto.2012.03.005

[6] Jobe, A.H. (2012) What Is RDS in 2012? *Early Human Development*, **88S2**, 42-44.

[7] Stevens, T.P., Blennow, M. and Soll, R.F. (2004) Early Surfactant Administration with Brief Ventilation vs Selective Surfactant and Continued Mechanical Ventilation for Preterm Infants with or at Risk for RDS. *Cochrane Database of Systematic Reviews*, **3**, Article ID: CD003063.

[8] Atarod, Z., Taghipour, M., Roohanizadeh, H., Fadavi, S. and Taghavipour, M. (2014) Effects of Single Course and Multicourse Betamethasone Prior to Birth in the Prognosis of the Preterm Neonates: A Randomized, Double-Blind Placebo-Control Clinical Trial Study. *Journal of Research in Medical Sciences*, **19**, 715-719.

[9] Niknafs, P., Faghani, A., Afjeh, A., Moradinazer, M. and Bahman-Bijari, B. (2014) Management of Neonatal Respiratory Distress Syndrome Employing ACoRN Respiratory Sequence Protocol versus Early Nasal Continuous Positive Airway Pressure Protocol. *Iranian Journal of Pediatrics*, **24**, 57-63.

[10] Jing, L., Hai Ying, C., Hua-Wei, W. and Xiang, Y.K. (2015) The Role of Lung Ultrasound in Diagnosis of Respiratory Distress Syndrome in Newborn Infants. *Iranian Journal of Pediatrics*, **25**, e323.

[11] Gortner, L. and Tutdibi, E. (2011) Respiratory Disorders in Preterm and term Neonates: An Update on Diagnostics and Therapy. *Zeitschrift für Geburtshilfe und Neonatologie*, **15**, 145-151. http://dx.doi.org/10.1055/s-0031-1285835

[12] Torchin, H., Ancel, P.Y., Jarreau, P.H. and Goffinet, F. (2015) Epidemiology of Preterm Birth: Prevalence, Recent Trends, Short- and Long-Term Outcomes. *Journal de Gynécologie Obstétrique et Biologie de la Reproduction* (*Paris*), **44**, 723-731. http://dx.doi.org/10.1016/j.jgyn.2015.06.010

[13] Arit, P., Nighat, H., Zubair, A.K. and Abdul Sattar, Sh. (2015) Frequency, Causes and Outcome of Neonates with Respiratory Distress Admitted to Neonatal Intensive Care Unit, National Institute of Child Health, Karachi. *Journal Pakistan Medical Association*, **65**, 771-775.

[14] Caner, I., Tekgunduz, K.S., Temuroglu, A., Demirelli, Y. and Kara, M. (2015) Evaluation of Premature Infants Hospitalized in Neonatal Intensive Care Unit between 2010-2012. *The Eurasian Journal of Medicine*, **47**, 13-20. http://dx.doi.org/10.5152/eajm.2014.38

[15] Fidanovski, D., Milev, V., Sajkovski, A., Hristovski, A., Sofijanova, A., Kojić, L. and Kimovska, M. (2005) Mortality risk Factors in Premature Infants with Respiratory Distress Syndrome Treated by Mechanical Ventilation. *Srpski Arhiv za Celokupno Lekarstvo*, **133**, 29-35. http://dx.doi.org/10.2298/SARH0502029F

14

One Day Polyethylene Glycol-3350 for Bowel Preparation in Pediatrics: A Literature Review

Shristi Shakya[1], Sumisti Shakya[2], Zhongyue Li[1*]

[1]Department of Gastroenterology, Children's Hospital of Chongqing Medical University, Chongqing, China
[2]Department of Obstetrics and Gynaecology, The Second Affiliated Hospital of Chongqing Medical University, Chongqing, China
Email: shristi_shakya@hotmail.com, sumisti@hotmail.com, *lizhongyue1001@hotmail.com

Abstract

Bowel preparation for colonoscopy in children is a challenging procedure. Wide variety of preparation protocols exist, varying with the hospital. Unlike in adults, there is a lack of uniform bowel preparation protocol in children. Ideally, the bowel preparation agents are assessed by their safety, efficacy and tolerability. Unfortunately, none of the preparations currently available meets all of these criteria. However, since last decade, Polyethylene Glycol-3350 (PEG-3350) is gaining popularity for bowel preparation with reported safety, efficacy, and tolerability. The only major drawback of PEG-3350 without electrolyte was 4 days long preparation time thus raising the question if the duration of preparation time could be minimized and yet have same efficacy, safety, and tolerability of the medicine. Hence, one day PEG-3350 regimen was introduced eventually and is now being studied with increased dosage or combined with other laxatives. This is the first review which compiles the study so far conducted on one day PEG-3350 without electrolyte as colonoscopy bowel preparation in children and tries to summaries if this regimen can be commonly used in children for colonoscopy bowel preparation.

Keywords

Bowel Preparation, One Day Preparation, Pediatrics, PEG-3350

1. Introduction

Bowel preparation for colonoscopy in children is a challenging procedure. Over the years, a wide variety of bo-

*Corresponding author.

wel preparation regimens have been used in children [1]-[4]. Medication that has been used is high dose Polyethylene glycol (PEG) with electrolyte, which in published studies has shown high efficacy [5], but had poor palatability due to its distinctive unpleasant taste along with poor tolerability by children because of large volume that must be complete within a short period of time which frequently required nasogastric tube [2] [3] [6] [7]. Magnesium citrate, or combinations with stimulants had poor palatability and needed dietary restrictions [2] [8]. Oral sodium phosphate in children is limited because of serious adverse effects such as hyperphosphatemia, hypocalcemia [8]-[11], acute kidney injury [12] and can result in colonic mucosal changes that mimic inflammatory bowel disease [13]. Enemas alone or in combination with stimulants that required anal insertion [10]. Bisacodyl or senna alone required clear liquid diet for 2 - 3 days with multiple enemas before colonoscopies examination with still had high poor preparation rate requiring repeated examination [2].

Ideally bowel preparation agents are judged by their safety, efficacy and tolerability [14]-[16]. No bowel preparation regimen meets the ideal criteria for bowel cleansing [2]. Beside these three ideal criteria, the other aspects of bowel preparation in pediatrics are ease of administration, palatability, dietary restriction, and daily routine disruption minimization [1].

Since last decade, Polyethylene glycol-3350 (PEG-3350), an osmotic laxative is commonly used as bowel preparation and has recently gained popularity [6] [14] [15] [17] [18]. PEG-3350 as a bowel preparation in children was first reported by Pashanker *et al.* [14] with administration dose of 1.5 g/kg/day for 4 days. It has shown to be effective and safe. Because of its tasteless character, it can be mixed with various types of drinks according to patient's choice. PEG 3350 is reported palatable and hence the compliance is excellent [14]. The only major drawback of this regimen is long preparation procedure time which led the parents to miss working days and absent school days for children. Hence raising the question if the duration of time could be minimised and still have same efficacy, safety, and tolerability of the medicine. Hence, one day PEG-3350 regimen was introduced and is studied with increased dose [17] [19]-[21] or combined with other laxatives [22]. The number of published studies investigating efficacy, safety and tolerability of one day PEG-3350 is relatively less. These studies were all single centered and varied widely in their design and only a few were prospective and randomized (**Table 1**) [17] [19]-[22]. This is the first review which tries to compile the studies so far on one day PEG-3350 without electrolyte as colonoscopy bowel preparation in children and attempts to summaries if this regimen can be commonly used in children for colonoscopy bowel preparation.

2. Efficacy

Efficacy of the bowel preparation is the clinical priority in high quality bowel preparation. The studies uses different outcome measures to define the success of the preparation 1. The intubation success rate to cecal and terminal ileum 2. Non-standard bowel preparation rating Scale "excellent", "good", "fair", or "poor" 3. Boston Bowel Preparation Scale (BBPS). So far, one day PEG-3350 without electrolyte studies reported adequate and effective bowel preparation range from 77% - 100% [17] [19] [21], cecum intubated range from 97% - 100% [17] [19] and terminal ileum reached range from 84% - 100% [19] [20]. Grading system graded by endoscopist in a prospective study showed excellent and good bowel preparation in 75% [20]. Sorser *et al.* [21] in their prospective RCT comparing one day vs three days administering PEG-3350 without electrolyte showed no significant difference among the two groups with excellent and good 100% in one day vs 93% in three days. 77% of patients in a prospective study showed BBPS score of at least 5 [19]. When BBPS was compared between one day vs two days administration of PEG-3350 without electrolyte, there was no significant difference between excellent and good BBPS score of 70% in one day and 72% in two days [22].

3. Safety

All colonoscopy preparation are associated with adverse effects. Clinical adverse effects include nausea, vomiting, abdominal pain/cramping, bloating, fatigue, weakness, headache, and dizziness. In all the studies there are mild to moderate degree of above symptoms but none of these reported to have clinically significant need of intervention [13]-[19]. Interestingly, when the studies compared one day with two days [22] and one day with three days [21] administration PEG-3350 without electrolyte; nausea, vomiting, abdominal pain were comparatively same between both groups with no statistically significant difference between these groups.

Metabolic disturbance includes electrolytes imbalance and change in osmolarity. PEG-3350 preparation without electrolyte was commonly used with sports drinks. The mixture of these two when compared with PEG

Table 1. One day PEG-3350 pediatrics colonoscopy preparation studies.

Author, years	Study design	No. of subject	Age of patients (years)	No. of patients completed dose	Efficacy	Safety	Tolerability/ acceptability	Need of enema	Diet
Adamiak *et al.*, 2010 [17]	Retrospective, 1 arm: PEG-3350, 238 or 255 g in 1.9 L of sport drink within 2 hours	272	13.7[a], (1.08 - 17.92)[b]	NA	Cecum reached 97.4%, procedure cancelled 1.1%	NA	NA	19/253	Regular meal for breakfast and lunch the day before the colonoscopy and clear liquids up to 3 hrs prior to their schedule
Abbas *et al.*, 2013 [19]	Prospective, open label trial: PEG-3350, 238 g with 1.5 L Gatorade in a few hours	46	14.50 ± 2.9[c] (8 - 18)[b]	43/46	Cecum reached 100%, terminal ileum 84%; BBPS 6.16[d] and BPPS score of least 5 in 33 (77%)	Nausea/ vomiting 60%, abdominal pain/ cramping 44%, fatigue/ weakness 40%, call on call provider 11%; K^+, BUN, CO_2 statistically decreased[#]	Likert scale acceptable (3) 64%, palatable (≥3) 73%, volume (≤2) 62%, unacceptable (≤2) 31%	2/46	Clear liquid after 1200 hrs the day before
Walia *et al.*, 2013 [20]	Prospective, 1 arm: PEG-3350 without electrolyte, <45 kg 136 g mixed in 32 ounces of Gatorade >45 kg 255 g mixed in 64 ounces of Gatorade	45	14 ± 3[c], (7 - 20)[b]	40/45	Terminal ileum 100%; *excellent 23%, good 52%, fair 23%, poor 21%	Nausea 34%, abdominal pain 23%, vomiting 16%, abdominal distension 20%, bloating 23%, dizziness 7%; serum glu-cose and CO_2 significantly decrease[#]	*Tolerability 39% or easy 61%, palatable good 14%, Ok 75%, bad 9%, yucky 2%	NA	Clear liquid the day before and NPO 3 hrs prior procedure
Najafi *et al.*, 2014 [22]	Randomised control trial, 2 arm: PEG, 2 g/kg (17 g in 240 ml of water or another beverage with 5 mg bisacodyl BD × 1 day PEG-3350, 1.5 g/kg with fruit juice for 2 days with 5 mg bisacodyl BD × 2 days	100	6.9 ± 31[c] vs 8 ± 3[c] (2 - 14)[b]	46/50 vs 47/50	Boston score excellent 7 vs 7, good 28 vs 29, fair 11 vs 11, poor 4 vs 3	^Nausea 1 vs 3, bloating 1 vs 1, abdominal pain 2 vs 4, headache 1 vs 2	*Full easy and tasty 20 vs 28, easy and tasty 26 vs 20, some tasteless and hard 3 vs 2, tasteless and hard 1 vs 0 ^no significantly difference	^6/50 vs 9/50	Fruit juice were allowed

Continued

Sorser *et al.*, 2014 [21]	Randomised control trial, 2 arm: PEG-3350, 4.5 g/kg/day max. 255 g × 1 day PEG-3350, 1.5 g/kg/day max. per day 85 g, max. total 255 g × 3 days	32	13.6[d] vs 11.6[d] (2 - 21)[b]	13/18 vs 13/14	*Excellent 89% vs 85%, good 11% vs 15%	^Nausea 44% vs 22%, vomiting 6% vs 14%, abdominal pain 22% vs 21%	Tolerability 89% vs 100%	NA	Clear liquids day before procedure with sips of water up to 3 hrs then NPO

BBPS: Boston Bowel Preparation Scale, BUN: Blood urea nitrogen, max.: maximum, NPO: nil per oral, PEG: Polyethylene glycol. [a]median, [b]range, [c]mean ± SD, [d]mean. *Non standard evaluation. #p < 0.05. ^p > 0.05. BPPS uses 10 point efficacy scale rating 0 - 3 in 3 section colon (right side, transverse side and left side) where 0 = "unprepared colon due to solid stool", 1 = "portion of mucosa not seen", 2 = "minor amount of residual staining", and 3 = "entire mucosa seen well with no staining". The sum of all 3 sections was added a total score from 0 to 9. Likert scale from 1 to 5 with 1 = "hated it", 2 = "didn't like it", 3 = "Ok", 4 = "good" and 5 = "excellent".

with electrolyte (PEG-ELS) contained about 9 times less sodium, 4 times less potassium and 6 times less chloride [1]. Low sodium can lead to net absorption of free water resulting in hyponatremia [23], specially in patients with impaired kidney function. The carbohydrate in sports drinks may lead to bacterial fermentation and hence production of combustable gases [24]. However, till date there is no reported major adverse event of Gatorade mixed with PEG-3350 in the pediatrics literature [1] [25]. In a prospective studies, the post bowel preparation serum potassium, blood urea nitrogen (BUN), carbon dioxide were significantly low when compared to pre bowel preparation but these were reported clinically insignificant [19]. On the other hand, in other prospective study, electrolytes (sodium, potassium, chloride), BUN, creatinine has no significant pre and post procedure changes but had statistically significantly decrease in serum glucose and carbon dioxide [20]. Small changes in serum osmolarity was found in both one day and three days PEG-3350 without electrolyte administration but it was not clinically and statistically significant difference between both groups [21].

4. Ease of Use

PEG-3350 without electrolyte is palatable due to its tasteless character and can be mixed with any drink of patient choice. However, in order to decrease the duration of administration time, the volume of medicine has to be increased. Hence, one day PEG-3350 regimen has to be administered in large volume in limited period of time and therefore had unacceptable volume rating [19]. Despite this, when the children were asked if they would take this regimen again, all patients of a prospective study stated that they would like to take same bowel preparation again in future [20]. Among those patients, 9 patients had undergone colonoscopy bowel preparation in the past with alternate bowel preparation regimen. Unlike PEG-ELS, in PEG-3350 without electrolytes there is no such report of use of nasogastric tube for administration of the assigned amount.

5. Quality of Evidence

The major advantage of this regimen is its short duration over a few hours hence reducing preparation time, decreasing the working hours of parents and missed school days for children with same efficacy and safety as that of three-days and two-days PEG-3350 regimen. However, studies from which these conclusions are drawn are a small number of trials, which all have certain study bias. The data are collected from small sample size, tertiary centre, and the grading system they used to grade the efficacy of the bowel preparation is non-standardised. The study conducted by Adamiak *et al.* [17] is a retrospective study without proper controls, which cannot be compared to other preparation due to lack of investigation which was not done at the beginning (serum electrolytes). The author also mentions lack of standard dose of PEG-3350. Although the parents were advice to mixed specific dose of PEG-3350, it was not clear the exact amount of PEG-3350 consume by patients. Furthermore, it lacks standard scale to assess the bowel preparation quality. In other hand, even though Abbas *et al.* [19] used BBPS in their prospective study and Najafi *et al.* [22] in their RCT study to assess the bowel preparation quality, this scoring system has not been validated or previously used in children. In both prospective studies [17] [19] and RCT conducted by Sorser *et al.* [21] have mentioned there may be performance bias due to lack of blinding to the endoscopist during procedure. None of the study has reported the method of recruiting the patient hence having a selection bias as well.

6. Conclusions

One day PEG-3350 without electrolyte has been shown to be safe, effective with acceptable adverse effects but with low acceptance rate due to large volume that needs to be ingested in limited time.

So far the cumulative mean age of one day PEG-3350 is 12.5 years. Hence, there is less use of these regimen in younger children. Therefore, we cannot conclude if this regimen can be safely used among younger children.

The commercially available drinks that have been used to mix with PEG-3350, the components of electrolytes are not stated. Therefore, the true level of electrolyte in the mixture to be ingested is unknown and we suggest this should be noted in future studies.

Due to small number of studies conducted in this field we cannot precisely conclude that one day PEG-3350 can be routinely use on daily basis for colonoscopy bowel preparation in children. However, in emergency cases with limited time frame, who urgently needed colonoscopy and the patients who are unwilling to complete a longer duration preparation dose, this regimen could be considered. Physician should be vigilant and should consider adjusting the dose and duration of drug according to each child's condition. Further large, prospective, multi centre, high quality randomised control trial is needed.

References

[1] Hunter, A. and Mamula, P. (2010) Bowel Preparation for Pediatric Colonoscopy Procedures. *Journal of Pediatrics Gastrointestinal and Nutrition*, **51**, 254-261. http://dx.doi.org/10.1097/MPG.0b013e3181eb6a1c

[2] Dahshan, A., Lin, C., Peters, J., Thomas, R. and Tolia, V. (1999) A Randomized, Prospective Study to Evaluated the Efficacy and Acceptance of Three Bowel Preparations for Colonoscopy in Children. *American Journal of Gastrointestinal*, **94**, 3497-3501. http://dx.doi.org/10.1111/j.1572-0241.1999.01613.x

[3] da Silva, M.M., Briars, G.L., Patrick, M.K., Cleghorn, G.J. and Shepherd, R.W. (1997) Colonoscopy Preparation in Children: Safety, Efficacy, and Tolerance of High- versus Low-Volume Cleansing Methods. *Journal of Gastroenterology and Nutrition*, **24**, 33-37. http://dx.doi.org/10.1097/00005176-199701000-00009

[4] Pinefield, A. and Stringer, M.D. (1999) Randomised Trail of Two Pharmacological Methods of Bowel Preparation for Day Case Colonoscopy. *Archives of Disease on Childhood*, **80**, 181-183. http://dx.doi.org/10.1136/adc.80.2.181

[5] Tuner, D., Benchimol, E.I., Dunn, H., Griffiths, A.M., Frost, K., Scaini, V., Avolio, J. and Ling, S.C. (2009) Picosalax versus Polyethylene Glycol for Bowel Clean out before Colonoscopy in Children: A Randomized Controlled Trail. *Endoscopy*, **41**, 1038-1045. http://dx.doi.org/10.1055/s-0029-1215333

[6] Safder, S., Demintieva, Y., Rewalt, M. and Elitsur, Y. (2008) Stool Consitency and Stool Frequency Are Excellent Clinical Markers for Adequate Colon Preparation after Polyethylene Glycol 3350 Cleansing Protocol: A Prospective Clinical Study in Children. *Gastrointestinal Endoscopy*, **68**, 1131-1135. http://dx.doi.org/10.1016/j.gie.2008.04.026

[7] Schanz, S., Kruis, W., Mickisch, O., Kuppers, B., Berg, P., Frick, B., Heiland, G., Schenck, B., Horstkotte, H. and Winkler, A. (2008) Bowel Preparation for Colonoscopy with Sodium Phosphate Solution versus Polyethylene Glycol-Based Lavage : A Multicenter Trail. *Diagnostic and Therapeutic Endoscopy*, **2008**, Article ID: 713521. http://dx.doi.org/10.1155/2008/713521

[8] El-Baba, M.F., Padilla, M., Houstan, C., MAdani, S., Lin, C.H., Thomas, R. and Yolia, V. (2006) A Prospective Study Comparing Oral Sodium Phosphate Solution Phosphate Solution to a Bowel Cleansing Preparation with Nutrition Food Package in Children. *Journal of Pediatric Gastroenterology and Nutrition*, **42**, 174-177. http://dx.doi.org/10.1097/01.mpg.0000189353.40419.31

[9] Gremse, D.A., Sacks, A.I. and Raines, S. (1996) Comparison of Oral Sodium Phosphate to Polyethylene Glycol-Based Solution for Bowel Preparation for Colonoscopy in Children. *Journal of Pediatric Gastroenterolgy and Nutrition*, **23**, 586-590. http://dx.doi.org/10.1097/00005176-199612000-00013

[10] Ehrenpreis, E.D. (2009) Increased Serum Phosphate Levels and Calcium Fluxes Are Seen in Smaller Individuals after a Single Dose of Sodium Phosphate Colon Cleansing Solution: A Pharmacokinetic Analysis. *Alimentary Pharmacology and Therapeutics*, **29**, 1201-1211. http://dx.doi.org/10.1111/j.1365-2036.2009.03987.x

[11] Shaoul, R., Wolff, R., Seligman, H., Tal, Y. and Jaffe, M. (2001) Symptoms of Hyperphosphatemia, Hypocalcemia, and Hypomagnesemia in an Adolescent Colonoscopy. *Gastrointestinal Endoscopy*, **53**, 650-652. http://dx.doi.org/10.1067/mge.2001.112712

[12] Hasall, E. and Lobe, T.E. (2007) Risky Business: Oral Sodium Phosphate for Preparation Colonoscopy Bowel Prepara-

tion in Children. *Journal of Pediatric Gastroenterology and Nutrition*, **45**, 268-269. http://dx.doi.org/10.1097/MPG.0b013e318064c85e

[13] Zwas, F.R., Cirillo, N.W., El-Serag, H.B. and Eisen, R.N. (1996) Colonic Mucosal Abnormalities Associated with Oral Soduim Phosphate Solution. *Gastrointestinal Endoscopy*, **43**, 463-466. http://dx.doi.org/10.1016/S0016-5107(96)70286-9

[14] Pashankar, D.S., Uc, A. and Bishop, W.P. (2004) Polyethylene Glycol 3350 without Electrolyte: A New Safe, Effective, and Palatable Bowel Preparation for Colonoscopy in Children. *The Journal of Pediatric*, **144**, 358-362. http://dx.doi.org/10.1016/j.jpeds.2003.11.033

[15] Phatak, U.P., Johnson, S., Husain, S.Z. and Pashankar, D.S. (2011) Two-Day Bowel Preparation with Polyethylene Glycol 3350 and Bisacodyl: A New, Safe, and Effective Regimen for Colonoscopy in Children. *Journal of Pediatric Gastrointestinal and Nutrition*, **51**, 71-74. http://dx.doi.org/10.1097/MPG.0b013e318210807a

[16] Kerkus, J., Horvath, A., Szychta, M., Woynarowski, M., Wegner, A., Wiernicka, A., Dadalski, M., Teisseyre, M. and Dziechciarz, P. (2013) High- versus Low-Volume Polyethylene Glycol plus Laxative versus Sennosides for Colonoscopy Preparation in Children. *Journal of Pediatrics Gastrointestinal and Nutrition*, **57**, 230-235. http://dx.doi.org/10.1097/MPG.0b013e3182950ef5

[17] Adamiak, T., Altaf, M. and Jensen, M.K. (2010) One-Day Bowel Preparation Glycol 3350: An Effective Regimen for Colonoscopy in Children. *Gastrointestinal Endoscopy*, **71**, 573-577. http://dx.doi.org/10.1016/j.gie.2009.10.042

[18] Jibaly, R., LaChance, J., Lecea, N., Ali, N. and Weber, J.E. (2011) The Utility of PEG3350 without Electrolytes for 2-Day Colonoscopy Preparation in Children. *European Journal of Pediatric Surgery*, **21**, 318-321. http://dx.doi.org/10.1055/s-0031-1280822

[19] Abbas, M.I., Nylund, C.M., Bruch, C.J., Nazareno, L.G. and Rogers, P.L. (2013) Prospective Evaluation of 1-Day Polyethylene Glycol-3350 Bowel Preparation Regimen in Children. *Journal of Pediatric Gastrointestinal and Nutrition*, **56**, 220-224. http://dx.doi.org/10.1097/MPG.0b013e31826630fc

[20] Walia, R., Steffen, R., Feinberg, L., Worley, S. and Mahajan, L. (2013) Tolerability, Safety, and Efficacy of PEG-3350 as a 1-Day Bowel Preparation in Children. *Journal of Pediatric Gastrointestinal and Nutrition*, **56**, 225-228. http://dx.doi.org/10.1097/MPG.0b013e3182758c69

[21] Sorser, S.A., Konanki, V., Hursh, A., Hagglund, K. and Lyons, H. (2014) 1-Day Bowel Preparation with Polyethylene Glycol 3350 Is as Effective and Safe as a 3-Day Preparation for Colonoscopy in Children. *BMC Research Notes*, **15**, 648. http://dx.doi.org/10.1186/1756-0500-7-648

[22] Najafi, M., Fallahi, G.H., Motamed, F., Farahmand, F., Khodadad, A., Ghajarzadeh, M., Rezaei, N. and Mehrabani, S. (2015) Comparision of One and Two-Day Bowel Preparation with Polyethylene Glycol in Pediatric Colonoscopy. *Turkish Journal of Gastroenterology*, **26**, 232-235. http://dx.doi.org/10.5152/tjg.2015.6837

[23] Nagler, J., Poppers, D. and Turetz, M. (2006) Severe Hyponatremia and Seizure Following a Polyethylene Glycol-Based Bowel Preparation for Colonoscopy. *Journal of Clinical Gastroenterology*, **40**, 558-559. http://dx.doi.org/10.1097/00004836-200607000-00017

[24] Werner, S.D. (1996) Preoperative Preparation Prior to Colorectal Surgery. *Gastrointestinal Endoscopy*, **43**, 530-531. http://dx.doi.org/10.1016/S0016-5107(96)70305-X

[25] Parakkal, D., Humberto, S., Muhammed, S. and Ehrenpreis, E.D. (2011) Preparing for Colonoscopy. In: Da Rocha, J.R., Ed., *Endoscopic Procedures in Colon and Rectum*, InTech, Winchester, 17-42. http://www.intechopen.com/books/endoscopic-procedures-in-colon-and-rectum/preparing-for-colonoscopy-2

15

Neurofibromatosis Type 1 Revealed by Ophthalmologic Complications: A Report of One Case in Ouagadougou, Burkina Faso

Caroline Yonaba*, **Aichatou Djibo, Chantal Zoungrana, Angèle Kalmogho, Ousseine Diallo, Patrice Tapsoba, Noufounikoun Méda, Ludovic Kam**

Centre Hospitalier Universitaire Yalgado Ouedraogo, Ouagadougou, Burkina Faso
Email: *caroyonaba@yahoo.fr

Abstract

Type 1 neurofibromatosis is an inherited multisystem neurocutaneous disease predisposing to tumors development. Serious skin and ophthalmologic complications, although rare, can occur throughout life. Furthermore in children, unawareness of early symptoms may delay diagnosis. We report the case of A.T. 8 years old, admitted for exophthalmosis and facial deformity dating back to the age of 2 years. The diagnosis of neurofibromatosis was suspected in the presence of light brown skin spots scattered all over the body and subcutaneous nodules. Ophthalmologic examination revealed bilateral exophthalmosis, eyelids neurofibromas, blepharoptosis, Lisch nodules, corneal edema, and optic atrophy. Head CT scan clarified the nature and the extent of ophthalmologic lesions. Treatment was symptomatic. Neurofibromatosis is rarely reported in children in our setting; it is probably under diagnosed. Clinicians should think of this diagnosis in presence of certain specific symptoms and make a clinical assessment.

Keywords

Neurofibromatosis, Eye, Complications, Children, Burkina Faso

1. Introduction

Neurofibromatosis (NF) includes two autosomal dominant diseases: neurofibromatosis type 1 (NF1) or Von Recklinghausen disease and neurofibromatosis type 2 [1] [2]. The NF1 is the most common, with an incidence of approximately one case per 3500 births [1] [3] [4] worldwide. It is a genetic autosomal dominant disease,

*Corresponding author.

whereas *de novo* mutations affect 50% of patients [3]. The mutation of the NF1 genes is located at the pericentromeric region of chromosome 17 [2] [3]. In our context, the rarity of the diagnosis is probably due to ignorance of NF1 clinical signs in children and the delay to seek care.

Clinical signs of NF1 are very diverse and increase in number and size as the individual grows older. The café au lait spots (CLS), visible at birth, are usually the first symptoms. As for eye complications, they can appear anywhere on the eye and at any age [5]. In most cases, symptoms of NF1 are mild, and children live normal live. In some cases, however, NF1 may cause cosmetic and psychological issues. Surgery is often recommended to remove the tumors.

We report a case of neurofibromatosis type 1 in an 8 year old girl revealed by eye complications in the pediatric department of the Yalgado Ouédraogo Teaching Hospital in Ouagadougou, Burkina Faso. Informed consent was obtained from the patient's family to report this case.

2. Observation

The eight years old girl was admitted at our department for eyelids blepharoptosis and facial deformity. The onset of symptoms goes back to the age of two years with gradual swelling of the cheeks and protrusion of the eyes. This has led to a series of consultations in their home region.

In October 2012, with the increasing eye protrusion and eyelids blepharoptosis, parents consulted for investigation.

The girl had a history of right upper eyelid tumor since birth. She was not known to have any other diseases other than the current abnormalities. She is second in a family of four siblings. Her growth (weight and height) and psychomotor development were normal. Clinical examination of the biological parents and siblings was unremarkable: no body spots, no deformity. The family had no history of similar diseases and there was no consanguinity between parents.

Examination of the head noted:

- Bilateral eyelid swelling consisting of tender numbs with blepharoptosis more pronounced on the right eye. (**Figure 1**)
- Bilateral exophthalmosis (**Figure 1**)
- Hypertrophy of the right hemi face and facial asymmetry
- Bilateral multinodular parotid swelling, compressing ear canals

Examination of the skin showed:

- Light brown spots (café au lait spots), numerous, scattered all over the body, diameter > 5 mm (**Figure 2**).
- Small hyperpigmented freckels (axillary freckles) about 2 to 3 mm in diameter.
- Tumors located on the back, some of them were only palpable, while others seemed to lift the skin above (subcutaneous neurofibromas) as shown on **Figure 3**
- A soft sessile tumor about 3 cm diameter with hypertrichosis (plexiform neurofibroma), located on the back,

Ophthalmologic examination gave details of the eye lesions:

- Bilateral plexiform neurofibromas of the upper eyelids
- Lisch nodules (**Figure 4**)

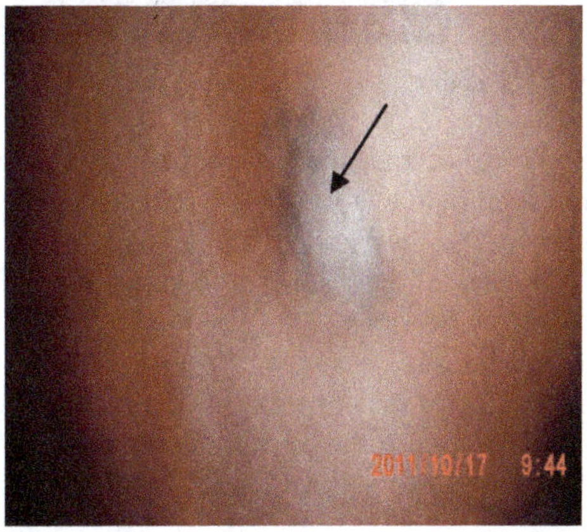

Figure 1. Neurofibroma with hypertrichosis on the back.

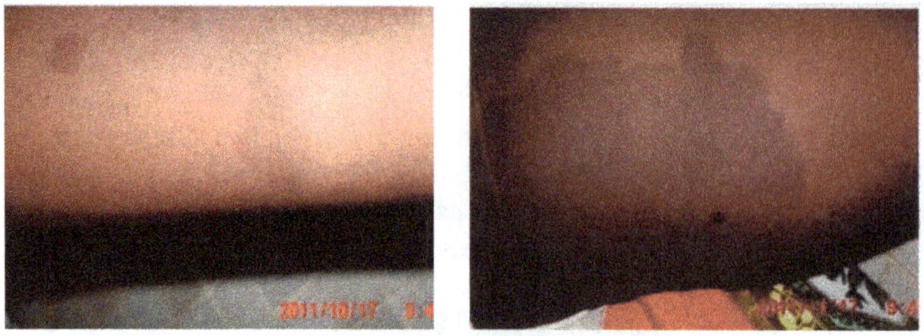

(a) (b)

Figure 2. Coffee milk colored spots (café au lait spots). (a) Left arm; (b) left thigh.

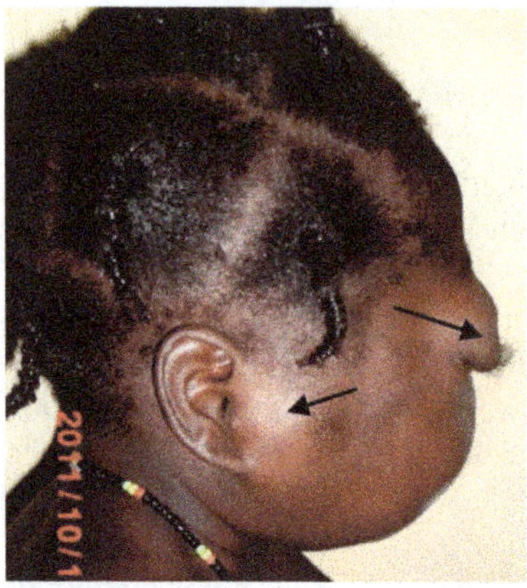

Figure 3. Parotid swelling + blepharoptosis + exophtalmosis of the right eye.

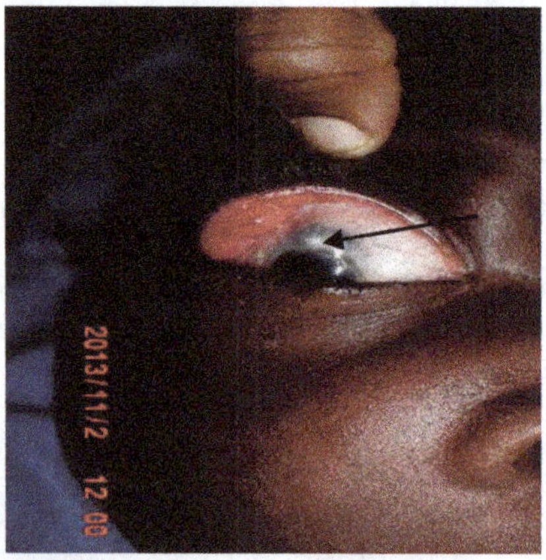

Figure 4. Lisch nodule.

- A thinning of the sclera, corneal edema, and optic atrophy of the right eye. The left eye was healthy.
- The intraocular pressure of the right eye was 41 cm and of the left eye 26 cm Hg (normal value: 10 - 20 cm Hg).The visual acuity was 4/10 on the right eye and 7/10 on the left eye.

Computed Tomography (CT scan) of the skull and brain specified the extent of the lesions (**Figure 5**):

- Left temporal parenchymal calcifications ,
- A bilateral grade III exophthalmosis,
- Thickening of the initial portions of the optic nerves and eye muscles

Histological examination of a biopsy of the parotid mass confirmed the diagnosis of NF1. It showed fusiform cell cytoplasm and sometimes undulating pyknotic nucleus with myxoid or "onion bulb" territories compatible with neurofibroma.

Molecular biology in search of genetic anomalies could not be performed.

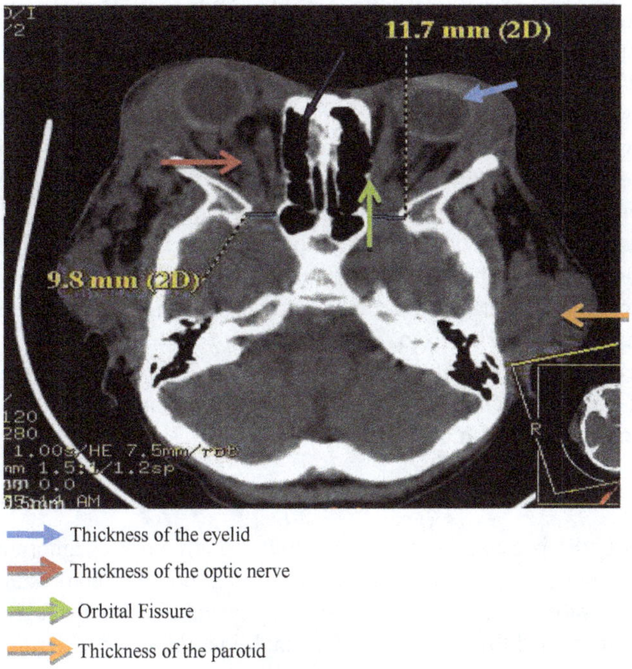

Figure 5. Computed tomography (C.T) scan of the skull and brain.

Treatment was symptomatic consisting of antibiotics, antiseptic and anti-inflammatory eye drops.

The course of the disease was marked by the gradual increase of blepharoptosis, of facial hypertrophy, and of the size of the plexiform neurofibroma on the back. One year later, the patient lost the sight of the right eye.

3. Discussion

Diagnosis of neurofibromatosis at a very late stage with severe orbital complications, in our patient, is due to unawareness of the first symptoms of the disease in children.

The café au lait spots are usually the first symptoms of NF. They are often congenital and rarely appear after the age of two [1]-[4]. Our patient had these spots since birth, they were certainly under diagnosed. The spots were scattered all over the body hence the difference with other common skin spots in infants. Literature does precise that they are ubiquity in neurofibromatosis [6].

Neurofibromas rarely appear in early childhood, except plexiform neurofibromas which are often congenital and still can be seen before the age of five years [3].The dermal or cutaneous neurofibromas appear only during puberty period and are almost always seen in adults [2] [5]. We did not notice any cutaneous neurofibromas in our case this is due to the young age of our patient who was only 8 years old.

Our patient had a lot of subcutaneous neurofibromas scattered on the right hemi face responsible for the hypertrophy. The plexiform neurofibromas, in their important form called "royal tumor" consist of skin and subcutaneous soft swellings with uneven consistency. The overlying skin is often thick and may be the site of hypertrichosis and a brown hyperpigmentation as in our patient. They predominate in the territory of the trigeminal nerve (eyelid and orbital) [2] [3].

There was an important ophthalmologic involvement in our patient. Ophthalmologic manifestations may occur at an early age or later and eyelid disorders are the most common in NF1 [5] [7]. Plexiform neuroma is the classic disorder of the eyelid which is generally unilateral and affects mostly the upper eyelid [5]. The plexiform neuroma in our patient affects both upper eyelids and is marked by a significant distorting blepharoptosis especially on the right eyelid. Blepharoptosis is a common opthalmologic manifestation of neurofibromatisis and is linked to an eyelid thickening due to the presence of the neurofibromas [7]-[9].

Dysplasia of the sphenoid is the most common cause of exophthalmosis in children with enlargement of the orbit [10] [11]. Cases of exophthalmosis during meningoencephalocele due to the destruction of the large wing of sphenoid had also been described [11] [12].

Lisch nodules are iris hamartomas which can sometimes be seen with the naked eye. They are pathognomonic of NF1 and are part of the diagnostic criteria [2] [3].

A decrease in visual acuity usually affects the eye on the affected side of the head, sometimes associated with other abnormalities such as deterioration of visual field, or glaucoma [7] [9] [13] [14]. In our patient the loss of visual acuity was associated with bilateral glaucoma and bilateral buphthalmosis.

Other ophthalmologic complications have also been described: thinning of the sclera, optic atrophy [15]. All these ophthalmic signs are probably linked to gliomas of symptomatic optic pathways [15].

Genetic tests performed on the patient and his parents could have showed if this was *de novo* mutation or inherited transmission [16] [17]. These tests are not available in our working environment.

Surgery is the main treatment and must take into account the unpredictability of the disease [8]. This treatment is not yet available in Burkina Faso.

In the end, the course of the disease is classically characterized by deterioration of symptoms during puberty or during an event such as pregnancy. Throughout life various tumors can occur [11]. It is still difficult to predict the prognosis of this long-term illness.

4. Conclusion

Clinical diagnosis of NF1 is usually easy. In our study, health workers ignorance of early clinical signs certainly explains the long delay of diagnosis and numerous ophthalmologic manifestations observed. The unforeseeable development of NF1 warrants early diagnosis and regular monitoring throughout life. Molecular diagnostic methods would have determined the etiology of this condition and so consider genetic counseling. This study highlights the need for inter-disciplinary collaboration; without doubt surgery could have improved the quality of life of our patient.

References

[1] Allanore, L. and Wolkenstein, P. (2009) Neurofibromatosis in Dermatology and Sexual Transmitted Diseases. 5ème édition, Masson, Paris, 485-488.

[2] Wolkenstein, P., Zeller, J. and Ismaïli, N. (2002) Neurofibromatosis. Encyclopédie Médico-Chirurgicale, Paris Editions Scientifiques et Médicales Elsevier SAS Dermatologie Pédiatrie, 4-092-C-10, 98-755-A-10, Elsevier SAS, Paris, 10.

[3] Pinson, S., Créange, A. and Barbarot, S. (2002) Recommandations for the Management of Type 1 Neurifibromatosis. *Journal Français d'Ophtalmologie*, **25**, 423-433.

[4] Wolkenstein, P. (2005) Neurofibromatosis and Bourneville's Tuberous Sclerosis. *Journal of Neuroradiology*, **32**, 174-179.

[5] Ferner, R. (2010) The Neurofibromatosis. *Practical Neurology*, **10**, 82-93. http://dx.doi.org/10.1136/jnnp.2010.206532

[6] Bonnemaison, E., Roze-Abert, B., Lorette, G., Sirinelli, D., Boscq, S., Mazjoub, M., *et al.* (2006) Type 1 Neurofibromatosis in Children: A Report of 100 Cases. *Archives de Pédiatrie*, **13**, 1009-1014. http://dx.doi.org/10.1016/j.arcped.2006.03.149

[7] Fany, A. and Gbe, K. (2002) Isolated Palpebral Tumor Revealing Von Recklinghausen's Neurofibromatosis: A Case Report. *Journal Français d'Ophtalmologie*, **8**, 822-825.

[8] Altan-Yayciogl, R. and Hintschich, C. (2010) Clinical Features and Surgical Management of Orbitotemporal Neurofibromatosis: A Retrospective Interventional Case Series. *Orbit*, **29**, 232-238. http://dx.doi.org/10.3109/01676831003660689

[9] Khairallah, M., Messaoud, R., Ladjimi, A., Hmisdi, K. and Chaouch, K. (1999) Association of Spheno-Orbital Dysplasia with Plexiform Neuroma in von Recklinghausen's Neurofibromatosis. *Journal Français d'Ophtalmologie*, **22**, 975-978.

[10] Farris, S.R. and Grove Jr., A.S. (1996) Orbital and Eyelid Manifestations of Neurofibromatosis: A Clinical Study and Literature Review. *Ophthalmic Plastic & Reconstructive Surgery*, **12**, 245-59. http://dx.doi.org/10.1097/00002341-199612000-00006

[11] Gotzamanis, A., Ducasse, A., Niederlender, P., *et al.* (2000) Unilateral Exophthalmos Is Revealing Agenesia of the Greater Wing of the Sphenoid. *Journal Français d O'phtalmologie*, **7**, 683-687.

[12] Abouchadi, A., Nassih, M., Rzin, A. and Elgbouri, H. (2005) Orbito-Temporal Plexiform Neurofibroma: 6 Cases. *Revue de Stomatologie et de Chirurgie Maxillo-faciale*, **106**, 272-275.

[13] Boulanger, J.M. and Larbrisseau, A. (2005) Neurofibromatosis Type 1 in Pediatric Population/Ste-Justine's Experience. *Canadian Journal of Neurological Sciences*, **32**, 225-231. http://dx.doi.org/10.1017/S0317167100004017

[14] Mejdoubi, M., Arne, J.L. and Sevely, A. (2007) Orbital Tumors in Children: CT and MR Imaging Features. *Journal de Radiologie*, **88**, 1855-1864. http://dx.doi.org/10.1016/S0221-0363(07)78363-4

[15] Chateil, J.F., Brun, M., Le Manh, C., Diard, F. and Labrèze, C. (2000) Phacomatosis in Children. Encyclopédie Médico-Chirurgicale, 4-092-B-10.54, Elsevier SAS, Paris.

[16] Bahuau, M., Vidaud, M. and Vidaud, D. (1997) Neurofibromatosis: Genetics and Molecular Physiopathology of NF1. *Médecine Thérapeutique*, **8**, 623-628.

[17] Huson, S.M., Compston, D.A., Clark, P. and Harper, P.S. (1989) A Genetic Study of von Recklinghausen Neurofibromatosis in South East Wales. I. Prevalence, Fitness, Mutation Rate, and Effect of Parental Transmission on Severity. *Journal of Medical Genetics*, **26**, 704-711. http://dx.doi.org/10.1136/jmg.26.11.704

16

Diarrhea and Hypokalemic Rhabdomyolysis Due to Apoptotic Colitis as the Initial Manifestation of Common-Variable Immunodeficiency in an Adolescent

David Green[1], Nina Dave[2], Hua Liu[3], Charu Subramony[4], Michael J. Nowicki[3]

[1]School of Medicine, University of Mississippi Medical Center, Jackson, USA
[2]Division of Pediatric Allergy-Immunology, University of Mississippi Medical Center, Jackson, USA
[3]Division of Pediatric Gastroenterology, University of Mississippi Medical Center, Jackson, USA
[4]Department of Pathology, University of Mississippi Medical Center, Jackson, USA
Email: mnowicki@umc.edu

Abstract

We present the case of an adolescent who presented with rhabdomyolysis due to severe hypokalemia arising from chronic diarrhea. Initial evaluation for celiac disease, known to present in this manner, was negative. Further evaluation with colonoscopy showed a normal appearing colon but biopsies showed a significant number of apoptotic cells in the mucosal crypts supporting a diagnosis of apoptotic colitis. Investigation into the cause of apoptotic colitis resulted in a diagnosis of common variable immune deficiency due to a defect in the inducible T-cell costimulator (ICOS) gene. Physicians should be aware of this uncommon condition and the importance of mucosal biopsy despite the presence of normal appearing mucosa.

Keywords

Apoptotic Colitis, Common-Variable Immune Deficiency, Hypokalemia, Rhabdomyolysis

1. Introduction

The patient described herein exemplifies the complex manner in which immunodeficiency states can present, pointing out the need for persistence and diligence in order to secure the correct diagnosis. Initial presentation of hypokalemia-induced rhabdomyolysis in an adolescent with chronic diarrhea, stunted growth, and weight loss prompted evaluation for an intestinal cause of the findings, in particular celiac disease. When the initial evaluation failed to secure a diagnosis, further investigation employing colonoscopy discovered the rare finding of apoptotic colitis. Causes of apoptotic colitis are few, providing a narrowed differential diagnosis from which the final diagnosis of CVID was made. Below is a detailed description of the evaluation of the patient, presented to point out the interplay of the various uncommon clinical features and laboratory findings seen in this case. Also, we offer a review of apoptotic colitis, a rare finding in children. Finally, a brief review of the diagnosis of CVID is presented.

2. Case Report

A 14-year-old white male presented to his local emergency department with fatigue, diffuse muscle pain, and severe weakness. The patient reported a life-long history of diarrhea, typically occurring twice per day, described as loose to watery in consistency, without blood or mucus. He denied abdominal pain, anal pain, nausea, vomiting, and nocturnal stooling. He reported a long history of poor growth, exacerbated by a recent ten pound weight loss. Past medical history was significant for repeated skin infections requiring oral antibiotics and incision and drainage; pneumonia twice; sinus infections (2 - 3/year); and recurrent otitis media as an infant requiring placement of pressure equalizer tubes. Family history was positive for peptic disease and negative for celiac disease, inflammatory bowel disease, and malabsorption disorders. Examination showed a weight of 38.7 kg (< 5th %ile), height of 156 cm (10th %ile), and body mass index of 15.9 kg/M^2 (<5th %ile). There was no scleral icterus. His heart and lung examinations were normal. His abdomen was soft, non-tender, without hepatosplenomegaly or masses. He had a diffuse psoriatic rash involving his scalp, trunk, and extremities. Mild digital clubbing was noted. Perianal examination showed no fissures, fistulae, or skin tags. Rectal examination showed normal position and tone with liquid, occult-blood negative stool in the vault. Laboratory evaluation was significant for severe hypokalemia (K^+ = 1.9 mmol/L, nl = 3.5 - 5.2) necessitating hospitalization for correction with intravenous fluids and potassium administration. Upon discharge from the hospital he was referred to gastroenterology for concerns of celiac disease due to poor nutrition, long-standing diarrhea, and hypokalemia.

The patient was seen in clinic where serum immunoglobulin (Ig) A and anti-tissue transglutaminase (TTG) IgA were obtained. The TTG-IgA was normal (<4 U/L), however, the serum IgA was low (17 mg/dl, normal = 70 - 400) making the results of the TGG-IgA unreliable. He returned for diagnostic esophagogastrodoudenoscopy (EGD) one week later, at which time he was again experiencing fatigue, weakness, and muscle pain. Laboratory evaluation showed hypolkalemia (1.6 mmol/L, nl = 3.5 - 5.1), hypocalcemia (6.9 mg/dl, nl = 9.4 - 10.2), mild transaminitis (alanine aminotransferase (ALT) = 63 U/L, nl = 0 - 40; aspartate aminotransferase level (AST) = 46 U/L, nl = 0 - 39), elevated creatinine kinase (1979 U/L, nl = 38 - 174), normal albumin (4.4 g/dl, nl = 3.5 - 5.1), and normal magnesium (1.6 mEq/l, nl = 1.3 - 2.0). EGD showed chronic gastritis and mild duodenitis, but no histological evidence for celiac disease. He was admitted for treatment of the electrolyte disorder. As the electrolytes corrected the serum creatinine kinase also normalized and he experienced improvement in his all symptoms, except for diarrhea. Colonoscopy was performed to evaluate for colitis as an etiology of the persistent diarrhea. The colonic mucosa was visually normal in appearance (**Figure 1**). Biopsies revealed no inflammation or crypt distortion, but did show an increased number of apoptotic cells within the mucosal crypts (**Figure 2**) from the transverse colon to the rectum, consistent with a diagnosis of apoptotic colitis.

The differential diagnosis for apoptotic colitis is limited, including drug-related colonopathy, graft-versus-host disease (GVHD), and immunodeficiency disorders, including human immunodeficiency virus (HIV) infection. The patient had a past history of recurrent infections and was shown to have low IgA levels as part of the initial evaluation for celiac disease, so an immunodeficiency evaluation was initiated. The findings of the immune work up are found in **Table 1**. The patient was diagnosed with common variable immunodeficiency (CVID). Genetic testing was done for the common underlying defects including transmembrane activator, calcium-modulator, and cycophilin ligand interactor (TACI), B-cell activating factor receptor (BAFF-R), and inducible T-cell costimulatory (ICOS); he was found to have ICOS deficiency. Treatment was initiated with monthly immunoglobulin replacement (Gamunex® 10%).

He continued to have ongoing intermittent bouts of weakness due to hypokalemia despite oral replacement therapy prompting evaluation for other potential causes. Evaluation for renal loss of electrolytes was normal. Hypokalemia periodic paralysis was ruled out by normal sequencing of the commonly involved genes (CACNL1A3 gene and SCN4A gene).

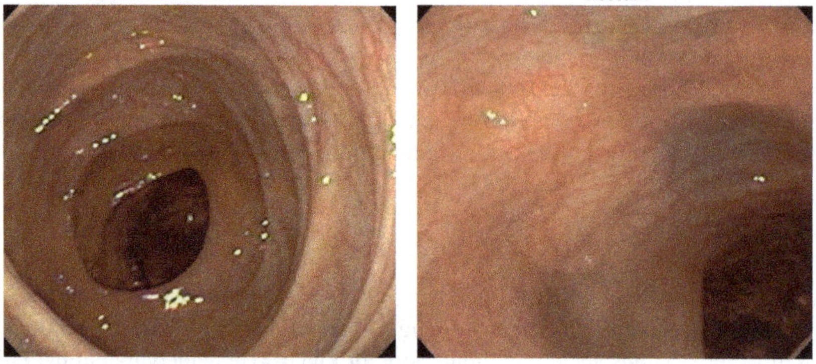

Figure 1. Endoscopic findings. The colonic mucosa appeared normal throughout as shown in photographs from the transverse colon and rectum.

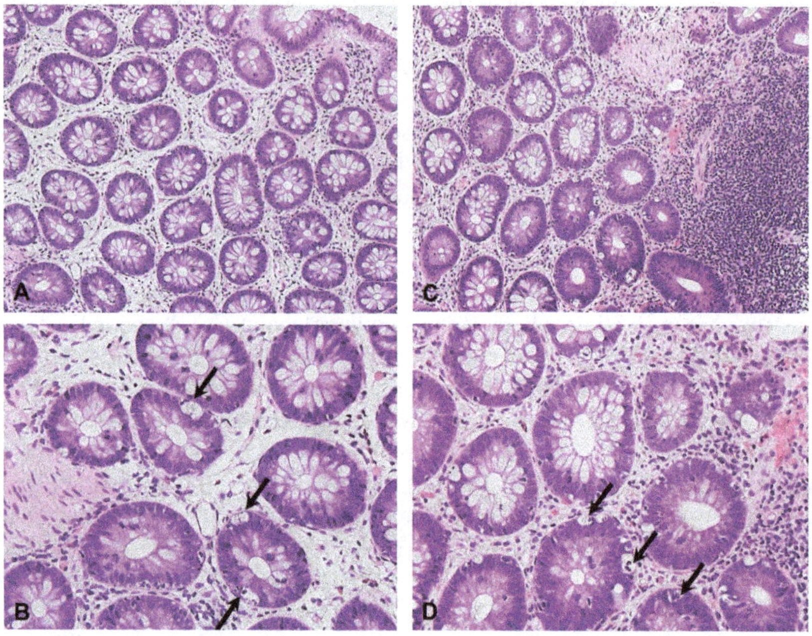

Figure 2. Histological findings. Biopsies from the transverse colon (A and B) and the rectum (C and D) revealed no inflammation or crypt distortion. An increased number of apoptotic cells were seen within the mucosal crypts (B and D; arrows) consistent with a diagnosis of apoptotic colitis (A and B, 20× magnification; C and D, 40× magnification).

Repeat colonoscopy was performed 9 months after initiation of immunoglobulin therapy again revealed normal appearing mucosa but persistence of apoptosis. He continued to have loose stools and intermittent bouts of hypokalemia, but both had improved significantly. The patient also had marked improvement in his psoriatic skin lesions.

3. Discussion

At initial presentation to our institution, the patient was noted to have severe hypokalemia and rhabdomyolysis. Rhabdomyolysis may result from a wide variety of causes, including primary muscle disease (metabolic and muscular dystrophy), infection, trauma, connective tissue disease, strenuous exercise, drug overdose, drug reaction, seizures, ischemia, and electrolyte derangements [1]. Electrolyte abnormalities associated with rhabdomyolysis include hypokalemia, hypocalcemia, hypophosphatemia, hyponatremia, hypernatremia, of which hypokalemia

Table 1. Results of the patient's immunological testing.

	Result	Normal values
Human immunodeficiency virus (HIV) antibody	Negative	Negative
C3	113 mg/dl	90 - 180 mg/dl
C4	27 mg/dl	10 - 40 mg/dl
CH50	51 U/ml	23 - 60 U/ml
CD2 (T cells)	78%	71% - 81%
CD3 (T cells)	76%	60% - 74%
CD4 (T cells)	44%	37% - 48%
CD8 (T cells)	26%	25% - 31%
4:8 ratio (T cells)	1.67	1.05 - 2.61
CD 56 NK cell	2%	3% - 10%
CD19 (B cell)	21%	2% - 11%
IgA	17 mg/gl	70 - 400 mg/dl
IgG 1	260 mg/dl	315 - 855 mg/dl
IgG 2	16 mg/dl	64 - 495 mg/dl
IgG 3	14 mg/dl	23 - 196 mg/dl
IgG 4	<1 mg/dl	11 - 157 mg/dl
IgG total	328 mg/dl	842 - 2013 mg/dl
IgM	28 mg/dl	40 - 230 mg/dl
IgE	4.5 mg/dl	0 - 200 mg/dl

is the most common, accounting for 14% - 28% of cases of rhabdomyolysis due to electrolyte abnormalities [2]. However, hypokalemia may go unrecognized as the cause of rhabdomyolysis due to the release of potassium from damaged muscle into the circulation [3]. Conversely, subclinical rhabdomyolysis may be missed; biochemical evidence of rhabdomyolysis was documented in 32% of hypokalemic patients in one study [4]. As exemplified in our patient, hypokalemia can result secondary to potassium loss in the stool due to diarrhea. The chronic nature of our patient's complaints of diarrhea, stunted growth, and weight loss prompted an evaluation for celiac disease, as hypokalemic myopathy is a rarely reported complication of celiac disease [2] [5] [6]. Screening serology was not useful, as the patient was deficient for immunoglobulin A (IgA), which occurs in about 2% of individuals with celiac disease [7]. Subsequent endoscopy documented normal duodenal histology, excluding celiac disease.

As the initial suspicion for celiac disease was excluded by upper endoscopy, colonoscopy was performed to assess for colonic causes of persistent diarrhea. Although the colon appeared grossly normal, biopsies showed a significant number of apoptotic cells in the colonic mucosa, extending from the transverse colon to the rectum. The finding of small numbers of apoptotic cells in normal colonic mucosa is expected as "physiological" apoptosis results in loss of senescent colonocytes without release of inflammatory cytokines. Apoptotic cells can also be seen as nuclear dust within the lamina propria of the colon, being more commonly found in patients with colitis (84%) than patients with normal colons (11%) [8]. Colitis due to Crohn's disease and ulcerative colitis is associated with an increased apoptotic rate, while lymphocytic colitis has apoptotic rates similar to that of normal colon [9]. Although apoptosis related to normal cell turnover does not alter epithelial barrier, apoptosis due to inflammation does lead to epithelial dysfunction. The proinflammatory cytokines tumor necrosis factor-α (TNFα) and interleukin (IL)-13 increase the apoptotic rate and increase apoptotic conductivity, compared to physiologic apoptosis. The increased conductance leads to a loss of electrolytes and water into the intestinal lu-men resulting in diarrhea [9].

The differential diagnosis for apoptotic colitis includes GVHD, HIV infection, drug-induced colonopathy, and immunodeficiency syndromes. In our patient GVHD was excluded by history and HIV infection was excluded by serological testing. Medications associated with apoptotic colitis include proton-pump inhibitors, non-steroidal anti-inflammatory drugs, and the immunosuppressant mycophenolate mofetil [10] [11]. Apoptotic colitis accounts for 2% of drug-related colitides, often mimicking GVHD [11]. The patient described herein was receiving no medications prior to onset of symptoms, ruling out a drug-related process. Subsequent testing showed that the patient had common variable immunodeficiency (CVID) due to a defect in inducible costimulator (ICOS).

Clinical presentation of CVID is heterogenous, gastrointestinal manifestations include sprue-like syndrome, intestinal nodular lymphoid hyperplasia, colitis, small bowel lymphoma, gastric atrophy, and achlorhydria. Similarly, the histological findings of the gastrointestinal tract in CVID are highly variable; the findings may mimic inflammatory bowel disease, granulomatous inflammation, GVHD, lymphocytic colitis, collangenous colitis, and apoptotic colitis [12]. In a small study addressing gastrointestinal pathology in patients with CVID, significant apoptotis was found in the colons of 50% of the patients. Smaller percentage of patients had apoptosis in the stomach (33%), small intestine (20%), and esophagus (5%) [12].

CVID is defined by a decrease in serum IgG and at least one other immunoglobulin isotype (usually IgA or IgM), functional defect in IgG response to immunizations, reduced numbers of memory B-cells, onset > 2 year of age, and exclusion of other causes of hypogammaglobulinemia [13] [14]. CVID is the second most common primary immunodeficiency, having a prevalence rate of 1:25,000; specific IgA deficiency is the most common, having a prevalence rate of 1:600. The age of onset of CVID has two major peaks, childhood (5 to 10 years) and early adulthood (20 to 30 years) [14]-[17].

Most cases of CVID are sporadic, with only 10% - 20% having a positive family history [18]. CVID can arise from a number of different gene defects. Defects in TACI are inherited in an autosomal dominant fashion and account for less than 10% - 15% of individuals with CVID. Autosomal recessive defects include CD19 deficiency, BAFF-R deficiency, and ICOS deficiency; each account for <1% of individuals with CVID [19].

The ICOS belongs to the family of costimulatory T cell molecules, which also includes CD28 and cytotoxic T-lymphocyte antigen-4. ICOS is only expressed on activated T cells where it co-induces the secretion of cytokines (IL-4, IL-5, IL-6, GM-CSF, TNF-α, and IFN-γ) and the superinduction of IL-10. IL-10 is a key cytokine for antibody production and germinal center B-cell survival [20]. Highest expression of ICOS is found within the T cell zones of secondary lymphoid organs and in the apical light zones of germinal centers. This expression pattern and the cytokines induced by ICOS point to an important role of ICOS:ICOS-ligand interaction in mediating T-B cell cooperation and promoting the terminal differentiation of B cells into memory cells and plasma cells [21] [22].

4. Conclusion

In conclusion, we present a young man who presented with hypokalemic-induced rhabdomyolysis resulting from potassium loss from chronic diarrhea. Investigation led to a diagnosis of apoptotic colitis, an uncommon cause of colitis with a limited differential diagnosis. The etiology of apoptotic colitis in this young man was CVID. Physicians should be aware of this rare association, and consider evaluation for immune deficiency when apoptotic colitis is identified at colonoscopy.

References

[1] Mannix, R., Tan, M.L., Wright, R. and Baskin, M. (2006) Acute Pediatric Rhabdomyolysis: Causes and Rates of Renal Failure. *Pediatrics*, **118**, 2119-2125. http://dx.doi.org/10.1542/peds.2006-1352

[2] Barta, Z., Miltenyi, Z., Toth, L. and Illes, A. (2005) Hypokalemic Myopathy in a Patient with Gluten-Sensitive Enteropathy and Dermatitis Herpetiformis Duhring: A Case Report. *World Journal of Gastroenterology*, **11**, 2039-2040.

[3] Vanholder, R., Sever, M.S., Erek, E., *et al.* (2000) Rhabdomyolysis. *Journal of the American Society of Nephrology*, **11**, 1553-1561.

[4] Singhal, P.C., Abramovici, M., Venkatesan, J., *et al.* (1991) Hypokalemia and Rhabdomyolysis. *Mineral and Electrolyte Metabolism*, **17**, 335-339.

[5] Ertekin, V., Selimoğlu, M.A., Tan, H. and Kiliçaslan, B. (2003) Rhabdomyolysis in Celiac Disease. *Yonsei Medical Journal*, **44**, 328-330.

[6] Williams, S.G., Davison, A.G. and Glynn, M.J. (1995) Hypokalaemic Rhabdomyolysis: An Unusual Presentation of Coeliac Disease. *European Journal of Gastroenterology and Hepatology*, **7**, 183-184.

[7] Chow, M.A., Lebwohl, B., Reilly, N.R. and Green, P.H. (2012) Immunoglobulin: A Deficiency in Celiac Disease. *Clinical Gastroenterology*, **46**, 850-854. http://dx.doi.org/10.1097/MCG.0b013e31824b2277

[8] Shichijo, K., Shin, T., Wen, C.Y., *et al.* (2007) Expression of Apoptotic Epithelial Cells in Biopsy Specimens of Patients with Colitis. *Digestive Diseases and Science*, **52**, 2037-2043. http://dx.doi.org/10.1007/s10620-006-9263-5

[9] Schulzke, J.D., Bojarski, C., Zeissig, S., *et al.* (2006) Disrupted Barrier Function through Epithelial Cell Apoptosis. *Annals of the New York Academy of Sciences*, **1072**, 288-299. http://dx.doi.org/10.1196/annals.1326.027

[10] Shepard, N.A. (2000) Muciphages and Other Mucosal Accumulations in the Colorectal Mucosa. *Histopathology*, **36**, 559-562.

[11] Villanacci, V., Casella, G. and Bassotti, G. (2011) The Spectrum of Drug-Related Colitides: Important Entities, though Frequently Overlooked. *Digestive and Liver Disease*, **43**, 523-528. http://dx.doi.org/10.1016/j.dld.2010.12.016

[12] Daniels, J.A., Lederman, H.M., Maitra, A. and Montgomery, E.A. (2007) Gastrointestinal Tract Pathology in Patients with Common Variable Immunodeficiency (CVID): A Clinicopathologic Study and Review. *American Journal of Surgical Pathology*, **31**, 1800-1812. http://dx.doi.org/10.1097/PAS.0b013e3180cab60c

[13] Conley, M.E., Notarangelo, L.D. and Etzioni, A. (1999) Diagnostic Criteria for Primary Immunodeficiencies. Representing PAGID (Pan-American Group for Immunodeficiency) and ESID (European Society for Immunodeficiencies). *Clinical Immunology*, **93**, 190-197. http://dx.doi.org/10.1006/clim.1999.4799

[14] Cunningham-Rundles, C. and Bodian, C. (1999) Common Variable Immunodeficiency: Clinical and Immunological Features of 248 Patients. *Clinical Immunology*, **92**, 34-48. http://dx.doi.org/10.1006/clim.1999.4725

[15] Spickett, G.P., Farrant, J., North, M.E., *et al.* (1997) Common Variable Immunodeficiency: How Many Diseases? *Immunology Today*, **18**, 325-328. http://dx.doi.org/10.1016/S0167-5699(97)01086-4

[16] Morimoto, Y. and Routes, J.M. (2008) Immunodeficiency Overview. *Primary Care*, **35**, 159-173. http://dx.doi.org/10.1016/j.pop.2007.09.004

[17] Yarmohammadi, H., Estrella, L., Doucette, J., *et al.* (2006) Recognizing Primary Immune Deficiency in Clinical Practice. *Clinical and Vaccine Immunology*, **13**, 329-332. http://dx.doi.org/10.1128/CVI.13.3.329-332.2006

[18] Kralovicova, J., Hammarstrom, L., Plebani, A., *et al.* (2003) Fine-Scale Mapping at IGAD1 and Genome-Wide Genetic Linkage Analysis Implicate HLA-DQ/DR as a Major Susceptibility Locus in Selective IgA Deficiency and Common Variable Immunodeficiency. *Journal of Immunology*, **170**, 2765-2775. http://dx.doi.org/10.4049/jimmunol.170.5.2765

[19] Scharenberg, A.M., Hannibal, M.C., Torgerson, T., *et al.* (1993-2003) In: Pagon, R.A., Adam, M.P., Bird, T.D., Dolan, C.R., Fong, C.T. and Stephens, K., Eds., *Common Variable Immune Deficiency Overview*, GeneReviews™ [Internet]. University of Washington, Seattle.

[20] Hutloff, A., Dittrich, A.M., Beier, K.C., *et al.* (1999) ICOS Is an Inducible T-Cell Costimulator, Structurally and Functionally Related to CD28. *Nature*, **397**, 263-266. http://dx.doi.org/10.1038/16717

[21] Beier, K.C., Hutloff, A., Dittrich, A.M.C., *et al.* (2000) Induction, Binding Specificity and Function of Human ICOS. *European Journal of Immunology*, **30**, 3707-3717. http://dx.doi.org/10.1002/1521-4141(200012)30:12<3707::AID-IMMU3707>3.0.CO;2-Q

[22] Rousset, F., Garcia, E., Defrance, T., *et al.* (1992) Interleukin 10 Is a Potent Growth and Differentiation Factor for Activated Human B Lymphocytes. *Proceedings of the National Academy of Science USA*, **89**, 1890-1893. http://dx.doi.org/10.1073/pnas.89.5.1890

Abbreviations

BAFF-R: B-Cell Activating Factor Receptor
CVID: Common-Variable Immunodeficiency
GVHD: Graft-Versus-Host Disease
ICOS: Inducible T-Cell Costimulator
TACI: Transmembrane Activator, Calcium-Modulator, and Cycophilin Ligand Interactor

17

TBXA2R rSNPs, Transcriptional Factor Binding Sites and Asthma in Asians

Norman E. Buroker

Department of Pediatrics, University of Washington, Seattle, USA
Email: nburoker@u.washington.edu

Abstract

Four regulatory single nucleotide polymorphisms (rSNPs) (rs2238631, rs2238632, rs2238633 and rs2238634) in intron one, two rSNPs (rs1131882 and rs4523) in exon 3 and one rSNP (rs5756) in the 3'UTR of the thromboxane A2 receptor (TBXA2R) gene have been associated with childhood-onset asthma in Asians. These rSNP alleles alter the DNA landscape for potential transcriptional factors (TFs) to attach resulting in changes in transcriptional factor binding sites (TFBS). These TFBS changes are examined with respect to asthma which has been found to be significantly associated with the rSNPs.

Keywords

***TBXA2R*, rSNPs, TFBS, Asthma**

1. Introduction

Asthma is a chronic inflammatory condition of the airways characterized by recurrent episodes of reversible airway obstruction and increased bronchial hyper-responsiveness which results from the interactions between genes and environmental factors [1]-[3]. Asthma causes episodes of wheeze, cough, and shortness of breath [4]. Recent studies indicate that the genetic factors of childhood-onset asthma differ from those of adult-onset asthma [3] [5]. Childhood asthma is a major clinical and public health problem as it affects nearly one in eight children in the USA [6] and worldwide [7]. The disease is genetically heterogeneous and genome-wide association studies (GWAS) have identified a group of loci at chromosome 17q21 that are strongly associated with childhood-onset asthma in Caucasians [5] [8]. The genetic origins of asthma are diverse where some disease pathways are specific to wheezing syndromes while others are shared with atopy and bronchial hyper-responsiveness [5]. To that end another gene has recently surfaced in Asian populations that have been found to be associated with lung function childhood-onset asthma [9].

The thromboxane A2 receptor (TBXA2R) gene which is located at chromosome 19p13.3 is a member of the seven-transmembrane G-protein-coupled receptor super family, which interacts with intracellular G proteins, regulates different downstream signaling cascades, and induces many cellular responses including the intracellular calcium influx, cell migration and proliferation, and apoptosis [10]. This gene is abundantly expressed in tissues at the mRNA and protein levels targeted by the TBXA2R ligand thromboxane A2 (TXA2) that include erythroleukaemia cells, vascular and bronchial smooth muscle, uterus and placental tissue, endothelium, epithelium, trophoblasts, thymus, liver and small intestine [11]. The activation of TBXA2R in bronchial smooth muscle cells by its ligand results in intercellular calcium mobilization with subsequent bronchoconstriction, which contributes to bronchial smooth muscle hyperplasia and airway remodeling, which occurs in response to chronic airway inflammation in asthma [12].

Four linked *TBXA2R* single nucleotide polymorphisms (SNPs, rs2238631, rs2238632, rs2238633 and rs2238634) which span a 431bp region of intron one have been found to be in linkage disequilibrium (LD) with two exon 3 SNPs [rs11318632, (c.795 T > C) and rs4523 (c.924 T > C)] [9], which are approximately 8.4 kb downstream from the intron one SNPs. The rs11318632 and rs4523 SNPs from exon 3 are synonymous and unlikely to influence the characteristics of the receptor protein. The exon 3 SNPs have been associated with asthma and its related phenotypes in Asian populations, where rs4523 SNP was found to be associated with adult asthma in a Japanese population [13] and childhood atopic asthma in a Chinese population [14], while the rs11318632 SNP was found to be associated with atopic asthma in a Korean population [15]. Two haplotypes (H2 & H4) involving the four linked *TBXA2R* SNPs from intron one where found to influence *TBXA2R* transcriptional activity and were also associated with asthma-related phenotypes [9]. This suggests that these SNPs may be part of a regulatory network for the *TBXA2R* gene in Asian populations. To follow up on this possibility these SNPs were examined for associations to potential transcription factor binding sites (TFBS).

Single nucleotide changes that affect gene expression by impacting gene regulatory sequences such as promoters, enhances, and silencers are known as regulatory SNPs (rSNPs) [16]-[19]. A rSNPs within a transcriptional factor binding site (TFBS) can change a transcriptional factor's (TF) ability to bind its TFBS [20]-[23] in which case the TF would be unable to effectively regulate its target gene [24]-[28]. This concept is examined for the above *TBXA2R* SNPs and their allelic association with TFBS. In this report, these SNP associations have been discussed with changes in potential TFBS and their possible relationship to childhood-onset asthma in Asians.

2. Materials and Methods

Identifying TFBS

The JASPAR CORE database [29] [30] and ConSite [31] were used to identify the TFBS in this study. JASPAR is a collection of transcription factor DNA-binding preferences used for scanning genomic sequences where ConSite is a web-based tool for finding cis-regulatory elements in genomic sequences. The Vector NTI Advance 11 computer program (Invitrogen, Life Technologies) was used to locate the TFBS in the *TBXA2R* gene (NCBI Ref Seq NM_201636) from 9.4 kb upstream of the transcriptional start site to 1.4 kb past the 3'UTR which represents a total of 17.1 Kbp. The JASPAR CORE database was also used to compute each nucleotide occurrence (%) within the TFBS where upper case lettering indicate that the nucleotide occurs 90% or greater and lower case less than 90%. The occurrence of each SNP allele in the TFBS is also computed from the database (**Table & Supplement**).

3. Results

TBXA2RrSNPs and TFBS

The *TBXA2R* gene encodes a member of the G protein-coupled receptor family and the protein interacts with thromboxane A2 to induce platelet aggregation and regulate hemostasis. The activity of this receptor is mediated by a G-protein that activates a phosphatidylinositol-calcium second messenger system. The four *TBXA2R*rSNPs [rs2238631 (A/G), rs2238632 (C/T), rs2238633 (T/G) and rs2238634 (G/T)] in intron one have been found to be in moderate LD with the exon 3 SNP [rs1131882 (C/T), c.795T > C] while the other exon 3 SNP [rs4523 (C/T), c.924T > C] has been found to be in strong LD with a 3'UTR SNP (rs5756 (C/T) [9]. Since the exon 3 SNPs have been found to be associated with asthma in Asian populations [10]-[12] and certain haplotypes of the intron one SNPs have an effect on the transcriptional activity of the *TBXA2R* gene [9], the potential TFBS for alleles of each of the seven SNPs were examined (**Table 1 & Supplement**).

The intron one rs2238631 SNP *TBXA2R*-A allele creates six unique TFBS for the ELK1 & 4, ETS1, GATA2, HAND1:TCFC2α and SPZ1 TFs which are involved in the mitogen-activate protein kinase signaling pathway, repression, controlling development, proliferation of hematopoietic and endocrine cell lineages, and initiation of B lymphopoiesis (**Table 1**). The intron one rs2238631 SNP *TBXA2R*-G allele creates two unique TFBS for the FOXC1 and TFAP2α TFs which are involved in cell viability and resistance to oxidative stress and activating transcription of some genes while inhibiting the transcription of other genes, respectively (**Table & Supplement**). Only one TFBS have been conserved between the two rs2238631 alleles which is for the EN1 TF which plays a role in development (**Table 1**).

Table 1. The TBXA2R SNPs that were examined in this study where the minor allele is in red. Also listed are the transcriptional factors (TF), their potential binding sites (TFBS) containing these SNPs and DNA strand orientation. TFs in red differ between the SNP alleles. Where upper case nucleotide designates the 90% conserved BS region and red is the SNP location of the alleles in the TFBS. Below the TFBS is the nucleotide occurrence (%) obtained from the Jaspar Core database. Also listed are the number (#) of binding sites in the gene for the given TF. Note: TFs can bind to more than one nucleotide sequence.

SNP	Allele	TFs	Protein name	# of Sites	TFBS	Strand
rs2238631	A	ELK1	ELK1, member of ETS oncogene family	1	aagccgGAta	minus
(A/G)					A = 96%	
Intron 1		ELK4	ELK4, ETS-domain protein	1	gCCGGAtac	minus
					A = 100%	
		EN1	Engrailed homeobox 1	1	acagggtatcc	plus
					t = 30%	
		ETS1	Protein C-ets-1	1	taTCCg	plus
					T = 98%	
		GATA2	GATA binding protein 2	10	gGATa	minus
					A = 98%	
		HAND1:TCFE2α	Heart- and neural crest derivatives-expressed protein 1: transcription factor E2A	1	tatCcGgctt	plus
					t = 83%	
		SPZ1	spermatogenicleucine zipper 1	1	aggGtatccgg	plus
					t = 34%	
	G	EN1	Engrailed homeobox 1	1	acagggtaccc	plus
					c = 30%	
		FOXC1	Forkhead box C1	1	gccggGTA	minus
					G = 100%	
		TFAP2α	Transcription factor AP-2 alpha (activating enhancer binding protein 2 alpha)	1	GCCgggtac	minus
					g = 49%	
rs2238632	C	MAFB	v-mafmusculoaponeuroticfibrosarcoma oncogene homolog B (avian)	1	Ggtgacgc	minus
(C/T)					c = 34%	
Intron 1		PAX2	Paired box gene 2	1	ggtgacgc	minus

Continued

					c = 35%	
	T	ARNT	aryl hydrocarbon receptor nuclear translocator	5	gACGTG	minus
					T = 100%	
		ARNT	aryl hydrocarbon receptor nuclear translocator	6	cACGTc	plus
					A = 95%	
		CREB1	cAMP responsive element binding protein 1	1	gcAcGtca	plus
					A = 100%	
		HIF1α:ARNT	Hypoxia-inducible factor 1:Aryl hydrocarbon receptor nuclear translocator	1	tgaCGTGc	minus
					T = 100%	
		MAFB	v-mafmusculoaponeuroticfibrosarcoma oncogene homolog B (avian)	1	Ggtgacgt	minus
					t = 20%	
		MAX	MYC associated factor X	1	gagCACGTca	plus
					A = 94%	
		PAX2	Paired box gene 2	1	ggtgacgt	minus
					t = 26%	
		USF1	Upstream transcription factor 1	3	CACGTca	plus
					A = 100%	
rs2238633	**G**	KLF4	Krueppel-like factor 4	1	aGGGtGgggt	minus
(T/G)					g = 90%	
Intron 1		MZF1_1-4	Myeloid zinc finger 1	21	tGGGGA	minus
					G = 95%	
		SP1	Specificity Protein 1	2	CcCcacCctg	plus
					c = 86%	
		ZNF354C	Zinc finger protein 354C	31	cccCAC	plus
					c = 38%	
	T	BRCA1	breast cancer 1, early onset	5	acAccac	plus
					A = 95%	
		EN1	Engrailed homeobox 1	1	gggtggtgtcg	minus
					t = 70%	
		KLF4	Krueppel-like factor 4	1	aGGGtGgtgt	minus
					t = 3%	
		ZNF354C	Zinc finger protein 354C	37	cacCAC	plus
					a = 44%	
rs2238634	**T**	HLTF	Helicase-like transcription factor	1	gagCtTagca	minus

Continued

(G/T)					T = 100%	
Intron 1		HNF4α	Hepatocyte nuclear factor 4, alpha	1	gGtgCtaAGctca a = 79%	plus
		NR2F1	Nuclear receptor subfamily 2, group F, member 1	1	tGAgCttagcaccc t = 85%	minus
		NR2E3	Nuclear receptor subfamily 2, group E, member 3	3	tgAGCTT T = 100%	minus
		NR2E3	Nuclear receptor subfamily 2, group E, member 3	2	tAAGCTC A = 100%	plus
		NR4A2	Nuclear receptor subfamily 4, group A, member 2	1	aAGctCAg a = 57%	plus
		ZFX	Zinc finger X-chromosomal protein	1	taagctcaGGCCTc a = 12%	plus
	G	ZFX	Zinc finger X-chromosomal protein	1	tcagctcaGGCCTc c = 35%	plus
rs1131882 **(C/T)**	**C**	GATA2	GATA binding protein 2	10	cGATg G = 91%	plus
c.795T > C **Exon 3**		GATA3	GATA binding protein 3	3	cGATga G = 98%	plus
		INSM1	Insulinoma-associated 1	1	tgtctGGGcgat g = 67%	plus
		NFE2L1:MAFG	Nuclear factor erythroid 2-related factor 1 Transcription factor MafG	4	gaTGAa g = 29%	plus
		NFIC	Nuclear factor 1 C-type	24	tgGGcg g = 17%	plus
	T	MZF1_1-4	Myeloid zinc finger 1	14	tGGGcA A = 90%	plus
		MZF1_5-13	Myeloid zinc finger 1	2	gtctGGGcaa a = 63%	plus
		NFIC	Nuclear factor 1 C-type	14	tgGGca a = 48%	plus
		NKX2-5	Natural killer 2 homeobox 5	2	ttcAttg t = 65%	minus
		Nobox	NOBOX oogenesis homeobox	1	TcATtgcc	minus

Continued

					t = 84%	
		PAX2	Paired box gene 2	1	cttCattg	minus
					t = 32%	
		SOX17	SRY (sex determining region Y)-box 17	1	ttcaTTGcc	minus
					T = 100%	
rs4523	**C**	AR	Androgen receptor	1	gggtGtACatcctGttCcgccg	minus
(C/T)					C = 100%	
c.924T > C		ELF5	E74-like factor 5	1	tacaTCCtg	minus
Exon 3					c = 45%	
		ELK1	ELK1, member of ETS oncogene family	1	gaacagGAtg	plus
					g = 50%	
		ELK4	ELK4, ETS-domain protein	1	aCaGGAtgt	plus
					g = 75%	
		ETS1	Protein C-ets-1	15	caTCCt	minus
					c = 40%	
		FEV	ETS oncogene family	1	caGGAtgt	plus
					g = 46%	
		FOXC1	Forkhead box C1	2	aggatGTA	plus
					G = 100%	
		GATA2	GATA binding protein 2	32	gGATg	plus
					g = 28%	
		NR3C1	Nuclear receptor subfamily 3, group C, member 1 (glucocorticoid receptor)	1	gtgtacAtcctGTtCcgc	minus
					c = 67%	
		SPI1	Spleen focus forming virus (SFFV) proviral integration oncogene spi1	3	aGGATgt	plus
					g = 79%	
	T	ELF5	E74-like factor 5	1	tataTCCtg	minus
					t = 45%	
		ELK1	ELK1, member of ETS oncogene family	1	gaacagGAta	plus
					a = 50%	
		ETS1	Protein C-ets-1	3	taTCCt	minus
					t = 14%	
		FEV	ETS oncogene family	1	caGGAtat	plus
					a = 54%	
		FOXL1	Forkhead box L1	1	aggatATA	plus
					A = 91%	

Continued

		GATA2	GATA binding protein 2	10	gGATa a = 28%	plus
		GATA3	GATA binding protein 3	2	gGATat a = 62%	plus
		KLF4	Krueppel-like factor 4	1	tGGGtGtata t = 7%	minus
		ZNF354C	Zinc finger protein 354C	4	ataCAC a = 44%	plus
rs5756 (C/T)	**C**	ARNT:AHR	aryl hydrocarbon receptor nuclear translocator aryl hydrocarbon receptor	28	gGCGTG G = 96%	plus
3'UTR		BRCA1	breast cancer 1, early onset	22	ccAccac c = 51%	minus
		EN1	Engrailed homeobox 1	5	gcgtggtggcg g = 70%	plus
		HIF1α:ARNT	Hypoxia-inducible factor 1: Aryl hydrocarbon receptor nuclear translocator	10	gggCGTGg G = 100%	plus
		KLF4	Krueppel-like factor 4	4	cGGGcGtggt G = 98%	plus
		PAX2	Paired box gene 2	9	cacCacgc c = 55%	minus
		TFAP2A	Transcription factor AP-2 alpha (activating enhancer binding protein 2 alpha)	8	GCCaccacg c = 9%	minus
		TFAP2A	Transcription factor AP-2 alpha (activating enhancer binding protein 2 alpha)	5	GCCgggcgt g = 74%	plus
		ZNF354C	Zinc finger protein 354C	37	caCCAC C = 94%	minus
	T	NFIC	Nuclear factor 1 C-type	18	cgGGca a = 48%	plus
		NFE2L1:MAFG	Nuclear factor erythroid 2-related factor 1 Transcription factor MafG	20	caTGcc T = 100%	minus
		TFAP2A	Transcription factor AP-2 alpha (activating enhancer binding protein 2 alpha)	8	GCCaccatg t = 7%	minus
		ZEB1	Zinc finger E-box binding homeobox 1	22	cACCat t = 34%	minus
		YY1	YY1 transcription factor	22	aCCATg T = 100%	minus

The intron one rs2238632 SNP *TBXA2R*-C allele creates no unique TFBS while the *TBXA2R* -T allele creates five unique TFBS which are for the ARNT, CREB1, HIF1α:ARNT, MAX and USF1 TFs which are involved with xenobiotic metabolism, circadian rhythmicity, cellular and systemic responses to hypoxia, transcriptional regulator and a cellular TF, respectively (**Table & Supplement**). Two TFBS have been conserved between the two alleles which are the MAFB and PAX2 TFs that are involved with the transcription of erythroid-specific genes in myeloid cells and plays a role in kidney cell development, respectively (**Table 1**).

The intron one rs2238633 SNP *TBXA2R*-G allele creates two unique TFBS for the MZF1_1-4 and SP1 TFs which are involved in transcriptional regulation and the regulation of genes involved in cell growth, apaoptosis, differentiation and immune responses, respectively (**Table & Supplement**). The intron one rs2238633 SNP *TBXA2R*-T allele also creates two unique TFBS for the BRCA1 and SP1 TFs which are involved in maintaining genomic stability and controlling development, respectively (**Table & Supplement**). Two TFBS have been conserved between the two alleles which are the KLF4 and ZNF354C TFs that are involved with the regulation of key transcription factors during embryonic development, activation and repression, respectively (**Table & Supplement**).

The intron one rs2238634 SNP *TBXA2R*-T allele creates five unique TFBS for the HLTF, HNF4α, NR2F1, NR2E3 and NR4A2 TFs which are involved with altering chromatin structure, regulates the expression of hepatic genes, initiation of transcription, signaling pathways and transcription regulation, respectively (**Table & Supplement**). The intron one rs2238634 SNP *TBXA2R*-G allele creates no unique TFBS. One TFBS has been conserved between the two alleles which is the ZFX TF which is a probable transcription activator.

The exon 3 rs1131882 SNP *TBXA2R*-C allele creates four unique TFBS for the GATA2, GATA3, INSM1 and NFE2L.1: MAFG TFs which are involved with regulation of genes for development and proliferation of hematopoietic and endocrine cell lineages, endothelial cell biology, neuroendocrine differentiation of human lung tumors, and up-regulation of cytoprotective genes via the antioxidant response element, respectively (**Table & Supplement**). The exon 3 rs1131882 SNP *TBXA2R*-T allele creates six unique TFBS for the MZF1_1-4, MZF1_5-13, NKX2-5, Nobox, PAX2 and SOX17 TFs which are involved with transcription regulation, negative regulator of chondrocyte maturation, oogenesis and kidney cell differentiation (**Table & Supplement**). One TFBS has been conserved between the two alleles which is the NFIC TF which is involved with activating transcription and replication.

The exon 3 rs4523 SNP *TBXA2R*-C allele creates five unique TFBS for the AR, ELK4, FOXC1, NR3C1 and SPI1 TFs which are involved with the regulation of eukaryotic gene expression, transcriptional activation and repression, viability and resistance to oxidative stress, regulation of carbohydrate, protein and fat metabolism as well as activating gene expression during myeloid and B-lymphoid cell development, respectively (**Table & Supplement**). The exon 3 rs4523 SNP *TBXA2R*-T allele creates four unique TFBS for the FOXL1, GATA3, KLF4 and ZNF354C TFs which are involved with the regulation of multiple processes including metabolism, cell proliferation and gene expression during ontogenesis, endothelial cell biology, embryonic development and transcription repression, respectively (**Table & Supplement**). Five TFBS have been conserved between the two alleles which are the ELF5, ELK1, ETS1, FEV and GATA2 TFs that are involved with regulation epithelium-specific genes, the mitogen-activate protein kinase signaling pathway, the TTRAP, UBE2I and Death associated protein, transcriptional repression and genes for development and proliferation of hematopoietic and endocrine cell lineages (**Table & Supplement**).

The 3'UTR rs5756 SNP *TBXA2R*-C allele creates seven unique TFBS for the ARNT:AHR, BRCA1, EN1, HIF1α:ARNT, KLF4, PAX2 and ZNF354C TFs which are involved with xenobiotic metabolism, genomic stability, controlling development, hypoxia, embryonic development, kidney cell differentiation and repression, respectively (**Table & Supplement**). The 3'UTR rs5756 SNP *TBXA2R*-T allele creates four unique TFBS for the NFIC, NFE2L1:MAFG, ZEB1 and YY1 TFs which are involved with activating transcription and replication, up-regulation of cytoprotective genes, transcription repression and control of transcription, respectively (**Table & Supplement**). Only one TFBS has been conserved between the two alleles which is the TFAP2α that is involved with controlling transcription.

4. Discussion

GWAS over the last decade have identified nearly 6500 disease or trait-predisposing SNPs where only 7% of these are located in protein-coding regions of the genome [32] [33] and the remaining 93% are located within non-coding areas [34] [35] such as regulatory or intergenic regions. SNPs which occur in the putative regulatory region of a gene where a single base change in the DNA sequence of a potential TFBS may affect the process of gene expression are drawing more attention [16] [18] [36]. A SNP in a TFBS can have multiple consequences. Often the SNP does not change the TFBS interaction nor does it alter gene expression since a transcriptional factor (TF) will usually recognize a number of different binding sites in the gene. In some cases the SNP may increase or decrease the TF binding which results in allele-specific gene expression. In rare cases, a SNP may eliminate the natural binding site or generate a new binding site. In which cases the gene is no longer regulated by the original TF. Therefore, functional rSNPs in TFBS may result in differences in gene expression, phenotypes and susceptibility to environmental exposure [36]. Examples of rSNPs associated with disease susceptibility are numerous and several reviews have been published [36]-[39].

GWAS have also identified many potential rSNPs and candidate genes associated with the asthma [5] [8] [40] [41], which indicates that the genetic origins of the disease are extremely diverse [5]. The EVE consortium conducted a meta-analysis of North American GWAS including individuals of European American, African American or African Caribbean and Latino ancestry. The study revealed that previously identified loci on chromosome 17q21 (encoding *ORMDL3* and *GSDMB*) [8] and the nearby *IL1RL1*, *TSLP* and *IL33* genes were robust to ethnic differences and had significant associations in all three ethnic groups [42]. The same study also identified another asthma susceptibility locus at *PYHIN1*, with the association being specific to individuals of African descent. The associated SNPs in *PYHIN1* occur with a minor allele frequencies of 0.26 - 0.29 in African-Americans and African-Caribbean controls, less than 0.05 in the Latino populations and not polymorphic in European Americans [42]. Yet another asthma susceptibility locus at *TBXA2R* has been associated with childhood-onset in Asians [9] which has been the focus of this report.

In this study the intron one rs2238631 *TBXA2R*-A minor allele [T (+ strand) or A (-strand)] located in the ELK1, ELK4, ETS1 and HAND1:TCFE2α TFBS has a 96%, 100%, 98% and 83% occurrence, respectively, in humans. These BS occurs only once in the gene and therefore a change in these TFBS created by this rSNP would probably have any impact on the regulation of the gene (**Table & Supplement**). In contrast, the intron one rs2238631 TBXA2R-A allele located in the SPZ1 TFBS has a 34% occurrence and also only occurs once in the gene which might not have much of an impact on the regulation of the gene since other nucleotides can be substituted at this position. Also, the intron one rs2238631 TBXA2R-A allele located in the GATA2 TFBS has a 98% occurrence but occurs nine other times in the gene; therefore, it might not have much of an impact on gene regulation. The rs2238631 *TBXA2R*-G common allele [C (+ strand) or G (-strand)] located in the FOXC1 and TFAP2α TFBS has a 100% and 49% occurrence in humans and these BS occur only once in the gene and therefore a change in these TFBS created by this rSNP would probably have any impact on the regulation of the gene for the FOXC1 TF but not much impact for the TFAP2α TF (**Table & Supplement**). The arrangement of these TFBS within various haplotypes might explain the LD found between these *TBXA2R* rSNPs [9].

Similar logic can be used to evaluate the potential TFBS within the other *TBXA2R* rSNPs found in the table. It should be noted that the minor alleles in the intron 1 rSNPs create more unique TFBS than do the common alleles by a ratio of 18 to 4, respectively (**Table 1**) while the same ratio for the exon 3 and 3'UTR rSNPs is 13 to 17. Unique TFBSs that would be expected to have an impact on asthma are ELK1 and SPZ1 created by the minor allele of rs2238631, HIF1α:ARNT created by the minor allele of rs2238632, INSM1 created by the minor allele of rs1131882 and FOXC1 created by the minor allele of rs4523. Other unique TFBS that would be expected to have an impact on asthma which are created by the rSNP common alleles would be FOXC1 (rs2238631) and HIF1α:ARNT (rs5756). The two haplotypes (H2 & H4) involving the four linked *TBXA2R* SNPs from intron one found to influence *TBXA2R* transcriptional activity and were also associated with asthma-related phenotypes [9] involving the minor alleles of rs2238631 and rs2238632 which create the unique TFBS for the ELK1, SPZ1 and HIF1α:ARNT, respectively. Also that worth mentioning would be the minor allele of rs2238634 which creates the NR2E3 TFBS whose TF is involved with signaling pathways (**Table & Supplement**).

The changes in biological and physiological conditions that have been associated with these rSNPs of the *TBXA2R* gene are shown in the table and supplement along with rSNP allele-specific TFBS. What a change in the rSNP alleles can do is to alter the DNA landscape around the SNP for potential TFs to attach and regulate a gene. This change in the DNA landscape can alter gene regulation which in turn can result in a change of a biological process or signaling pathway resulting in disease or illness. In this report, the seven rSNPs of the *TBXA2R* gene which have been examined illustrate that a change in rSNP alleles can provide different TFBS which in turn could also be associated with asthma.

Conflict of Interest

Author declares that there is no conflict of interests.

References

[1] Martinez, F.D. and Vercelli, D. (2013) Asthma. *Lancet*, **382**, 1360-1372. http://dx.doi.org/10.1016/S0140-6736(13)61536-6

[2] Dijk, F.N., de Jongste, J.C., Postma, D.S. and Koppelman, G.H. (2013) Genetics of Onset of Asthma. *Current Opinion in Allergy & Clinical Immunology*, **13**, 193-202. http://dx.doi.org/10.1097/ACI.0b013e32835eb707

[3] Mantzouranis, E., Papadopouli, E. and Michailidi, E. (2014) Childhood Asthma: Recent Developments and Update. *Current Opinion in Pulmonary Medicine*, **20**, 8-16. http://dx.doi.org/10.1097/MCP.000c0000000000014

[4] Papadopoulos, N.G., Arakawa, H., Carlsen, K.H., Custovic, A., Gern, J., Lemanske, R., Le Souef, P., Makela, M., Roberts, G., Wong, G., Zar, H., Akdis, C.A., Bacharier, L.B., Baraldi, E., van Bever, H.P., de Blic, J., Boner, A., Burks, W., Casale, T.B., Castro-Rodriguez, J.A., Chen, Y.Z., El-Gamal, Y.M., Everard, M.L., Frischer, T., Geller, M., Gereda, J., Goh, D.Y., Guilbert, T.W., Hedlin, G., Heymann, P.W., Hong, S.J., Hossny, E.M., Huang, J.L., Jackson, D.J., de Jongste, J.C., Kalayci, O., Ait-Khaled, N., Kling, S., Kuna, P., Lau, S., Ledford, D.K., Lee, S.I., Liu, A.H., Lockey, R.F., Lodrup-Carlsen, K., Lotvall, J., Morikawa, A., Nieto, A., Paramesh, H., Pawankar, R., Pohunek, P., Pongracic, J., Price, D., Robertson, C., Rosario, N., Rossenwasser, L.J., Sly, P.D., Stein, R., Stick, S., Szefler, S., Taussig, L.M., Valovirta, E., Vichyanond, P., Wallace, D., Weinberg, E., Wennergren, G., Wildhaber, J. and Zeiger, R.S. (2012) International Consensus on (ICON) Pediatric Asthma. *Allergy*, **67**, 976-997. http://dx.doi.org/10.1111/j.1398-9995.2012.02865.x

[5] Spycher, B.D., Henderson, J., Granell, R., Evans, D.M., Smith, G.D., Timpson, N.J. and Sterne, J.A. (2012) Genome-Wide Prediction of Childhood Asthma and Related Phenotypes in a Longitudinal Birth Cohort. *Journal of Allergy and Clinical Immunology*, **130**, 503-509.

[6] Akinbami, L. (2006) The State of Childhood Asthma, United States, 1980-2005. *Advanced Data*, **381**, 1-24.

[7] Lai, C.K., Beasley, R., Crane, J., Foliaki, S., Shah, J. and Weiland, S. (2009) Global Variation in the Prevalence and Severity of Asthma Symptoms: Phase Three of the International Study of Asthma and Allergies in Childhood (ISAAC). *Thorax*, **64**, 476-483. http://dx.doi.org/10.1136/thx.2008.106609

[8] Moffatt, M.F., Kabesch, M., Liang, L., Dixon, A.L., Strachan, D., Heath, S., Depner, M., von Berg, A., Bufe, A., Rietschel, E., Heinzmann, A., Simma, B., Frischer, T., Willis-Owen, S.A., Wong, K.C., Illig, T., Vogelberg, C., Weiland, S.K., von Mutius, E., Abecasis, G.R., Farrall, M., Gut, I.G., Lathrop, G.M. and Cookson, W.O. (2007) Genetic Variants Regulating ORMDL3 Expression Contribute to the Risk of Childhood Asthma. *Nature*, **448**, 470-473. http://dx.doi.org/10.1038/nature06014

[9] Takeuchi, K., Mashimo, Y., Shimojo, N., Arima, T., Inoue, Y., Morita, Y., Sato, K., Suzuki, S., Nishimuta, T., Watanabe, H., Hoshioka, A., Tomiita, M., Yamaide, A., Watanabe, M., Okamoto, Y., Kohno, Y., Hata, A. and Suzuki, Y. (2013) Functional Variants in the Thromboxane A2 Receptor Gene Are Associated with Lung Function in Childhood-Onset Asthma. *Clinical & Experimental Allergy*, **43**, 413-424. http://dx.doi.org/10.1111/cea.12058

[10] Huang, J.S., Ramamurthy, S.K., Lin, X. and Le Breton, G.C. (2004) Cell Signalling through Thromboxane A2 Receptors. *Cell Signal*, **16**, 521-533. http://dx.doi.org/10.1016/j.cellsig.2003.10.008

[11] Miggin, S.M. and Kinsella, B.T. (1998) Expression and Tissue Distribution of the mRNAs Encoding the Human Thromboxane A2 Receptor (TP) Alpha and Beta Isoforms. *Biochimica et Biophysica Acta*, **1425**, 543-559. http://dx.doi.org/10.1016/S0304-4165(98)00109-3

[12] Rolin, S., Masereel, B. and Dogne, J.M. (2006) Prostanoids as Pharmacological Targets in COPD and Asthma. *European Journal of Pharmacology*, **533**, 89-100. http://dx.doi.org/10.1016/j.ejphar.2005.12.058

[13] Unoki, M., Furuta, S., Onouchi, Y., Watanabe, O., Doi, S., Fujiwara, H., Miyatake, A., Fujita, K., Tamari, M. and Nakamura, Y. (2000) Association Studies of 33 Single Nucleotide Polymorphisms (SNPs) in 29 Candidate Genes for Bronchial Asthma: Positive Association a T924C Polymorphism in the Thromboxane A2 Receptor Gene. *Human Genetics*, **106**, 440-446. http://dx.doi.org/10.1007/s004390000267

[14] Leung, T.F., Tang, N.L., Lam, C.W., Li, A.M., Chan, I.H. and Ha, G. (2002) Thromboxane A2 Receptor Gene Polymorphism Is Associated with the Serum Concentration of Cat-Specific Immunoglobulin E as Well as the Development and Severity of Asthma in Chinese Children. *Pediatric Allergy and Immunology*, **13**, 10-17. http://dx.doi.org/10.1034/j.1399-3038.2002.01033.x

[15] Shin, H.D., Park, B.L., Jung, J.H., Wang, H.J., Park, H.S., Choi, B.W., Hong, S.J., Lee, Y.M., Kim, Y.H. and Park, C.S. (2003) Association of Thromboxane A2 Receptor (TBXA2R) with Atopy and Asthma. *Journal of Allergy and Clinical*

Immunology, **112**, 454-457. http://dx.doi.org/10.1067/mai.2003.1641

[16] Knight, J.C. (2003) Functional Implications of Genetic Variation in Non-Coding DNA for Disease Susceptibility and Gene Regulation. *Clinical Science*, **104**, 493-501. http://dx.doi.org/10.1042/CS20020304

[17] Knight, J.C. (2005) Regulatory Polymorphisms Underlying Complex Disease Traits. *Journal of Molecular Medicine*, **83**, 97-109. http://dx.doi.org/10.1007/s00109-004-0603-7

[18] Wang, X., Tomso, D.J., Liu, X. and Bell, D.A. (2005) Single Nucleotide Polymorphism in Transcriptional Regulatory Regions and Expression of Environmentally Responsive Genes. *Toxicology and Applied Pharmacology*, **207**, 84-90. http://dx.doi.org/10.1016/j.taap.2004.09.024

[19] Wang, X., Tomso, D.J., Chorley, B.N., Cho, H.Y., Cheung, V.G., Kleeberger, S.R. and Bell, D.A. (2007) Identification of Polymorphic Antioxidant Response Elements in the Human Genome. *Human Molecular Genetics*, **16**, 1188-1200. http://dx.doi.org/10.1093/hmg/ddm066

[20] Claessens, F., Verrijdt, G., Schoenmakers, E., Haelens, A., Peeters, B., Verhoeven, G. and Rombauts, W. (2001) Selective DNA Binding by the Androgen Receptor as a Mechanism for Hormone-Specific Gene Regulation. *The Journal of Steroid Biochemistry and Molecular Biology*, **76**, 23-30.

[21] Hsu, M.H., Savas, U., Griffin, K.J. and Johnson, E.F. (2007) Regulation of Human Cytochrome P450 $4F_2$ Expression by Sterol Regulatory Element-Binding Protein and Lovastatin. *Journal of Biological Chemistry*, **282**, 5225-5236. http://dx.doi.org/10.1074/jbc.M608176200

[22] Takai, H., Araki, S., Mezawa, M., Kim, D.S., Li, X.Y., Yang, L., Li, Z.Y., Wang, Z.T., Nakayama, Y. and Ogata, Y. (2008) AP1 Binding Site Is Another Target of FGF2 Regulation of Bone Sialoprotein Gene Transcription. *Gene*, **410**, 97-104. http://dx.doi.org/10.1016/j.gene.2007.11.017

[23] Buroker, N.E., Huang, J.Y., Barboza, J., Ledee, D.R., Eastman Jr., R.J., Reinecke, H., Ning, X.H., Bassuk, J.A. and Portman, M.A. (2012) The Adaptor-Related Protein Complex 2, Alpha 2 Subunit (AP2α2) Gene Is a Peroxisome Proliferator-Activated Receptor Cardiac Target Gene. *The Protein Journal*, **31**, 75-83. http://dx.doi.org/10.1007/s10930-011-9379-0

[24] Huang, C.N., Huang, S.P., Pao, J.B., Hour, T.C., Chang, T.Y., Lan, Y.H., Lu, T.L., Lee, H.Z., Juang, S.H., Wu, P.P., Huang, C.Y., Hsieh, C.J. and Bao, B.Y. (2012) Genetic Polymorphisms in Oestrogen Receptor-Binding Sites Affect Clinical Outcomes in Patients with Prostate Cancer Receiving Androgen-Deprivation Therapy. *Journal of Internal Medicine*, **271**, 499-509. http://dx.doi.org/10.1111/j.1365-2796.2011.02449.x

[25] Huang, C.N., Huang, S.P., Pao, J.B., Chang, T.Y., Lan, Y.H., Lu, T.L., Lee, H.Z., Juang, S.H., Wu, P.P., Pu, Y.S., Hsieh, C.J. and Bao, B.Y. (2012) Genetic Polymorphisms in Androgen Receptor-Binding Sites Predict Survival in Prostate Cancer Patients Receiving Androgen-Deprivation Therapy. *Annals of Oncology: Official Journal of the European Society for Medical Oncology/ESMO*, **23**, 707-713.

[26] Yu, B.L., Lin, H.L., Yang, L.X., Chen, K., Luo, H.H., Liu, J.Q., Gao, X.C., Xia, X.F. and Huang, Z.F. (2012) Genetic Variation in the Nrf2 Promoter Associates with Defective Spermatogenesis in Humans. *Journal of Molecular Medicine*, **90**, 1333-1342. http://dx.doi.org/10.1007/s00109-012-0914-z

[27] Wu, J.M., Richards, M.H., Huang, J.H., Al-Harthi, L., Xu, X.L., Lin, R., Xie, F.L., Gibson, A.W., Edberg, J.C. and Kimberly, R.P. (2011) Human *FasL* Gene Is a Target of β-Catenin/T-Cell Factor Pathway and Complex *FasL* Haplotypes Alter Promoter Functions. *PLoS ONE*, **6**, Article ID: e26143. http://dx.doi.org/10.1371/journal.pone.0026143

[28] Alam, M., Pravica, V., Fryer, A.A., Hawkins, C.P. and Hutchinson, I.V. (2005) Novel Polymorphism in the Promoter Region of the Human Nerve Growth-Factor Gene. *International Journal of Immunogenetics*, **32**, 379-382. http://dx.doi.org/10.1111/j.1744-313X.2005.00541.x

[29] Bryne, J.C., Valen, E., Tang, M.H., Marstrand, T., Winther, O., da Piedade, I., Krogh, A., Lenhard, B. and Sandelin, A. (2008) JASPAR, the Open Access Database of Transcription Factor-Binding Profiles: New Content and Tools in the 2008 Update. *Nucleic Acids Research*, **36**, D102-D106.

[30] Sandelin, A., Alkema, W., Engstrom, P., Wasserman, W.W. and Lenhard, B. (2004) JASPAR: An Open-Access Database for Eukaryotic Transcription Factor Binding Profiles. *Nucleic Acids Research*, **32**, D91-D94.

[31] Sandelin, A., Wasserman, W.W. and Lenhard, B. (2004) ConSite: Web-Based Prediction of Regulatory Elements Using Cross-Species Comparison. *Nucleic Acids Research*, **32**, W249-W252.

[32] Pennisi, E. (2011) The Biology of Genomes. Disease Risk Links to Gene Regulation. *Science*, **332**, 1031. http://dx.doi.org/10.1126/science.332.6033.1031

[33] Kumar, V., Wijmenga, C. and Withoff, S. (2012) From Genome-Wide Association Studies to Disease Mechanisms: Celiac Disease as a Model for Autoimmune Diseases. *Seminars in Immunopathology*, **34**, 567-580. http://dx.doi.org/10.1007/s00281-012-0312-1

[34] Hindorff, L.A., Sethupathy, P., Junkins, H.A., Ramos, E.M., Mehta, J.P., Collins, F.S. and Manolio, T.A. (2009) Potential Etiologic and Functional Implications of Genome-Wide Association Loci for Human Diseases and Traits. *Pro-*

ceedings of the National Academy of Sciences of the United States of America, **106**, 9362-9367. http://dx.doi.org/10.1073/pnas.0903103106

[35] Kumar, V., Westra, H.J., Karjalainen, J., Zhernakova, D.V., Esko, T., Hrdlickova, B., Almeida, R., Zhernakova, A., Reinmaa, E., Vosa, U., Hofker, M.H., Fehrmann, R.S., Fu, J., Withoff, S., Metspalu, A., Franke, L. and Wijmenga, C. (2013) Human Disease-Associated Genetic Variation Impacts Large Intergenic Non-Coding RNA Expression. *PLoS Genetics*, **9**, Article ID: e1003201. http://dx.doi.org/10.1371/journal.pgen.1003201

[36] Chorley, B.N., Wang, X.T., Campbell, M.R., Pittman, G.S., Noureddine, M.A. and Bell, D.A. (2008) Discovery and Verification of Functional Single Nucleotide Polymorphisms in Regulatory Genomic Regions: Current and Developing Technologies. *Mutation Research*, **659**, 147-157. http://dx.doi.org/10.1016/j.mrrev.2008.05.001

[37] Prokunina, L. and Alarcon-Riquelme, M.E. (2004) Regulatory SNPs in Complex Diseases: Their Identification and Functional Validation. *Expert Reviews in Molecular Medicine*, **6**, 1-15. http://dx.doi.org/10.1017/S1462399404007690

[38] Buckland, P.R. (2006) The Importance and Identification of Regulatory Polymorphisms and Their Mechanisms of Action. *Biochimica et Biophysica Acta*, **1762**, 17-28. http://dx.doi.org/10.1016/j.bbadis.2005.10.004

[39] Sadee, W., Wang, D., Papp, A.C., Pinsonneault, J.K., Smith, R.M., Moyer, R.A. and Johnson, A.D. (2011) Pharmacogenomics of the RNA World: Structural RNA Polymorphisms in Drug Therapy. *Clinical Pharmacology & Therapeutics*, **89**, 355-365. http://dx.doi.org/10.1038/clpt.2010.314

[40] Wan, Y.I., Shrine, N.R., Soler Artigas, M., Wain, L.V., Blakey, J.D., Moffatt, M.F., Bush, A., Chung, K.F., Cookson, W.O., Strachan, D.P., Heaney, L., Al-Momani, B.A., Mansur, A.H., Manney, S., Thomson, N.C., Chaudhuri, R., Brightling, C.E., Bafadhel, M., Singapuri, A., Niven, R., Simpson, A., Holloway, J.W., Howarth, P.H., Hui, J., Musk, A.W., James, A.L., Brown, M.A., Baltic, S., Ferreira, M.A., Thompson, P.J., Tobin, M.D., Sayers, I. and Hall, I.P. (2012) Genome-Wide Association Study to Identify Genetic Determinants of Severe Asthma. *Thorax*, **67**, 762-768. http://dx.doi.org/10.1136/thoraxjnl-2011-201262

[41] Perin, P. and Potocnik, U. (2014) Polymorphisms in Recent GWA Identified Asthma Genes *CA*10, *SGK*493, and *CTNNA*3 Are Associated with Disease Severity and Treatment Response in Childhood Asthma. *Immunogenetics*, **66**, 143-151. http://dx.doi.org/10.1007/s00251-013-0755-0

[42] Torgerson, D.G., Ampleford, E.J., Chiu, G.Y., Gauderman, W.J., Gignoux, C.R., Graves, P.E., Himes, B.E., Levin, A.M., Mathias, R.A., Hancock, D.B., Baurley, J.W., Eng, C., Stern, D.A., Celedon, J.C., Rafaels, N., Capurso, D., Conti, D.V., Roth, L.A., Soto-Quiros, M., Togias, A., Li, X., Myers, R.A., Romieu, I., Van Den Berg, D.J., Hu, D., Hansel, N.N., Hernandez, R.D., Israel, E., Salam, M.T., Galanter, J., Avila, P.C., Avila, L., Rodriquez-Santana, J.R., Chapela, R., Rodriguez-Cintron, W., Diette, G.B., Adkinson, N.F., Abel, R.A., Ross, K.D., Shi, M., Faruque, M.U., Dunston, G.M., Watson, H.R., Mantese, V.J., Ezurum, S.C., Liang, L., Ruczinski, I., Ford, J.G., Huntsman, S., Chung, K.F., Vora, H., Calhoun, W.J., Castro, M., Sienra-Monge, J.J., del Rio-Navarro, B., Deichmann, K.A., Heinzmann, A., Wenzel, S.E., Busse, W.W., Gern, J.E., Lemanske Jr., R.F., Beaty, T.H., Bleecker, E.R., Raby, B.A., Meyers, D.A., London, S.J., Gilliland, F.D., Burchard, E.G., Martinez, F.D., Weiss, S.T., Williams, L.K., Barnes, K.C., Ober, C. and Nicolae, D.L. (2011) Meta-Analysis of Genome-Wide Association Studies of Asthma in Ethnically Diverse North American Populations. *Nature Genetics*, **43**, 887-892. http://dx.doi.org/10.1038/ng.888

Supplement

Table 1. Transcriptional factor (TF) descriptions.

TFs	TF description
AR	Steroid hormone receptors are ligand-activated transcription factors that regulate eukaryotic gene expression and affect cellular proliferation and differentiation in target tissues.
ARNT	Involved in the induction of several enzymes that participate in xenobiotic metabolism.
ARNT:AHR	The dimer alters transcription of target genes. Involved in the induction of several enzymes that participate in xenobiotic metabolism.
BRCA1	This gene encodes a nuclear phosphoprotein that plays a role in maintaining genomic stability, and it also acts as a tumor suppressor.
CREB1	This gene encodes a transcription factor that is a member of the leucine zipper family of DNA binding proteins
ELF5	A member of an epithelium-specific subclass of the Ets transcritpion factor family.
ELK1	The protein encoded by this gene is a nuclear target for the ras-raf-MAPK signaling cascade.
ELK4	Involved in both transcriptional activation and repression.
EN1	Homeobox-containing genes are thought to have a role in controlling development.
ETS1	The protein encoded by this gene belongs to the ETS family of transcription factors and has been shown to interact with TTRAP, UBE2I and Death associated protein.
FEV	It functions as a transcriptional repressor.
FOXC1	This gene belongs to the forkhead family of transcription factors which is characterized by a distinct DNA-binding forkhead domain. An important regulator of cell viability and resistance to oxidative stress.
FOXL1	FOX transcription factors are characterized by a distinct DNA-binding forkhead domain and play critical roles in the regulation of multiple processes including metabolism, cell proliferation and gene expression during ontogenesis.
GATA2	A member of the GATA family of zinc-finger transcription factors that are named for the consensus nucleotide sequence they bind in the promoter regions of target genes and play an essential role in regulating transcription of genes involved in the development and proliferation of hematopoietic and endocrine cell lineages.
GATA3	Plays an important role in endothelial cell biology.
HAND1:TCFE2α	Hand1 belongs to the basic helix-loop-helix family of transcription factors. The Tcfe2a gene encodes the transcription factor E2A, a member of the "class I" a family of basic helix-loop-helix (bHLH) transcription factors (also known simply as "E-proteins"). The transcription factor E2A controls the initiation of B lymphopoiesis.
HIF1α:ARNT	HIF1 is a homodimeric basic helix-loop-helix structure composed of HIF1a, the alpha subunit, and the aryl hydrocarbon receptor nuclear translocator (Arnt), the beta subunit. The protein encoded by HIF1 is a Per-Arnt-Sim (PAS) transcription factor found in mammalian cells growing at low oxygen concentrations. It plays an essential role in cellular and systemic responses to hypoxia.
HLTF	This gene encodes a member of the SWI/SNF family. Members of this family have helicase and ATPase activities and are thought to regulate transcription of certain genes by altering the chromatin structure around those genes.
HNF4α	The encoded protein controls the expression of several genes, including hepatocyte nuclear factor 1 alpha, a transcription factor which regulates the expression of several hepatic genes
INSM1	This gene is a sensitive marker for neuroendocrine differentiation of human lung tumors.
KLF4	Transcription factor that can act both as activator and as repressor. Regulates the expression of key transcription factors during embryonic development.
MAFB	The encoded nuclear protein represses ETS1-mediated transcription of erythroid-specific genes in myeloid cells.
MAX	The protein encoded by this gene is a member of the basic helix-loop-helix leucine zipper (bHLHZ) family of transcription factors
MZF1_1-4	Binds to target promoter DNA and functions as trancription regulator. May be one regulator of transcriptional events during hemopoietic development. Isoforms of this protein have been shown to exist at protein level.
MZF1_1-5-13	Binds to target promoter DNA and functions as trancription regulator. May be one regulator of transcriptional events during hemopoietic development. Isoforms of this protein have been shown to exist at protein level.
NFE2L1:MafG	Nuclear factor erythroid 2-related factor (Nrf2) coordinates the up-regulation of cytoprotective genes via the antioxidant response element (ARE). MafG is a ubiquitously expressed small maf protein that is involved in cell differentiation of erythrocytes. It dimerizes with P45 NF-E2 protein and activates expression of a and b-globin.

Continued

NFIC	Recognizes and binds the palindromic sequence 5'-TTGGCNNNNNGCCAA-3' present in viral and cellular promoters and in the origin of replication of adenovirus type 2. These proteins are individually capable of activating transcription and replication.
NKX2-5	This gene encodes a member of the NK family of homeobox-containing proteins. Transcriptional repressor that acts as a negative regulator of chondrocyte maturation.
NOBOX	This homeobox gene encodes a transcription factor that is thought to play a role in oogenesis.
NR2E3	This protein is part of a large family of nuclear receptor transcription factors involved in signaling pathways.
NR2F1	Coup (chicken ovalbumin upstream promoter) transcription factor binds to the ovalbumin promoter and, in conjunction with another protein (S300-II) stimulates initiation of transcription.
NR3C1	Glucocorticoids regulate carbohydrate, protein and fat metabolism, modulate immune responses through suppression of chemokine and cytokine production and have critical roles in constitutive activity of the CNS, digestive, hematopoietic, renal and reproductive systems.
NR4A2	Transcriptional regulator which is important for the differentiation and maintenance of meso-diencephalic dopaminergic (mdDA) neurons during development.
PAX2	Probable transcription factor that may have a role in kidney cell differentiation.
SOX17	Acts as transcription regulator that binds target promoter DNA and bends the DNA.
SP1	Can activate or repress transcription in response to physiological and pathological stimuli. Regulates the expression of a large number of genes involved in a variety of processes such as cell growth, apoptosis, differentiation and immune responses.
SPI1	This gene encodes an ETS-domain transcription factor that activates gene expression during myeloid and B-lymphoid cell development.
SPZ1	This gene encodes a bHLH-zip transcription factor which functions in the mitogen-activate protein kinase (MAPK) signaling pathway.
TFAP2A	The protein encoded by this gene is a transcription factor that binds the consensus sequence 5'-GCCNNNGGC-3' and activates the transcription of some genes while inhibiting the transcription of others.
USF1	This gene encodes a member of the basic helix-loop-helix leucine zipper family, and can function as a cellular. transcription factor.
YY1	Multifunctional transcription factor that exhibits positive and negative control on a large number of cellular and viral genes by binding to sites overlapping the transcription start site
ZEB1	This gene encodes a zinc finger transcription factor. Acts as a transcriptional repressor.
ZFX	A member of the kruеppel C2H2-type zinc-finger protein family and probable transcriptional activator.
ZNF354C	May function as a transcription repressor.

18

Overview of Intervention Programs for Parents of Young Children (0 - 6)

Merav Goldblatt, Rivka Yahav, Tsameret Ricon

Faculty of Social Welfare & Health Sciences, University of Haifa, Haifa, Israel
Email: tricon@univ.haifa.ac.il

Abstract

In most of the world's societies and cultures, the biological mother and father bear primary responsibility to care for their child's needs and to guide him or her through the process of entry into society [1]. The parent serves, for the most part, as the significant figure with the greatest amount of influence over the child's life. Through his parent, the child learns the skills necessary to experience the world and function in it, whether the skills are in relation to survival needs such as eating, washing and mobility or developmental and social needs such as forming social relationships and developing the capacity to think and learn through play and supervision [2]. Thus the parent plays a critical but complex role in the development of his or her child, a role that requires development of a wide range of new behavioral, communicational, cognitive and emotional skills and capabilities in order to understand and cope with the challenges of child-rearing. Similarly, parenting styles and characteristics are influenced by a number of variables: The parent, the child, the interaction between them, and environmental variables such as culture, socio-economic status, and the existing family unit [2]. When children who suffer from behavioral difficulties do not receive the parental care they need, there is reasonable cause for concern that difficulties will develop in adulthood in a range of life areas that will have an impact on their lives and well-being and on their ability to adapt to society and contribute to it [3]. Accordingly, over the past 50 years parent-training programs have been developed to strengthen parents through learning and providing tools of experience and developmental knowledge, for the purpose of promoting the child's sense of wellbeing and quality of life [2] [4]. Objective: The purpose of this review is to provide an overview of evidence-based interventions for parents of young children (0 - 6), programs that are currently active in Israel and in the world, and to explicate the significant characteristics common to them that contribute to their effectiveness and success.

Keywords

Interventions for Parents, Early Development, Young Children, Review

1. Introduction

Raising a child in a nurturing and enriching environment while providing warmth, love and encouragement, in secure boundaries, is one of the parent's main functions [5]. When children who suffer from various difficulties do not receive the parental care they need, there is a reasonable cause for concern that difficulties will develop in adulthood in a range of life areas that will have an impact on their lives and well-being and on their ability to adapt to society and contribute to it [6]. Accordingly, over the past 50 years parent training programs have been developed to strengthen parents through learning and providing tools of experience and developmental knowledge, for the purpose of promoting the child's sense of wellbeing and quality of life [2] [4].

The purpose of this document is to provide an overview of evidence-based interventions currently active in Israel and in the world for parents of young children (0 - 6), and to explicate the significant common characteristics that contribute to their effectiveness and success.

1.1. Parent's Role and Early Detection

In most of the world's societies and cultures, the biological mother and father bear primary responsibility to care for their child's needs and to guide him or her through the process of his entry into society [1]. The parent serves, for the most part, as the most significant and influential figure in the life of the child. The parent is also a medium for the child to learn problem-solving skills, as their lives together with the inevitable problems along the way provide endless opportunities for learning [2] [5].

The motor, cognitive, emotional and social development of children aged 0 - 6 influences and shapes their later lives [5]. Parenting itself is a necessary component in child development in all area of life. Through his parent the child learns the skills necessary to experience the world and function in it, whether the skills are in relation to survival needs such as eating, washing and mobility or developmental and social needs such as forming social relationships and developing the capacity to think and learn through play and supervision [2]. Good parenting has been found to be a predictor of positive social, behavioral, emotional and academic adjustment. In contrast, problematic parenting has been found to be a predictor of antisocial behavior and functional difficulties later on in life [7]. Thus the parent plays a critical but complex role in the development of his or her child, a role that requires development of a wide range of new behavioral, communicational, cognitive and emotional skills and capabilities in order to understand and cope with the challenges of child-rearing. Similarly, parenting styles and characteristics are influenced by a number of variables: The parent, the child, the interaction between them, and environmental variables such as culture, socio-economic status, and the existing family unit [2].

Parenting requires one to develop new skills in order to understand and cope with raising the child. For example, behavioral problems that disturb daily routines and include aggression, resistance and disobedience are regularly seen among children [8]. When children who suffer from these behavioral difficulties do not receive the required care there is reasonable cause for concern that difficulties will arise in adulthood in a range of life areas: learning, work, interpersonal relations, addictions (alcohol, drugs), as well as development of emotional difficulties and psychiatric diagnoses [9] [10]. In addition, one of the significant findings in longitudinal studies that examine antisocial and criminal behavior is that chronically antisocial behaviors that appear early in life usually lead to criminal behavior and lives of crime later on. In light of this, it is extremely important that policies for intervention and prevention should start in early childhood [3]. Early investment, in early childhood, empowers the child in the family context, increases the chances of successful integration in educational, social, and community frameworks, and prevents the need for intervention at later stages [2].

1.2. Parent Training Programs

Identification of the significant effect of parental behavior during early stages of life upon child development and behavior precipitated the need to develop modes of therapeutic work with parents [4] [5]). Therapeutic work with parents exists in a number of forms and models, including a number of types of intervention in which the parent is not the main focus, with therapy defined as "with" the parent (Parental therapy/guidance), and interventions in which therapeutic work focuses on the parent himself (Parenthood Therapy) [11]. Three types of common interventions with parents can be identified:

1) Meeting with parents in parallel to child therapy—The emphasis is on child therapy and the parent is accompanied and connected to the process the child is undergoing. The change in the parent will take place indirectly and especially as a result of his own independent work.

2) Parental guidance—The emphasis is upon changing patterns of parenting, with or without child therapy. This is a psycho-educational intervention that includes teaching models of child development as a basis for understanding the child's needs, and advice on effective parenting derived from both cognitive and dynamic schools of thought.

3) Therapeutic interventions with parents in the context of dyadic (relational) therapy or parent-child therapy—This intervention can sometimes have significant and deep, though indirect impact on parenting.

In this document we will focus on intervention programs with the parent (mostly 2 and 3 above). Beginning in the 1960's a number of research groups began to develop parent training programs which by now have a broad base of research [2]. This relates to programs that strengthen parenting through learning and provision of tools of experience and developmental knowledge [11], with the ultimate goal of promoting the child and parent's sense of wellbeing and quality of life [2] [4] [12].

The parent training programs developed over the years are many and diverse. The programs differ with regard to the models and methodologies that underlie them, so that while the emphasis in some of the programs is solely on didactic learning (technical transfer of structured knowledge via a lecture or watching a movie), others place an emphasis on learning through doing, where the parent learns skills by practicing with the child and the therapist in the clinic and in a natural setting [4] [13] [14]. Similarly, programs are characterized by a diverse range of content (developmental knowledge about the child, parental sense of agency, communication skills, strategies of behavioral management and more); turn to different target populations (special and regular populations); and include different settings (clinic, home visits, parent groups, and individual therapy). The programs also expanded to include not only behavioral problems but also to relate to and improve the child's cognitive development, anxieties, and general health [12].

1.3. Training Programs Characteristics

Despite the existing difference and diversity, training programs for parents include similar characteristics, with the most important being: 1) evaluating the problems and difficulties that the parents are facing; 2) training the parent to use new coping skills; 3) practicing use of these skills with the child; 4) feedback on implementation of the skills [15]. In most of the programs the primary work of the therapist with the parent(s) is identifying and interpreting the child's behavior and developing the skills required for coping accordingly.

The parents experience different techniques of role play, group or individual discussion, watching training movies and getting feedback in order to actively practice the use of strategies vis a vis the child. Many programs include homework in order to improve the likelihood of generalization and transfer of the knowledge and experience gained in the clinic under controlled conditions, to the dynamic environment in the home [2] [8].

1.4. Parent Training in the Light of Research

On the whole it seems that programs led by therapists have proven to be effective in promoting positive change in the behavior of both child and parent, in the communication between them, and in improving the self-image of the parent [2] [8] [12] [16]. Studies that examined the effectiveness of programs over time showed that the influence of these programs is maintained over time and can contribute to lessening the child's behavioral difficulties and antisocial and criminal behavior in his later life and in all areas of life [3].

2. Intervention Programs

Intervention programs can be divided into three main sections: 1) Interventions type; 2) Intervention categorized by professions (nursing, occupational therapy, nutrition, communication disorders and psychology); 3) Intervention directed to specific type of populations. Interventions for parents are surveyed with regard to the background, rationale and goals, in addition to a description of the process and effectiveness. In reviewing the current research we will address whole sections. We will also review two additional categories: Parent-child intervention programs prevalent in the world and popular intervention programs that are not evidence-based. A summary of the categorized intervention programs is added in **Table 1**.

2.1. Interventions Categorized by Professions

Parent-Child Interventions in Sleep Difficulties

Today it is well known that sleep fills important functions in the first years of development, including the de-

Table 1. List of the categorized intervention programs.

Interventions categorized by professions	Overview of parent-child intervention programs by population	Parent-child intervention programs prevalent in the world	Popular intervention programs that are not evidence-based
1) Parent-child interventions in sleep difficulties	1) Four parent-child intervention programs during pregnancy	1) Living with children	1) PET-Parent Effectiveness Training
2) Occupational therapy: Three Intervention Programs	2) Overview of mixed programs for single-parent mothers	2) The incredible years	2) STEP—Systematic Training for Effective Parenting
3) Physical therapy: Five intervention programs	3) Intervention programs for fathers	3) HNC—Helping The Noncompliant Child	3) Triple P: Positive Parenting Program (USA)
4) Communication disorders: Two intervention programs in the areas of language and literacy.	4) Healthy family America for at-risk populations	4) PCIT—Parent Child Interaction Therapy	4) EHS—Early Head Start (USA)
5) Nutrition: Community intervention to promote healthy life habits among children and youth			
6) Psychology: Three parent-child intervention programs focused on attachment			

velopment of the nervous systems, growth, motor development, behavioral and emotional regulation, and cognitive functioning [17]-[21]. Sleep disturbances at a young age are among the most common complaints presented by parents to pediatricians and other professionals, at a rate of 20% - 30% [22]. These complaints include difficulties falling asleep and waking up during the night, called in professional language "childhood behavioral insomnia" [23].

Sleep difficulties are a product of the interaction between parents and children and therefore any therapeutic intervention needs to be directed at changing the behaviors of parents and children. Since many parents have mistaken perceptions and lack knowledge about proper sleep patterns and habits among children, and this expresses itself in over-involvement and in difficulties in setting clear limits regarding sleep, interventions rely upon a cognitive-behavioral approach. The behavioral component is designed to extinguish the positive conditioning that was created when at the time parents, when putting their child to sleep, are busy trying to calm the child (for example: rocking the carriage, driving in a car, or falling asleep in the parent's bed) instead of allowing him to develop mechanisms for self-calming and the ability to fall asleep on his own.

Treatment of sleep disturbances at a young age is important not only from a developmental perspective [21]. Sleep disturbances tend to be maintained for years [24], and they have a significant impact on the emotional wellbeing and quality of life of the parents [25].

There is a great deal of evidence in the scientific literature about the effectiveness of parenting interventions for treating or preventing sleep disturbances among young children (0 - 6) [26]-[28]. These interventions include psycho-educational counseling to parents, behavioral extinction (full or gradual), and building a sleep routine. Cognitive Behavioral Therapy for Insomnia (CBT-I) is today considered the treatment of choice for insomnia among adults [29], and its long-term effectiveness is even greater than medication therapies [30]. This treatment has been found effective also for behavioral insomnia among children, with a success rate of 94% in reducing problems of falling asleep and wakening during the night, and 82% in follow-ups over periods of 3 - 6 months [31]. The physiological factors in early childhood sleep disorders are clear, including breathing disorders in sleep, asthma and disturbances in the digestive system. Treatments can be provided before or in parallel to cognitive-behavioral treatment.

The system of beliefs, expectations and interpretations of parents about their children's sleep are related to as a basis for leading to a change in behavior. These cognitions are often related to issues of setting limits, limiting parental involvement and the interpretation given to the meaning of the child's waking up at night. Parents enhance their knowledge and awareness about sleep and learn strategies for promoting healthy sleep habits in early childhood. The emotional component of the parents is also related to, including expression of fears about the child's resilience and his ability to manage with limited parental involvement during the night, as well as feelings of guilt, doubts and resistances to treatment. Cognitive treatment before beginning behavioral interventions often increases parental compliance.

Extinction of the positive conditioning that developed when parents were involved in calming the child during the night, by gradually decreasing parental involvement. According to this method, in the course of putting the child to bed, the parent gives the child a clear message that he is not alone, but that he must fall asleep on his own. The parent leaves the child in the bed and comes for a brief visit at fixed intervals (typically every 5 minutes), until the child falls asleep. This process lasts for a number of days until the child learns to fall asleep on his own without crying or protest. During visits the child should not be taken out of the bed, and the visit should be kept brief (one minute or less). In addition, parents should be helped to establish a fixed sleep routine every night and to be consistent with it over time. It should be taken into account that the child will express protest during the course of this process, and many parents will have difficulty coping with this resistance and maintaining the changes, fearing that they may be causing their child harm.

This treatment is found to be effective in many studies and to this day no negative effects have been reported regarding the behavioral method [21].

2.2. Occupational Therapy: Three Intervention Programs

Background: In recent decades pediatric occupational therapists have developed early intervention programs designed to improve parents' sense of competence, based on relationships of partnership with families and with an emphasis on the interaction between the parent and child [32]-[33].

Rationale and goals: In most of the early intervention programs the occupational therapists place an emphasis upon parent participation in play activities in order to teach them about the needs of the child and about their own needs as parents [34]. It is important to note that some of these intervention programs are in the consultation model of the occupational therapist and some include a model of direct intervention, even though no significant difference has been found in the effectiveness of either model [35]. The professional literature shows that the therapist's focus on strengthening the parent-child interaction and improving their attachment patterns leads to an improvement in additional developmental components, such as the child's cognitive development over the years [36]. Similarly an emphasis is placed in the interventions on the relationship between improved parental sensitivity to "signs" that the child transmits and an improvement in the level of "playfulness" and motivation of the child, the degree of the child's independence and inquiry, and his capacity for social interaction [37].

Modes of intervention:

1) A prevention program held for mothers of typical babies in lower socioeconomic neighborhoods in Jerusalem [33].

In this program mothers held meetings once every other month with an occupational therapist in the Tipot Halav, during the course of the child's first year. These meetings included providing information and modeling for the mother about sensory-motor, language and cognitive activities.

Effectiveness of the intervention: In a study of the effects of the program after about two years it was found that the mothers in the intervention group had more knowledge about child development, improved perceptions of their ability to contribute their child's wellbeing and development, and better implementation of developmental knowledge compared to a control group.

2) An early intervention program for mothers of typical young children (ages 2.5 - 3 years) [34] that was implemented in Australia.

The goal of this intervention program was to encourage mother-child interaction by means of play and to expand the mother's knowledge about child development. The intervention took place over the course of ten weekly meetings and was based on the activity of preparing a game or demonstrating games. In the program the following outcome measurements were taken before the intervention, at its conclusion, and after one and a half years: The way the mother relates to causality with regard to the child's behavior, the extent of parental tension, the mother's self-image as an educator, the child's temperament and behavior.

Effectiveness of the intervention: While no change was found in the quantitative outcome measures between the intervention group and the control group, participants were found to be satisfied with the intervention program, and they reported that they implemented the knowledge they had gained in initiating playgroups of mothers in the community.

3) A group intervention of occupational therapists on the issue of time management and improving mothers' occupational performance.

Mothers were given support and provided with various strategies for improving family time management (establishing family rules, delegating responsibility, managing time demands and more) [38].

Effectiveness of the intervention: Focus groups were held in which mothers reported on feelings of personal empowerment, wellbeing with regard to child care and the learning of strategies for coping with daily tasks and the burdensome routine [39].

Additional important principles for successful intervention:

- Focus on the parent-child interaction as a "therapeutic tool, evaluating the parents' perceptions and values, providing the parent with positive reinforcement and including him in the therapeutic process" [40]. Moreover, in terms of the strategies occupational therapists use during early interventions, it was found that the most effective strategies are creating joint interaction of the therapist with the parent and child, and taking advantage of the learning opportunities that present themselves during the course of the interaction [41].
- Occupational therapist's relating to the management of the mothers' time while designing early interventions [42] [43]. This in order that the interventions will fit in with family routines, will not place a burden on the already overburdened mothers of young children, and will contribute to the mother's quality of life and to the wellbeing of the family [44].
- Understanding the home environment and the objects in it in order to integrate intervention goals with the family routine and daily play situations [45]. In a study that examined the way in which mothers managed the home environment in order to encourage developmental play of typical babies aged 1 - 18 months [46] it was found that mothers had different strategies for managing play objects in the house and for organizing and maintaining the home environment so that it would support the infant's development.

2.3. Physical Therapy: Five Intervention Programs

Background: Around the 1980's professionals began to get a deep appreciation of the importance of early intervention programs, especially during early childhood. Most of the intervention programs in the field of physical therapy are hands-on programs, in other words the treatment is mostly performed by skilled physical therapists.

Rationale and goals: In the last decade there is an increased appreciation of the role and importance of the parent in treatment, and it subsequently has received a central place in research studies. Involving parents in treatment itself, whether as assistants to the therapist or as providers of treatment themselves, improves the parent's understanding and ability to help his child on both the motor and mental levels, promotes the child's development and achievement of developmental milestones, and helps the parents to create a safe environment adapted to their child [47].

Modes of intervention:

Studies chosen for the survey are examples of studies in which physical therapy counseling to parents, whether of children at risk or children with developmental disorders, is a core program component:

1) The effectiveness of mother-child counseling relative to learning the technique of NDT therapy, for mothers whose babies have been diagnosed with CP at the age of 8 - 32 months [48] (USA).

In the context of the intervention mothers in the experimental group were supervised by a physical therapist, and taught how to improve the mother-baby interaction with an emphasis on adjusted positioning, while mothers in the control group received NDT therapy and were supervised in only one technique in accordance with the baby's needs.

Effectiveness of the intervention: Outcomes showed significant success in changing the behavior of the mother and baby in the experimental group-mothers were more engaged in positive initiative/coaching and in face-to-face response, than mothers in the control group. In addition, babies in the experimental group responded better to their mothers. This change in the behaviors of mothers and babies is considered significant to the child's independent development in the rest of his life.

2) An intervention program for improving the motor abilities of premature infants [49] (Thailand).

A sample was taken from the intervention population of premature infants (born prior to week 37) with no genetic abnormal disorders, without bleeding in the brain, operations, hydrocephalus or Retinopathies. The intervention program included a total of 12 activities per child by the main therapist, from standard week 40. Every week until the age of 3 months, training and practice took place in the subjects' homes. Babies were checked by the TIMP test for neuro-motor behavioral assessment and the therapist was interviewed. In addition the therapists were asked to demonstrate the exercises and everything was documented on video.

Effectiveness of the intervention: While there was a significant improvement in the TIPM results in the experimental group in a measurement at 4 months of age, no difference was found between groups.

3) Counseling of new mothers with the goal of lessening the risk for postpartum depression, which is a risk factor for the baby's motor and emotional development [50] (Australia).

The intervention program lasted eight weeks and included an hour of joint physical activity for mothers and babies and a half hour lesson on healthy living. The intervention began in the 6th - 10th week after birth.

Effectiveness of the intervention: Researchers found a significant improvement in the rating of well-being and a decreased level of depression in the experimental group in comparison to the control group. This study shows that routine use of a program of exercise and healthy lifestyle education can reduce long-term problems such as postpartum depression.

4) An early intervention program called COPCA (Coping with and Caring for Infants with special needs) is focused on the family of a baby with CP in comparison with physical therapy using the NDT method [51] (Holland).

The study was performed with two groups, one of traditional physical therapy in accordance with the NDT, and the second with COPCA. Treatment was provided by licensed physical therapists once a week over the period of a year in the family's home.

Effectiveness of the intervention: Outcomes were not provided, but the researchers assume that COPCA will have positive outcomes because the program provides parents with positive strategies for coping with different situations, and consequently it should lead to better results on the child's motor and cognitive tests.

5) A para-professional home-visiting program for an at-risk, low socioeconomic population [52] (USA).

The program accompanies first-time parents, beginning during pregnancy, in the home. The goals of the program are to promote pregnancy health, child development, and mother's wellbeing. Home visits continued until the age of two, becoming more frequent as pregnancy advanced, and after birth visits were once a week and then every other week.

Effectiveness of the intervention: The study found lower percentages of child abuse, fewer immediate pregnancies, a higher quality of mother-child interaction, less behavioral problems among the children, and better language development among the research population.

2.4. Communication Disorders: Two Intervention Programs in the Areas of Language and Literacy

Background: Many studies show that language development, like the early signs of literacy, takes place long before the child meets the formal educational settings such as the daycare center, pre-school setting and school. Already in the first year of life, even before the appearance of the first words, there is a rich and complex communication between the baby and parent. Watching, making noises and use of gestures are the means at the baby's disposal, and their integration makes possible the development of reciprocal relations and communication with the environment [53]. In different studies it has been found that daily reading of stories and a reading style in which parents talk about the story and respond to the child's comments and questions, support the child's development of language, contribute to expanding his vocabulary and assist in improving his ability to understand and to express himself [53] [54]. It has also been found that reading stories encourages the child's awareness of the role and use of written language (Concept about Print) and awakens a positive attitude toward story reading [55]. Socio-interactive theories that seek to explain the process of language acquisition emphasize the importance of social support and contextual framing in the process of language development thereby highlighting the importance of reading stories in general and more specifically as part of an intervention program for children with language difficulties.

Rationale and goals: The concept underlying intervention programs in the area of language and literacy is that language is an important tool in the development of socialization in general and more specifically in the development of linguistic socialization. Active participation in verbal interactions promotes linguistic-social communication and shapes thinking and cultural values [56] [57]. In Israel there are many intervention programs sponsored by the Ministry of Education or various philanthropic organizations. These programs operate within the formal educational system only from the age of 3. Children from birth to age 3 who participate in formal frameworks under the auspices of organizations such as WIZO and NAAMAT, and under the supervision of the

Ministry of Industry and Commerce, are mostly exposed to philanthropic intervention programs (for example of the Caring Commission of UJA-Federation of New York). From among the variety of programs offered throughout the world (and whose documentation can be found in the literature) that deal with support of families in need, the focus will be on those that meet the following criteria: Programs built on the basis of collection of longitudinal data on a wide range of measures in the home and in educational frameworks, data taken from a representative sample that makes possible conclusions and generalizations, programs that examined their effectiveness with methods of Evidence Based Practice, those that clearly formulate the theoretical rationale underlying program design, and provide a detailed and comprehensive description of how it is carried out. The two programs that will be presented below begin with the assumption, proven in many studies, that development of linguistic capacity, the quality of verbal interaction between the child and his parents, and the nurturing of emergent literacy in pre-school years, are all strong predictors of school success [58] [59].

Modes of intervention:

1) The parent-child home program (USA) [60].
(http://www.cebc4cw.org/program/the-parent-child-home-program/detailed).

The target population is poor families, single-parent families, young parents, or immigrants. The program serves children aged 2 - 4 years, and places an emphasis upon the quality of linguistic interaction and communication between parents and children, on social and emotional development, and on nurturing emergent literacy as preparation for school. Work with families takes place in the home environment and the parents are exposed to a model of enriching interaction with the child. The goal of the intervention is to enhance the quality and quantity of verbal interactions, strengthening the parent's sense of self as a parent, developing language and literacy skills and increasing the child's social behavior. The program last for two years and the facilitators visit the family's home twice a week. Families receive books and toys that enrich the literacy environment in the home. The program does not offer the family activities beyond the time in which the facilitator is in the family's home. Facilitators undergo a sixteen-hour preparatory workshop and meet weekly in learning and support group (a detailed guide can be purchased with full details and recommendations for program implementation).

2) Home instruction for parents of preschool youngsters [61].
(http://www.cebc4cw.org/program/home-instruction-for-parents-of-preschool-youngsters/detailed).

This program is intended for children from birth to 5 years of age in families living in poverty whose home environments put them at high risk for developmental delay. The goal of the program is to foster language ability and emergent literacy in preparation for school. Program facilitators go into the family home but do not make direct contact with the children, rather they do role playing with the parents with regard to proposed activities and to how to establish communication with the child. Together with entry into the home the program also offers group meetings for parents in order to create a supportive and enriching parent group. The program last for three years but the frequency of meetings is not documented. In this program the families receive books and work books for activities with the children beyond the meetings with the facilitator (a guide can be purchased with all of the details and recommendations for program implementation).

2.5. Nutrition: Community intervention to Promote Healthy Life Habits among Children and Youth

Background: The project is intended to establish a community health promotion program in lower socio-economic neighborhoods in Haifa. The need for such a program is clear in light of the evidence that lifestyle in early life has implications for development of chronic illnesses, such as heart disease and diabetes, at a later age, as well as implications for social functioning and quality of life during childhood and adulthood. Improving the quality of nutrition and level of activity among children is particularly important in light of the increase in rates of obesity, primarily in the lower socio-economic strata. It is important to emphasize that weight loss among children is not one of the program's goals. Instead the aim is to help parents and their children to adopt healthier lifestyles.

In early childhood the family environment is particularly important to the development of food preferences, eating habits and style, and exercise routines. Children's food consumption is influenced by their preferences and by their sense of hunger and satiation, but also by the type of foods that their parents put before them and make accessible. It has been demonstrated that when children are offered a variety of healthy foods they choose a diet that meets the criteria for a healthy diet with no need of parental intervention. Of course this situation is the opposite to what actually happens in an environment in which there is an abundance of processed foods loaded with calories and an encouragement of a sedentary lifestyle [62].

Intervention processes: Behavioral therapy is considered the first line of treatment for child and adolescent obesity. Behavioral therapy includes teaching parents and children about goal setting, preventing relapse, problem solving and managing the surrounding environment such that it will encourage good nutrition and physical activity. All of the programs that involve young children the parents are also involved, since it is they that mostly control their child's nutrition. Findings from different programs show that an effective program needs to focus on instructions for parents designed to foster eating patterns and food choices that are suitable to a healthy diet. Instruction to parents needs to include an explanation of how children develop eating habits in the family context. Practical instruction for parents includes tools for fostering choice of healthy foods and encouraging children to accept new food. Similarly, parents should be provided with information that is practical and easily understood about the size of portions appropriate for children, and suggestions about the timing and frequency of meals and stacks [63].

The program "Tailor-made for me" of the Israel Ministry of Education (www.tafuralay.co.il) is implemented both in pre-school settings and schools in Israel. The advantage of the program is that it is adapted to the Israeli population and its effectiveness has been demonstrated through research [62] [63]. The nutritional intervention was planned especially to improve knowledge about nutrition and includes learning topics through lectures and discussions. All of the sessions are led by pre-school teachers and are adapted to their level. In addition, the children bring their parents monthly information sheets that discuss various issues related to nutrition. The children are encouraged to share their nutritional information with their parents, and the parents are asked to discuss the issue with their children.

The primary goals are promoting healthy eating habits, an active lifestyle among the children and their parents, and developing a program for preventing child obesity. The program has additional more specific goals such as encouraging nursing and eating breakfast, limiting "television time", and more.

2.6. Psychology: Three Parent-Child Intervention Programs Focused on Attachment

Background: An important aspect of parenting is helping the child by providing appropriate responses and creating safe attachment, to develop his internal regulatory systems in a manner appropriate to the requirements of the environment [64]. The mother's state of attachment during pregnancy is found to be related to the quality and degree of the infant's level of security in attachment [65].

Difficulty in internal regulation occurs when the parent has difficulty providing appropriate care and can be expressed on the emotional, behavioral and physiological levels. Children whose needs were not met are at a high level of risk to develop difficulties in the long term that are related to problems in emotional and behavioral self-regulation such as a tendency to use addictive substances and criminal behavior. Thus parents need to provide the child with a same, predictable and controllable environment that supports the child in his development of self-regulatory skills [66]. Similarly, studies show that the mother's capacity to reflect on her functioning is a central component in her ability to transmit and create attachment to the child [65]. These findings support the building of interventions that give tools for reflective functioning, thereby encouraging creation of secure attachment between mother and child.

1) Attachment and bio-behavioral catch-up intervention (ABC) [67] (USA).

Rationale and intervention goals: In order to narrow biological, behavioral and emotional gaps related to the child's primary relational systems (attachment), an intervention program was designed that focused upon counseling the parent on how to develop his capacities to provide adapted responses and a secure environment. This program focused on a population of toddlers in foster families in order to examine the extent to which it is possible to rehabilitate disturbances in the child's primary attachments with his main caretakers. An additional assumption underlying the study was that early intervention would have more significant and extensive impact than interventions done in later years.

Course of intervention: The program focuses on development of the child's self-regulatory capacities. It includes three main intervention areas: Helping the (foster) parent to interpret the child's rejection behaviors, counseling the parent how to overcome their own issues that prevent them from providing nurturing care, and on how to provide the child with an environment that encourages development of self-regulatory capacities (helping the child to identify emotions and express them appropriately, providing appropriate sensory stimuli). The intervention program has an organized guidebook, with topics divided over ten weekly meetings, held in the family's home by a professional therapist, and activities are adapted to a range of ages. Meetings are active and include hands-on counseling together with the child, joint discussions. Sessions are filmed so that they can later be jointly analyzed.

Intervention Effectiveness: A random controlled experiment (RCT) performed with 60 children to evaluate the program found positive outcomes showing that performance of a formal time-limited program promoted the development of self-regulatory capacity among children in foster care. In the experimental group that participated in the program the children produced more appropriate levels of cortizol in comparison to the control group. In addition, parents of children in the experimental group reported fewer behavioral problems.

2) The Circle of Security Intervention (COS) [68] (USA).

Rationale and intervention goals: There is a great deal of evidence that the quality of attachment between the parent and child in the first years of life has an important impact on his development and on his becoming an independent adult. Insecure attachment is found in the literature to be a risk factor for development of psychopathology later in life.

Accordingly the goal of the program is to counsel the parent on how to be more attentive to the child and to himself in order to develop secure attachment. In addition, an emphasis is placed on self-evaluation of the parent-child attachment existing prior to performance of the intervention, so that the therapist can know what the child has learned about how to participate in a relationship with the parent and direct the intervention to his unique needs.

The course of intervention: The program is comprised of a set protocol including 20 weekly group meetings (5 - 6 parents) an hour and a quarter each. Meetings include therapeutic and educational components, and are led by a licensed psychotherapist. The protocols are based on attachment theory and are appropriate for both intervention and prevention. The program has five key components: a) Establishing the group as a safe space in which the parent can reflect upon his relationship with his child; b) Improving the parent's ability to provide his child with adapted and sensitive responses by learning about the child's basic attachment needs; c) Improving the parent's ability to interpret manifest and latent signs that the child exhibits to make its needs known; d) Increasing the parent's ability to feel empathy through use of reflections on the child's and parent's behaviors; e) Increasing the parent's ability to understand how his own developmental history affects his current abilities as a parent.

The first meetings are devoted to educational and didactic aspects of the issue of attachment. During the following meetings the therapist, following a set protocol, focuses on each parent and generates active discussions on each topic through the use of short video films.

Intervention effectiveness: A longitudinal study with measurements before and after the intervention examined whether parents and children from at-risk populations who participated in the program transitioned between types of parent-child attachment. Findings of the study were positive and showed that the program could help to reduce characteristics of insecure attachment for young children. About 70% of the children categorized as belonging to the "disorganized" type of insecure attachment were categorized following the intervention as belonging to the secure attachment group. The researchers attributed this change to the contribution of the program to the parent's ability to identify and reflect upon his own defensive strategies that previously had prevented him from responding sensitively and appropriately to the child's needs.

3) Video feedback intervention to promote positive parenting (VIPP) [69].

Rationale and intervention goals: The parent's mental representation of the characteristics of attachment and his behavior toward the child are influenced by his own internal representations of attachment and affect the quality of attachment with the child. The goal of the intervention is to strengthen and encourage the parent's sensitive and adapted response to the child's signs by filming the parent and child and giving feedback (the parent in a sense serves as his own model).

Course of intervention: This program is based on attachment theory and includes a set protocol in which the parent-child dyad is filmed in their home, and later watches the videos together with the therapist. During intervention meetings, held with a psychologist once a month for an hour and a half, the parent is given feedback and support when they show positive responses to the child.

Effectiveness of intervention: In a study performed on this intervention with mothers and babies around one year of age, the program was found to have positive effects on the level of adapted/sensitive responses provided by mothers to the child. At the same time, characteristics of secure attachment were not found to increase in the research sample following the intervention.

3. Overview of Parent-Child Intervention Programs by Population

3.1. Four Parent-Child Intervention Programs during Pregnancy

Background: Stress and negative mood during pregnancy are risk factors for the baby's development, for the mother's mood after birth, and for development of secure attachment between the parents and the baby. Relevant studies have found effects on low birth weight, early birth and difficulties during birth, low APGAR scores, difficulties in varying facial expressions in accordance with stimuli and more [70]-[72]. In addition the literature shows that the mother's psychopathology before and during pregnancy increases the risk that the child will develop emotional difficulties and difficulties in self-regulation [73]. Hence there is a need for an appropriate intervention with expecting parents during pregnancy and following birth in order to help them establish the foundations that will continue to serve the parents, the child, and the family unit.

3.1.1. Psychodynamically Oriented Intervention [74] (USA)

Rationale and goals: Psychodynamic interventions directed at treating the person's different conflicting representations have a significant advantage as preventive treatment for women with affective disorders during pregnancy, which may be triggered by distorted or unadjusted internal representations. The assumptions underlying the intervention are that it is important to reach an understanding of the mother's inner world in order to later have an impact of the process of the child's growth and development [74].

Course of intervention: Individual therapy done by a trained psychodynamic therapist. Therapy dwells on the woman, her personal history and her experience of pregnancy. This process expands the psychological space in which the imaginary baby can grow and become distinguished from problematic representations that were the product of the mother's early painful or unsatisfying experiences with her own mother [74].

Intervention effectiveness: No evidence is provided as to the effectiveness of the intervention.

3.1.2. Mindful Motherhood Intervention [75]

Rationale and goals: Literature shows that the experience of stress and strain during pregnancy has a direct impact upon birth and child development. The Mindfulness Method is a means for developing the capacity for observation that can bring about a change in mental or physiological state [76].

Intervention course: Intervention meetings are weekly over a period of eight weeks and are held in a group of 12 - 20 women for two hours at a time. Meetings are facilitated by a clinical psychologist with specialized training in the method, and they include three main methodologies for observing emotions and thoughts: 1) Learning and practicing breathing techniques; 2) Using guided meditation and yoga exercises; 3) Using and understanding psychological concepts such as acceptance.

Program meetings include lectures, discussions and practical exercises such as awareness of the developing fetus, discussion of anxieties about birth, calming walks, and more. In addition participants are given a disc with guided meditation and reading material to supplement what they learn in the meetings.

Intervention effectiveness: In a random controlled pre- and post-intervention pilot study done with 31 women it was found that use of this intervention program during pregnancy reduced negative mood, anxiety, and depressive feelings. In addition it was found that the intervention helped to improve and raise the mood of participants. The effects on the period following birth and on the baby's subsequent development were not studied.

3.1.3. Family Foundations (FF) [76] (USA)

Rationale and goals: During and following pregnancy many changes take place in the composition and management of the family unit. A central aspect of family life is the way in which the parents work together and support one another in coping with conflicts that arise around the raising of the child. The main goal of the program is to strengthen this cooperation and to accompany the changes that the parents undergo during pregnancy and after the birth, by encouraging support and coordination in the relationship [76].

Course of intervention: The program is delivered in local hospital departments as part of a program of birth education, is intended for couples during pregnancy and after birth, and is open to the general public. The program focuses on giving tools for conflict management, problem-solving, communication and support that encourage collaborative parenting. These tools are learned by psycho-educationally oriented discussions of topics like sharing the burden and providing appropriate stimuli to the child. The program is comprised of a series of eight meetings, before and after birth, for both parents. Each group is made up 6 - 10 couples, and is facilitated by a male and female team of therapists who have undergone special training.

Intervention effectiveness: A random controlled study on 169 couples during the period of a first pregnancy found positive outcomes—a significant improvement in the level of cooperation between members of the couple, a decrease in the level of the mother's depression, the couple's anxiety, and the stress regarding the parent-child relationship. The study also showed an increase in the child's self-regulation and quality of sleep. A higher impact was found among the low socio-economic population. The researchers conclude that the cooperation program can have a positive impact especially for at-risk families.

Additional factors recommended when planning and designing intervention programs for the period of pregnancy:

- A planned approach including treatment of a number of parenting components has the greatest impact [76];
- A continuum of at least 11 meetings over 3 months, and supportive and sensitive accompaniment of staff operating the program [77].

3.2. Overview of Mixed Programs for Single-Parent Mothers

Background: There are four known studies that examined the effects of intervention programs for single-parent mothers of children with behavioral problems and children diagnosed with ADHD. Among these, the only study that included a Clinical Controlled Trial was performed by Chacko *et al.*, (2009) [78].

Intervention course: A behavioral program for single-parent mothers of children aged 5 - 12 diagnosed with Attention Deficit Hyperactivity Disorder (ADHD).

Intervention effectiveness: Study findings showed a significant reduction in dimensions of oppositional behavior and mother's stress level, and improved parent-child interaction and parental behavior. However a significant difference was not found between the experimental group and the control group with regard to dimensions related to symptoms of ADHD in the children and of depression in the mother.

3.3. Intervention Programs for Fathers

Background: In the past a greater emphasis was placed on the role of the mother in the process of the child's emotional development, but research today recognizes the importance of the father and even claims that under certain circumstances growing up without a father figure is associated with emotional difficulties in the child [79].

Intervention course: A meta-analysis of 26 studies analyzed the effect of father involvement in parent training programs on program success, and whether the father and mother benefit equally from the program [80].

Intervention effectiveness: The analysis found that studies that included programs in which the father was involved found better outcomes for child behavior and parental conduct that programs that did not include fathers. However there was no difference in the findings of the programs with regard to change in the parent's perception of parenting. In comparison with the mothers, fathers were less likely to implement what they practiced, and reported less on the child's achievements as a result of participation in the program. The researchers conclude that there is a need to involve fathers in parent intervention programs because this increases the likelihood of program success, and recommend further research to learn how to adapt the programs to meet the particular needs of fathers [81].

3.4. Healthy Family America for At-Risk Populations [82] (from the Program Web-Site http://www.healthyfamiliesamerica.org/home/index.shtml)

Target population: Families with children from birth to age 3 - 5 who live in poverty in the United States, and whose children are at risk of abuse and neglect.

The program is also suitable for families with histories of trauma, domestic violence, mental health or substance abuse.

Goals and rationale: Promoting positive parenting, strengthening health and child development and preventing child abuse and neglect by identifying families at risk and providing early intervention. The emphasis in the programs is on developing the parent's strengths rather than focusing on his weaknesses, and creating a healthy attachment between the parent and child. An additional emphasis is on providing families with culturally sensitive services.

Intervention course: HFA services are provided on a voluntary basis and begin during pregnancy. The program offers two primary components-evaluations that determine whether the family is likely to benefit from participation in the program, and weekly home visits to the target population. The program is intensive and long-term (3 to 5 years after the baby's birth). In addition, it provides the family and child with psychological testing and initial screening, support groups, parent training, and groups focused on father involvement. Service providers in the program undergo special training, but are not required to have any academic or therapeutic background.

Intervention effectiveness: Surveys of more than 15 evaluation studies of HFA in 12 states showed the following results: A reduction in poor treatment of children, improved parental care, a decline in premature and low-weight babies, improved parent-child interactions and school preparedness, decreased dependence upon welfare services, greater accessibility to health services and higher rates of vaccinations.

4. Parent-Child Intervention Programs Prevalent in the World

This section will survey evidence-based intervention programs.

1) Living with Children was the first parent training program developed by a group of researchers, led by Gerald Patterson of the Oregon Research Center in the United States [83].

Target population: Children between the ages of 3 - 14 who were referred due to behavior problems.

Treatment setting: Clinic, individual therapy opposite a single family.

Tools: Therapist guidebook: "A social learning approach to family intervention". The guidebook includes a pre-treatment interview with the parent, a questionnaire evaluating the parent's perception of the quality and frequency of his child's behavior, forms guiding the therapist in making telephone calls with parents and forms for the therapist.

The guidebook for parents: "Living with Children" that includes basic concepts and strategies for learning and behavioral management for the parent to learn on his own.

Length of program: An initial meeting of an hour and a half for gathering information and then 6 - 10 brief observations of 25 minutes in the home over a period of two weeks.

Program content: At the core of the program is the guidebook for parents that deal with how children and parents can learn and emphasizes how behavior can be changed through the use of positive reinforcement. The parent learns to perceive himself as the agent of these changes. The therapist teaches the parent to identify specific behaviors that are his targets and then how to build a plan of positive reinforcements (making eye contact, empowerment) and negative reinforcements to cope with this behavior. The plan usually includes a profit and loss table of points for behavior that took place or not, and the goal is that with time the points will themselves become a reward. The parent learns to use the "time out" technique in which the child is isolated from friends and from activities that he enjoys.

Mode of program delivery: Individual meetings with the parent, during which he is tested on the guidebook. In therapy meetings the therapist uses pre-structured scenarios and role plays in order to teach the parent how to build a behavioral plan with his child.

Unique program characteristics: Emphasis on the theoretical learning of behavioral theories in order to develop the capacity to perform transfer and independent building of a behavioral management plan for the child. In addition the program places an emphasis on observations and documentation of the child's behaviors by the parent, and uses a point system as a central tool for changing the child's behavior.

Research support: The program was researched in many controlled studies since 1976 that found that the program produces a significant decrease in undesired behaviors relative to control groups. Follow-up studies show maintenance of program outcomes a year after its completion [2].

Impressions and recommendations: The program is concrete, clear, accessible and detailed. As such, however, it narrows the therapist's therapeutic possibilities. It is appropriate for families that can experience a close connection and are capable of understanding the theoretical materials upon which the program is based.

2) The Incredible Years—the program was developed in 1984 by Carolyn Webster Stratton from the Washington University, USA [84] [85].

Target population: The basic program is intended for children age 2 - 8 with behavioral problems.

Therapeutic process: Parent groups in the clinic, without children.

Program materials: Can be purchased on the internet.

- Therapist guidebook including questions for guiding parents.
- Training videos, in a variety of languages and including more than 250 video clips of a variety of situations from a parent's day to day life, with guidance on how to behave and how not to behave.
- Guidebook for group leaders.
- Guidebook for parents including the contents of the entire basic program.

Length of program: About 10 - 14 weeks. Parents meet weekly in groups of 8 - 12 people for training meetings lasting about two hours.

Program contents: The program focuses first on teaching the parent how to play with his child in a way that the child leads in order to strengthen the relationship between them. The parent is instructed to use a behavioral points plan to encourage desirable behavior and to use the "time out" technique to cope with unwanted behaviors. In addition the parent is guided to teach his child a process of problem solving, and learns to use self-regulation strategies such as relaxation techniques for stopping negative thoughts and improving communication skills.

Means of program delivery: The therapist serves as an aid for the parent while he develops new attitudes, shares experiences and discusses problems and ways to resolve them. The group format and watching the video clips with a variety of common situations are used for this purpose. After watching videos role plays are done and homework is given out that encourages use of the learned skills in the natural environment.

Unique aspects of the program: Particular emphasis is placed on a participatory approach on the assumption that the therapist will help the parent bring to fruition his knowledge and abilities. In addition the program relies a great deal upon video clips and learning through role playing among parents, without the child being present. The program differs from other programs in its high costs and requirements for special training. A collection of the various books and the training workshops for therapists cost between $1300 and $1700.

Research support: Over the last 20 years many controlled and peer-reviewed studies have been performed (on different populations from a range of ethnic backgrounds). These studies showed that the program improves parent-child interactions and reduces children's violent behavior and parental rigidity. Studies are currently being performed to examine the program's effectiveness as a prevention program and initial findings show a positive impact on positive parental behaviors, but results are weaker in relation to the child's behavior [2].

Impression and recommendations: This program is evidence-based and provides accessible information supporting implementation by both therapists and parents. It has a significant advantage for therapists in that the video clips concretize the learning and facilitate communication between therapist and parent. The parent benefits from the group format which is less threatening while at the same time providing significant social support. The program's main limitation is its high cost.

3) HNC—Helping the Noncompliant Child

This program was developed during the 1980's by the researchers Rex Forehand and Robert McMahon from George Washington University in the United States.

Target population: Children ages 3 - 8 with inappropriate behavior a lack of compliance with parental demands.

Treatment process: Intensive parent-child sessions in the clinic.

Program materials:

- Therapist handbook (Helping the noncompliant Child: Family based treatment for oppositional behavior, 2003) that provides guidelines for performing an initial evaluation, observations of structured and free parent-child play, and session management. Reading the book alone is not enough in order to put the model into practice, as experience and developmental knowledge are required.
- Researchers developed an instrument for evaluating parents' knowledge about behavioral principles that has been found to be sensitive to the program's intervention, and its use is recommended.
- Self-help book for the parent (Parenting the Strong Willed Child).

Program duration: 12 weeks not including the evaluation process (interview and initial observations), with an average number of 10 weekly sessions of 60 - 90 minutes.

Program content: Phase 1—In this phase the parent is gradually guided in combining three skills (being attentive, reinforcing and ignoring) during the child's free play. The skills are learned during therapy sessions and practiced at home, and there are criteria that the parent must meet in order to show that he has learned.

Phase 2—In this phase the parent learns how to guide the child. He learns how to give clear positive instructions, how to reinforce the following of instructions, and how to use the "time out" technique when instructions are not followed.

In the end there are therapy sessions for practicing transference of the skills beyond the home environment.

Means of program delivery: The skills learned in the two phases are adopted in small steps, at the parent's pace, but there are criteria which the parent needs to meet with regard to each skill, and this enables the therapist to monitor the parent's progress and his readiness to move on to the next phase. The therapist uses role playing and feedback, and also shares the program components with the child.

Unique characteristics of the program: The child's level of participation in therapy sessions, the active role provided him and the rigid structure whereby the therapist decides when the parent moves from one phase to the next are unique to this program. A unique aspect of the program handbook is its extensive and detailed discussion on theory.

Research support: Controlled studies performed during the 1970's showed positive outcomes of behavioral change and maintenance of desired child and parent behavior. There were also positive findings of program generalization as well as an improvement in parents' perceptions of their child. Follow up studies performed about ten years after program end showed maintenance of the acquired habits and skills. Studies are currently being performed to examine the program's effectiveness as a prevention program with at-risk populations, and there are positive findings that support its use as a community-based prevention program [2].

Impression and recommendations: The program is composed of different components that have been studied in depth and found effective. The guidebook provides a great deal of background information but less specific practice guidelines, so the program is oriented to therapists with basic knowledge and experience in therapy based on behaviorist principles.

4) PCIT—Parent Child Interaction Therapy.

The program was developed in the 1980's by Sheila Eyberg from Oregon University, USA.

Target population: Children aged 2 - 8 displaying behavioral difficulties. The guidebook claims that the program can also help children with anxiety, low self-esteem, developmental difficulties related to intellectual disabilities, abuse, neglect, divorce and adoption.

Treatment course: Individual clinic-based format, usually together with the child.

Program materials:

- Therapist guidebook ("Parent Child Interaction Therapy") containing information about the program and detailed guidelines how to manage the evaluation process and the therapy sessions. The guidebook includes standardized scales for performing the evaluation, one of which was developed by the program.
- The program relies mostly on a training technique in which the therapist observes the parent and child through a one-way mirror, and gives the parent instructions through an earphone.

Program length: Between 8 - 14 weeks of weekly meetings lasting 90 minutes.

Program content: The program begins with an evaluation that includes observations of free and structured parent-child play. In the first phase, sessions are held only with the parents, who learn techniques for letting the child lead in free play. Through discussion, role plays and home exercises the parent is taught how to describe appropriate behavior, to imitate play and to give praise and reinforcements in the course of play. The condition for moving on to the next stage is an observation of the parent and the child in which the therapist evaluates according to pre-established criteria whether the parent has acquired the skills.

In the second phase the parent learns through practice in the clinic and at home-basic strategies for coping with the child's oppositional behavior: The parent is guided to gradually mediate and to break down instructions into small steps, first with simple play instructions, and later in real life situations.

Program delivery: Each session in a given phase has a chapter in the handbook with guidelines on how to teach the parent and a chapter with guidelines how to train the parent in real-time when he is practicing with the child. There is a structured and detailed protocol on how to use the "time out" technique and how to prepare a graph of parental progress for purposes of monitoring.

Characteristics unique to the program: The program is based on the topic of secure parent-child attachment and emphasizes imitation and reflection in the course of interaction, contributing to the creation of a secure atmosphere that is responsive and sensitive to the needs of the child. The program is unique in its use of observations and instructions from behind a one-way mirror. Similarly, the program describes in depth the way in which the parent can teach the child and places particular emphasis upon practicing situations of responsiveness and obedience at home.

Research support: The first controlled experiment evaluating the program found significant positive effects from the use of the two program phases upon the behavior of both child and parent, in contrast to didactic parenting groups or groups that received no intervention. Studies over the past 20 years that evaluated the program found additional positive results, including generalization of the improvement in skills to the learning environment (school) and its maintenance after conclusion of treatment [86].

Impression and recommendations: The program includes considerable detail on how and what to teach, making it ideal for the beginning therapist, but the observations and evaluations in the second program phase are not sufficiently uniform or clear.

Popular Intervention Programs That Are Not Evidence-Based

A number of programs that lack firm research support are nonetheless broadly implemented. The main ones are discussed below:

1) PET—Parent Effectiveness Training.

Target population: Children of all ages; Treatment setting-Provided by trained facilitators in either individual or group formats; Children over the age of 12 can participate in groups with the parents.

Program materials: Program materials can be purchased on the internet, including: Guidebook, audio-cassettes, and a basic course for parents and facilitators on how to transmit the program. It is also possible to undergo training workshops in order to become an authorized trainer in the program.

Program duration: Eight weeks during which the parents meet once a week in groups of 8 - 16, for three hours at a time.

Program content: At the heart of the program is the practicing of the "active listening" technique designed to create a warm and accepting relationship between the parent and child. The parent is taught to help the child find appropriate solutions to his needs, rather than to provide them himself. He learns to refrain from giving instruction, advice, or criticism, and instead to focus on active listening in which he reflects back to the child what he thinks the child is trying to express or do. In addition, the program suggests to the parent that he accommodate the environment in some ways, for instance by finding things for the child to do.

Means of program delivery: One needs to participate in a workshop that includes training.

Unique characteristics of the program: The theory that underlies the program is unique in that it gives equal space to the child vis a vis the parent, and encourages active listening and the child's independent finding of solutions. This is the only program in which there is no limitation on the age of participating children, including babies, and in which length of weekly meetings is three hours.

Research support: A meta-analysis performed during the 1990's and in 2001 found that the program had a positive influence on the parent's self-image, but this effect was not statistically significant. In recent years there has been no research support for the program, and it is problematic to compare the different studies that used different research methods. Shriver & Allen (2008) [2] recommend the program's continued evaluation.

Impression and recommendation: The program can be suitable for a parent interested in developing in the direction of allowing more space, listening and containing, and less in the use of control and limits. The program does not encourage allowing the child to do whatever he wants, and uses environmental adjustments in order to prevent undesirable behaviors. It can support a therapist in promoting positive change in the parent's self image, and there is partial research support for this, but there is no evidence regarding its ability to produce change in the child himself.

2) STEP—Systematic Training for Effective Parenting.

Target population: Primarily for ages 6 - 12 but there are also programs for ages 0 - 6 and adolescents. The program is for the general population and not for parents of children with special behavioral difficulties.

Treatment setting: Parent group without children. No recommendation is made as to the number of participants in a group.

Program materials: Guidebook for therapists (Leaders' Resource Guide) that includes detailed instructions how to lead each meeting, and videos and training books for parents.

Program duration: Recommends 7 weekly meetings lasting 1 - 2 hours.

Program content: At the heart of the program is a philosophy that one should refrain from the use of punishment or rewards of various kinds, and the strategies are identical to those in the PET program-active listening, "I statements", and encouraging a democratic family environment.

Program delivery: The user's guide includes detailed and extensive instructions as to how to manage the meeting with the parent, and the parent guidebook includes illustrations of possible scenarios, and suggestions for parents and children in similar situations.

Unique program aspects: The program emphasizes relating to the child as a small and equal adult with equal rights, but also encourages the parent to build behavioral tables and objectives.

Research support: An extensive evaluation was carried out on the program but it did not apply evidence-based methodologies. Some of the studies that met evidence-based methodological criteria found positive outcomes for parental self-image, and increased trust in the parent-child relationship. But other studies done in parallel did not find significant improvement [2].

Impression and recommendations: The program can be suitable when a therapist wants to encourage a parent to control the child less and to be more accepting and supportive. A significant advantage for the therapist is the guidebook that provides detailed guidelines. However, the assumption underlying the program that the child should be related to as a small adult with equal rights, is subject to controversy in light of developmental research that claims that the child should be related to in age-appropriate ways. In addition the program is oriented only toward the normal population, and does not offer a solution for coping with children with significant behavioral problems.

3) Triple P—Positive Parenting Program (USA).

The program is designed to prevent acute emotional and behavioral situations for children by strengthening their parents' knowledge, skills and confidence.

Target population: Ages 0 - 16, for both regular and at-risk populations.

Treatment setting: Individual or group sessions or self-learning by parent.

Program materials: Therapist guidebook that can be purchased on the program's website, aid and assistance through training material on the site and enrichment workshops for therapists.

Program duration: 8 - 10 meetings of one to one and a half hours.

Program content: Emphasis is placed on the parent's development of skills. The program includes five different levels of intervention: Information, selective intervention, focused parent training (up to four sessions for parents of children with minor behavior problems), expanded parent training (8 - 10 meetings alone/group/self-training).

Program delivery: A variety of media are used, from telephone consultations till family interventions. The therapist uses an active therapy approach that includes modeling, watching videos, role playing, practice, and homework.

Research support: A meta-analysis of 24 relevant studies performed in 2007 for interventions for 3 - 12 year olds concluded that the various interventions have a positive effect, depending on the length and type of intervention [2].

Impression and recommendations: The program is intended for families with children of a broad range of ages, from pre-school to high school. It is flexible and can be adapted to normative or high-risk populations. The program encourages the reduction of risk factors for children's developing behavioral and emotional problems by increasing knowledge, skills, and self-confidence of parents.

4) EHS—Early Head Start (USA).

Program description: A community program developed and financed by the United States federal government. The program began operating in 1995 and as of 2010 there are about 1008 programs implemented in states throughout the USA, in Columbia, Puerto Rico and the Virgin Islands, with services being provided to over 133,000 children under the age of three. The program focuses on promoting the development of infants and toddlers by strengthening the family, promoting parenting abilities among pregnant women and improving family functioning [87].

Target population: pregnant women and families with children up to the age of 3.

Treatment setting: Services are provided in child development centers and in home visits.

Program materials: No materials are specified but a great deal of educational and counseling information is available of the program's web-site (http://www.ehsnrc.org).

Program duration: Provided in the community until age 3 without limitation. Average family participation in the program is 20 - 23 months, with the child receiving an average of 1391 hours of care in the centers.

Program content: The program uses a variety of strategies such as medical and educational counseling to the parent, provision of information on child development, referral to para-medical services, emotional therapies and group activities coordinated by the family's case manager, and provision of ongoing support to the family [88]. All content must meet standards set by the program, and federal inspectors are sent every three years to every program site to review its implementation.

Program delivery: Following an evaluation of the needs of the locality the program directors decide whether to use the support center model, home visits, or a combination of the two. Treatments are given to the family itself. Support centers provide mostly child development services such as educational counseling and consultation to the parent and a minimum of two home visits per family per year. In the home visiting program developmental and counseling services are provided through weekly visits and at least two social activities for the parent each month [89]. Program counselors come from the areas of education, educational counseling and therapy, and undergo a special training in the program content and receive intensive supervision for as long as they work.

Unique program characteristics: The program provides a variety of services at a horizontal-community level, and focuses both on the developmental aspect and on the strengthening of the overall family unit in the community. The program is widely funded by the federal government and this has made widespread implementation possible. Regularly scheduled monitoring evaluates and oversees program implementation.

Research support: The program invests resources and attributes great importance to the performance of research. It was evaluated in a random study that included 3001 families in 17 different programs. The research population was diverse in relation to ethnicity, language, and other characteristics. Analysis of findings revealed higher performance and a higher level of cognitive and language development among three year old children who had participated in the program. Parents who had participated in the program were more emotionally supportive and provided more learning and language stimulation than a control group and used less physical punishment. The most significant effects were found in programs that offered a combination of home visits and center-based services [87]. A follow-up study done prior to entry in kindergarten on children who participated in the program from birth found positive effects of reduced depression among those children's mothers [90].

Impression and recommendations: The program is appropriate for implementation at the individual and community level in a variety of ways. It has research support and a great deal of encouragement for program research, professional training, and supportive accompaniment of the program staff.

5. Discussion

The purpose of this chapter has been to provide an overview of intervention programs for parents, mostly evidence-based, that operate today in Israel and in the world, and to examine meaningful shared characteristics that contribute to their effectiveness and success. It is evident that programs that strengthen parenting through learning and provision of tools of experience and developmental knowledge promote both the parent's and the child's sense of well-being and quality of life [11].

On the basis of the various programs reviewed according to profession, populations, degree of use and extent of research support, the following general components can be emphasized:

- Use of a model that combines **knowledge acquisition and active implementation** (demonstrating the activity of the adult with the child). For example: Work to improve parental sensitivity to "signs" that the child is transmitting promotes the child's degree of "playfulness", motivation, independence and inquiry, as well as his capacity for social interaction [37].
- **Frequency** of therapy/counseling sessions—most of the programs include at least 10 sessions at close intervals or community work over a year.
- **Intervention point of entry**—From early stages of development (including pregnancy). This refers to early detection and beginning of the intervention as early as possible. When the program is defined as a prevention program for couples during pregnancy and after birth it focuses on providing tools for conflict management, problem solving, communication and mutual support that encourage collaborative parenting [75]. Prevention programs demonstrated reductions in percentages of child abuse, child behavioral problems, and closely following pregnancies, as well as an increase in positive and high quality mother-child interactions and improved language development [52].
- Importance of **home visits**—For relationship and ongoing communication as well as for familiarity with the daily environment. Strengthening the basic structure by "co-parenting", strengthening the parents' capacity for open and empathic communication, for resolving disagreements and for working together in the home.

- **A varied and skilled staff** from a number of professional disciplines.
- **Multi-system care that includes community components**—A diverse multi-disciplinary staff relates to the entire family, with concern for all the physical needs and creation of a continuum of care through collaboration between all of the relevant systems and relating to broad environmental contexts such as: Integrating the intervention into the family routine so as not to create burden and role conflict, and to contribute to the parent's quality of life and the family's wellbeing [44]. The therapist should have a good understanding of the home environment and of the objects there, and should integrate intervention into the family routine and daily play situations [45].
- **Integrating interventions with daily life**—In a group intervention program of occupational therapists on the topic of time management and improving mothers' occupational behavior participants exhibited a high level of satisfaction from the support and various strategies they learned to improve time management in family day-to-day life (such as setting family rules, delegating responsibilities, juggling time demands and more [38]. It was found that routine use of programs of physical fitness and healthy living education can reduce long-term problems. It is evident that the family environment is particularly important in early childhood for developing food preferences, eating habits and style, and physical exercise habits.
- **Use of diverse media for training**: training videos, filming sessions and jointly viewing them. The goal of the primary intervention is to strengthen and encourage the parent's sensitive and accommodating response to signs that his child shows. This is accomplished by filming the parent and child and providing feedback (the parent essentially serves as his own model).
- **Accessibility-work "at eye level"**—Professionals "see" parents as whole people with needs and difficulties, with a need for mutual respect and egalitarian relationships; this is essential to creating a true parallel process at all levels that will lead to meaningful change (Packer, 2000; Rivkin & Yadgar, 2010). Clear and understandable language is used that is suitable and accessible to the specific population. As a rule, the intervention creates a "space" for sharing feelings, expressing frustration, developing reflective thinking, giving legitimacy and finding alternative client-focused solutions through a dynamic process. The closeness, the personal relating, and simulation of life situations, are the basis of program success (Katzir, 2008). Intervention processes expand the parents' repertoire of adaptive responses, and reinforce their strengths and abilities, as well as those of their children, while focusing on simple and easily applied psycho-educational principles.
- **Therapist discourse and supervision on supervision**—Structured supervision of professionals on multi-disciplinary staffs is essential as it provides a space to talk about the complexity of the work with parents and children (Packer, 2000; Katzir, 2008).

6. Conclusion

In summary it can be said that the central theme that arises from the study is that of the parent as a central figure who leads, feels, designs and educates his child. Parent training at the various levels, needs to be client-focused (parent, child) and situation-focused with an emphasis on learning and the need for consistency in managing parent-child interactions. Every intervention needs to begin with evaluating needs and choosing whether to use a center-based model to which parents come with their children, or home visiting or a combination of both, with treatment being family-focused. Below we will set out the intervention model itself in accordance with the central principles mentioned above which were found to be most effective in promoting both the parent and the child's sense of well-being and quality of life.

Acknowledgements

Thank all members of the Haifa University Interdisciplinary Clinical Center and the Faculty of Social Welfare & Health Sciences in Haifa University who contributed to this review article.

References

[1] Greenbaum, C.W. and Fried, D. (2011) Relations between the Family and the Early Childhood Education System (Preschool to Grade 3) Status Report and Recommendations. The Initiative for Applied Education Research.

[2] Shriver, M.D. and Allen, K.D., Eds. (2008) Working with Parents of Noncompliant Children: A Guide to Evidence-Based Parent Training for Practitioners and Students. American Psychological Association, Washington DC.

[3] Piquero, A.R., Farrington, D.P., Welsh, B.C., Tremblay, R. and Jennings, W.G. (2009) Effects of Early Family/Parent

Training Programs on Antisocial Behavior and Delinquency. *Journal of Experimental Criminology*, **5**, 83-120. http://dx.doi.org/10.1007/s11292-009-9072-x

[4] Thomas, R. and Zimmer-Gembeck, M.J. (2007) Behavioral Outcomes of Parent-Child Interaction Therapy and Triple P—Positive Parenting Program: A Review and Meta-Analysis. *Journal of Abnormal Child Psychology*, **35**, 475-495. http://dx.doi.org/10.1007/s10802-007-9104-9

[5] Scott, S., O'Connor, T. and Futh, A. (2006) What Makes Parenting Programmes Work in Disadvantaged Areas. The PALS Trial.

[6] Piquero, A.R., Farrington, D.P. and Blumstein, A. (2003) The Criminal Career Paradigm. In: Tonry, M., Ed., *Crime and Justice: A Review of Research*, University of Chicago Press, Chicago.

[7] Wade, S.L. (2004) Commentary: Computer-Based Interventions in Pediatric Psychology. *Journal of Pediatric Psychology*, **29**, 269-272. http://dx.doi.org/10.1093/jpepsy/jsh035

[8] Reyno, S.M. and McGrath, P.J. (2006) Predictors of Parent Training Efficacy for Child Externalizing Behavior Problems—A Metaanalytic Review. *Journal of Child Psychology and Psychiatry*, **47**, 99-111. http://dx.doi.org/10.1111/j.1469-7610.2005.01544.x

[9] Champion, L.A., Goodall, G. and Rutter, M. (1995) Behavior Problems in Children and Stressors in Early Adult Life. I. A 20 Year Follow-Up of London School Children. *Psychological Medicine*, **25**, 231-246. http://dx.doi.org/10.1017/S003329170003614X

[10] Moffitt, T.E. (1993) Life-Course-Persistent and Adolescence-Limited Antisocial Behavior: A Developmental Taxonomy. *Psychological Review*, **100**, 674-701. http://dx.doi.org/10.1037/0033-295X.100.4.674

[11] Oren, D. (2011) Parenthood Treatment. (In Hebrew)

[12] Wyatt Kaminski, J., Valle, L.A., Filene, J.H. and Boyle, C.L. (2008) A Meta-Analytic Review of Components Associated with Parent Training Program Effectiveness. *Journal of Abnormal Child Psychology*, **36**, 567-589. http://dx.doi.org/10.1007/s10802-007-9201-9

[13] Salas, E. and Cannon-Bowers, J.A. (2001) The Science of Training: A Decade of Progress. *Annual Review of Psychology*, **52**, 471-499. http://dx.doi.org/10.1146/annurev.psych.52.1.471

[14] Swanson, H.L. and Hoskyn, M. (2001) Instructing Adolescents with Learning Disabilities: A Component and Composite Analysis. *Learning Disabilities Research and Practice*, **16**, 109-119. http://dx.doi.org/10.1111/0938-8982.00012

[15] Barth, R.P., Landsverk, J., Chamberlain, P., Reid, J.B., Rolls, J.A., Hurlburt, M.S., *et al.* (2005) Parent-Training Programs in Child Welfare Services: Planning for a More Evidence-Based Approach to Serving Biological Parents. *Research on Social Work Practice*, **15**, 353-371. http://dx.doi.org/10.1177/1049731505276321

[16] Barlow, J. and Stewart-Brown, S. (2000) Behavior Problems and Group-Based Parent Education Programs. *Journal of Developmental and Behavioral Pediatrics*, **21**, 356-370. http://dx.doi.org/10.1097/00004703-200010000-00007

[17] Roffwarg, H.P., Muzio, J.N. and Dement, W.C. (1966) Ontogenetic Development of the Human Sleep-Dream Cycle. *Science*, **152**, 604-619. http://dx.doi.org/10.1126/science.152.3722.604

[18] Mindell, J.A., Kuhn, B., Lewin, D.S., Meltzer, L.J., Sadeh, A. and American Academy of Sleep Medicine (2006) Behavioral Treatment of Bedtime Problems and Night Wakings in Infants and Young Children. *Sleep*, **29**, 1263-1276.

[19] Ednick, M., Cohen, A.P., McPhail, G.L., Beebe, D., Simakajornboon, N. and Amin, R.S. (2009) A Review of the Effects of Sleep during the First Year of Life on Cognitive, Psychomotor and Temperament Development. *Sleep*, **32**, 1449-1458.

[20] Scher, A., Hall, W.A., Zaidman-Zait, A. and Weinberg, J. (2010) Sleep Quality, Cortisol Levels and Behavioral Regulation in Toddlers. *Developmental Psychobiology*, **52**, 44-53.

[21] Tikotzky, L. and Sadeh, A. (2010) The Role of Cognitive-Behavioral Therapy in Behavioral Childhood Insomnia. *Sleep Medicine*, **11**, 686-691. http://dx.doi.org/10.1016/j.sleep.2009.11.017

[22] Meltzer, L.J. and Mindell, J.A. (2006) Sleep and Sleep Disorders in Children and Adolescents. *Psychiatric Clinical North Amsterdam*, **29**, 1059-1076. http://dx.doi.org/10.1016/j.psc.2006.08.004

[23] American Academy of Sleep Medicine (2005) International Classification of Sleep Disorders: Diagnostic and Coding Manual. 2nd Edition, American Academy of Sleep Medicine, Westchester.

[24] Lam, P., Hiscock, H. and Wake, M. (2003) Outcomes of Infant Sleep Problems: A Longitudinal Study of Sleep, Behavior and Maternal Well-Being. *Pediatrics*, **111**, e203-e207. http://dx.doi.org/10.1542/peds.111.3.e203

[25] Bayer, J.K., Hiscock, H., Hampton, A. and Wake, M. (2007) Sleep Problems in Young Infants and Maternal Mental and Physical Health. *Journal of Paediatrics and Child Health*, **43**, 66-73. http://dx.doi.org/10.1111/j.1440-1754.2007.01005.x

[26] Wolfson, A., Lacks, P. and Futterman, A. (1992) Effects of Parent Training on Infant Sleeping Patterns, Parents' Stress and Perceived Parental Competence. *Journal of Consulting and Clinical Psychology*, **60**, 41-48.

http://dx.doi.org/10.1037/0022-006X.60.1.41

[27] Kerr, S.M., Jowett, S.A. and Smith, L.N. (1996) Preventing Sleep Problems in Infants: A Randomized Controlled Trial. *Journal of Advanced Nursing*, **24**, 938-942. http://dx.doi.org/10.1111/j.1365-2648.1996.tb02929.x

[28] Stremler, R., Hodnett, E., Lee, K., MacMillan, S., Mill, C., Ongcangco, L. and Willan, A. (2006) A Behavioral-Educational Intervention to Promote Maternal and Infant Sleep: A Pilot Randomized, Controlled Trial. *Sleep*, **29**, 1609-1615.

[29] Morin, C.M., Bootzin, R.R., Buysse, D.J., Edinger, J.D., Espie, C.A. and Lichstein, K.L. (2006) Psychological and Behavioral Treatment of Insomnia: Update of the Recent Evidence (1998-2004). *Sleep*, **29**, 1398-1414.

[30] Riemann, D. and Perlis, M.L. (2009) The Treatments of Chronic Insomnia: A Review of Benzodiazepine Receptor Agonists and Psychological and Behavioral Therapies. *Sleep Medicine Reviews*, **13**, 205-214. http://dx.doi.org/10.1016/j.smrv.2008.06.001

[31] Sadeh, A. (2005) Cognitive-Behavioral Treatment for Childhood Sleep Disorders. *Clinical Psychology Review*, **25**, 612-628. http://dx.doi.org/10.1016/j.cpr.2005.04.006

[32] Hanzlik, J.R. (1998) Parent-Child Relations: Interaction and Intervention. In: Case-Smith, J., Ed., *Pediatric Occupational Therapy and Early Intervention*, 2nd Edition, Butterworth-Heinemann, Boston, 207-222.

[33] Parush, S. and Hann-Markowitz, J. (1996) The Efficacy of an Early Prevention Program Facilitated by Occupational Therapists: A Follow-Up Study. *American Journal of Occupational Therapy*, **51**, 247-251. http://dx.doi.org/10.5014/ajot.51.4.247

[34] Esdaile, S.A. (1996) A Play-Focused Intervention Involving Mothers of Preschoolers. *American Journal of Occupational Therapy*, **50**, 113-123. http://dx.doi.org/10.5014/ajot.50.2.113.

[35] Dreiling, D.S. and Bundy, A.C. (2003) Brief Report—A Comparison of Consultative Model and Direct-Indirect Intervention with Preschoolers. *American Journal of Occupational Therapy*, **57**, 566-569. http://dx.doi.org/10.5014/ajot.57.5.566

[36] Sajaniemi, N., Mäkelä, J., Salokorpi, T., von Wendt, L., Hämäläinen, T. and Hakamies-Blomqvist, L. (2000) Cognitive Performance and Attachment Patterns at Four Years of Age in Extremely Low Birth Weight Infants after Early Intervention. *European Child & Adolescent Psychiatry*, **10**, 122-129. http://dx.doi.org/10.1007/s007870170035

[37] Okimoto, A.M., Bundy, A. and Hanzlik, J. (2000) Playfulness in Children with and without Disability: Measurement and Intervention. *American Journal of Occupational Therapy*, **54**, 73-82. http://dx.doi.org/10.5014/ajot.54.1.73

[38] VanLeit, B. and Crowe, T.K. (2002) Outcomes of an Occupational Therapy Program for Mothers of Children with Disabilities: Impact on Satisfaction with Time Use and Occupational Performance. *American Journal of Occupational Therapy*, **56**, 402-410. http://dx.doi.org/10.5014/ajot.56.4.402

[39] Helitzer, D.L., Cunningham-Sabo, L.D. VanLeit, B. and Crowe, T.K. (2002) Perceived Changes in Self-Image and Coping Strategies of Mothers of Children with Disabilities. *The Occupational Therapy Journal of Research*, **22**, 25-33.

[40] Mayer, M.L., White, B.P., Ward, J.D. and Barnaby, E.M. (2002) Therapists' Perceptions about Making a Difference in Parent-Child Relationships in Early Intervention Occupational Therapy Services. *American Journal of Occupational Therapy*, **56**, 411-421. http://dx.doi.org/10.5014/ajot.56.4.411

[41] Colyvas, J.L., Sawyer, L.B. and Campbell, P.H. (2010) Identifying Strategies Early Intervention Occupational Therapists Use to Teach Caregivers. *American Journal of Occupational Therapy*, **64**, 776-785. http://dx.doi.org/10.5014/ajot.2010.09044

[42] Crowe, T.K. (1993) Time Use of Mothers with Young Children: The Impact of a Child's Disability. *Developmental Medicine Child Neurology*, **35**, 621-630. http://dx.doi.org/10.1111/j.1469-8749.1993.tb11700.x

[43] Crowe, T.K. and Florez, S.I. (2006) Time Use of Mothers with School-Age Children: A Continuing Impact of a Child's Disability. *American Journal of Occupational Therapy*, **60**, 194-203. http://dx.doi.org/10.5014/ajot.60.2.194

[44] Segal, R. and Beyer, C. (2006) Integration and Application of a Home Treatment Program: A Study of Parents and Occupational Therapists. *American Journal of Occupational Therapy*, **60**, 500-510. http://dx.doi.org/10.5014/ajot.60.5.500

[45] Pierce, D., Munier, V. and Myers, C.T. (2009) Informing Early Intervention through an Occupational Science Description of Infant-Toddler Interactions with Home Space. *American Journal of Occupational Therapy*, **63**, 273-287. http://dx.doi.org/10.5014/ajot.63.3.273

[46] Pierce, D. (2000) Maternal Management of the Home as a Developmental Play Space for Infants and Toddlers. *American Journal of Occupational Therapy*, **53**, 290-299. http://dx.doi.org/10.5014/ajot.54.3.290

[47] Ketelaar, M., Vermeer, A., Helders, P.J.M. and Hart, H. (1989) Parental Participation in Intervention Programs for Children with Cerebral Palsy. *Topics in Early Childhood Special Education*, **18**, 108-117. http://dx.doi.org/10.1177/027112149801800206

[48] Hanzlik, R.J. (1989) The Effect of Intervention on the Free-Play Experience for Mothers and Their Infants with Deve-

lopmental Delay and Cerebral Palsy. *Physical & Occupational Therapy in Pediatrics*, **9**, 33-51. http://dx.doi.org/10.1300/J006v09n02_04

[49] Lekskulchai, R. and Cole, J. (2001) Effect of a Developmental Program on Motor Performance in Infants Born Preterm. *Australian Journal of Physiotherapy*, **47**, 169-176. http://dx.doi.org/10.1016/S0004-9514(14)60264-6

[50] Norman, E., Sherburn, M., Osborne, R.H. and Galea, M.P. (2010) An Exercise and Education Program Improves Wellbeing of New Mothers: A Randomized Controlled Trial. *Physical Therapy*, **90**, 348-355. http://dx.doi.org/10.2522/ptj.20090139

[51] Hielkema, *et al.* (2010) Learn 2 Move 0-2 Years: Effects of a New Intervention Program in Infants at Very High Risk for Cerebral Palsy; a Randomized Controlled Trial. *BMC Pediatrics*, **10**, 76. http://dx.doi.org/10.1186/1471-2431-10-76

[52] Olds, D.L., Kitzman, H.J., Cole, R.E., Hanks, C.A., Arcoleo, K.J., Anson, E.A., Luckey, D.W., Knudtson, M.D., Henderson Jr., C.R., Bondy, J. and Stevenson, A.J. (2010) Enduring Effects of Prenatal and Infancy Home Visiting by Nurses on Maternal Life Course and Government Spending: Follow-Up of a Randomized Trial among Children at Age 12 Years. *Archives of Pediatrics & Adolescent Medicine*, **164**, 419-424. http://dx.doi.org/10.1001/archpediatrics.2010.49

[53] Karmiloff, K. and Karmiloff-Smith, A. (2001) Pathways to Language. Harvard University Press, Cambridge, Massachusetts.

[54] Crain-Thoreson, C. and Dale, P.S. (1999) Enhancing Linguistic Performance: Parents and Teachers as Book Reading Partners for Children with Language Delays. *Topics in Early Childhood Special Education*, **19**, 28-39. http://dx.doi.org/10.1177/027112149901900103

[55] Whitehurst, G.J., Arnold, D.S., Epstein, J.N., Angell, A.L., Smith, M. and Fishcel, J.E. (1994) A Picture Book Reading Intervention in Day Care and Home for Children from Low-Income Families. *Developmental Psychology*, **30**, 679-689. http://dx.doi.org/10.1037/0012-1649.30.5.679

[56] Bruner, J.S. (1990) Acts of Meaning. Harvard University Press, Cambridge, Massachusetts.

[57] Vygotsky, L. (1978) Mind in Society: The Development of Higher Psychological Processes. Harvard University Press, Cambridge, Massachusetts.

[58] Bennett, K.K., Weigel, D.J. and Martin, S.S. (2002) Children's Acquisition of Early Literacy Skills: Examining Family Contributions. *Early Childhood Research Quarterly*, **17**, 295-317. http://dx.doi.org/10.1016/S0885-2006(02)00166-7

[59] Hood, M., Conlon, E. and Andrews, G. (2008) Preschool Home Literacy Practices and Children's Literacy Development: A Longitudinal Analysis. *Journal of Educational Psychology*, **100**, 252-271. http://dx.doi.org/10.1037/0022-0663.100.2.252

[60] The Parent-Child Home Program (2011). http://www.cebc4cw.org/program/the-parent-child-home-program/detailed

[61] Home Instruction for Parents of Preschool Youngsters (2011). http://www.cebc4cw.org/program/home-instruction-for-parents-of-preschool-youngsters/detailed

[62] Birch, L.L. and Davison, K.K. (2001) Family Environmental Factors Influencing the Developing Behavioral Controls of Food Intake and Childhood Overweight. *Pediatric Clinics of North America*, **48**, 893-907. http://dx.doi.org/10.1016/S0031-3955(05)70347-3

[63] Agency for Healthcare Research and Quality (2008) Effectiveness of Weight Management Programs in Children and Adolescents. Rockville, September 2008. Report No. 08-E014.

[64] Nemet, D., Geva, D. and Eliakim, A. (2011) Health Promotion Intervention in Low Socioeconomic Kindergarten Children. *Journal of Pediatrics*, **158**, 796-801.

[65] Field, T., Schanberg, S.M., Scafidi, F., Bauer, C.R., Vega-Lahr, N., Garcia, R., Nystrom, J. and Kuhn, C.M. (1986) Tactile/Kinesthetic Stimulation Effects on Preterm Neonates. *Pediatrics*, **77**, 654-658.

[66] Fonagy, P., Steele, M., Moran, G., Steele, H. and Higgitt, A. (1993) Measuring the Ghost in the Nursery: An Empirical Study of the Relation between Parents' Mental Representations of Childhood Experiences and Their Infants' Security of Attachment. *Journal American Psychoanalyze Association*, **41**, 957-989. http://dx.doi.org/10.1177/000306519304100403

[67] Dozier, M., Peloso, E., Lindhiem, O., Gordon, M.K., Manni, M., Sepulveda, S., Ackerman, J., Bernier, A. and Levine, S. (2006) Developing Evidence-Based Interventions for Foster Children: An Example of a Randomized Clinical Trial with Infants and Toddlers. *Journal of Social Issues*, **62**, 767-785. http://dx.doi.org/10.1111/j.1540-4560.2006.00486.x

[68] Dozier, M., Manni, M., Gordon, M.K., Peloso, E., Gunnar, M.R., Stovall-McClough, K., Eldreth, D. and Levine, S. (2006) Foster Children's Diurnal Production of Cortisol: An Exploratory Study. *Child Maltreatment*, **11**, 189-197. http://dx.doi.org/10.1177/1077559505285779

[69] Hoffman, K.T. and Marvin, R.S. (2006) Changing Toddlers' and Preschoolers' Attachment Classifications: The Circle of Security Intervention. *Journal of Consulting and Clinical Psychology*, **74**, 1017-1026. http://dx.doi.org/10.1037/0022-006X.74.6.1017

[70] Kalinauskiene, L., Cekuoliene, D., Van IJzendoorn, M.H., Bakermans-Kranenburg, M.J., Juffer, F. and Kusakovskaja, I. (2009) Supporting Insensitive Mothers: The Vilnius Randomized Control Trial of Video Feedback Intervention to Promote Maternal Sensitivity and Infant Attachment Security. *Child: Care, Health & Development*, **35**, 613-623. http://dx.doi.org/10.1111/j.1365-2214.2009.00962.x

[71] Nielsen Forman, D., Videbech, P., Hedegaard, M., Salvig, J.D. and Secher, N.J. (2000) Postpartum Depression: Identification of Women at Risk. *BJOG: An International Journal of Obstetrics & Gynaecology*, **107**, 1210-1217. http://dx.doi.org/10.1111/j.1471-0528.2000.tb11609.x

[72] Wadhwa, P.D., Culhane, J.F., Rauh, V., Barve, S.S., Hogan, V., Sandman, C.A., *et al.* (2001) Stresses, Infection and Preterm Birth: A Biobehavioural Perspective. *Paediatric and Perinatal Epidemiology*, **15**, 17-29. http://dx.doi.org/10.1046/j.1365-3016.2001.00005.x

[73] Bonari, L., Pinto, N., Ahn, E., *et al.* (2004) Perinatal Risks of Untreated Depression during Pregnancy. *Canadian Journal of Psychiatry*, **49**, 726-735.

[74] Dawson, G., Frey, K., Self, J., Panagiotides, H., Hessl, D. and Yamada, E. (1999) Frontal Brain Electrical Activity in Infants of Depressed and Nondepressed Mothers: Relation to Variations in Infant Behavior. *Child Development*, **70**, 1058-1066. http://dx.doi.org/10.1111/1467-8624.00078

[75] Bergner, S., Monk, C. and Werner, E.A. (2008) Dyadic Intervention during Pregnancy? Treating Pregnant Women and Possibly Reaching the Future Baby. *Infant Mental Health Journal*, **29**, 399-419. http://dx.doi.org/10.1002/imhj.20190

[76] Vieten, C. and Astin, J. (2008). Effects of a Mindfulness-Based Intervention during Pregnancy on Prenatal Stress and Mood: Results of a Pilot Study. *Archives of Women's Mental Health*, **11**, 67-74. http://dx.doi.org/10.1007/s00737-008-0214-3

[77] Feinberg, M.E. and Kan, M.L. (2008) Establishing Family Foundations: Intervention Effects on Coparenting, Parent/Infant Well- Being and Parent-Child Relations. *Journal of Family Psychology*, **22**, 253-263. http://dx.doi.org/10.1037/0893-3200.22.2.253

[78] Cowan, C.P. and Cowan, P.A. (1995) Interventions to Ease the Transition to Parenthood: Why They Are Needed and What They Can Do. *Family Relations*, **44**, 412-423. http://dx.doi.org/10.2307/584997

[79] Chacko, A., Wymbs, B.T., Wymbs, F.A., Pelham, W.E., Swanger-Gagne, M.S., Girio, E., *et al.* (2009) Enhancing Traditional Behavioral Parent Training for Single Mothers of Children with ADHD. *Journal of Clinical Child and Adolescent Psychology*, **38**, 13. http://dx.doi.org/10.1080/15374410802698388

[80] Harper, C.C. and McLanahan, S.S. (2004) Father Absence and Youth Incarceration. *Journal of Research on Adolescence*, **14**, 369-397. http://dx.doi.org/10.1111/j.1532-7795.2004.00079.x

[81] Lundahl, B.W., Tollefson, D., Risser, H. and Lovejoy, M.C. (2008) A Meta-Analysis of Father Involvement in Parent Training. *Research on Social Work Practice*, **18**, 97-102. http://dx.doi.org/10.1177/1049731507309828

[82] Healthy Family America (2011). http://www.healthyfamiliesamerica.org/home/index.shtml

[83] Patterson, G.R. (1982) Coercive Family Process. Castalia, Eugene.

[84] Webster-Stratton, C. and Hammond, M. (1998) Conduct Problems and Level of Social Competence in Head Start Children: Prevalence, Pervasiveness and Associated Risk Factors. *Clinical Child Psychology and Family Psychology Review*, **1**, 101-124.

[85] Webster-Stratton, C. and Herbert, M. (1994) Troubled Families—Problem Children: Working with Parents: A Collaborative Process. John Wiley & Sons, Oxford.

[86] Hood, K.K. and Eyberg, S.M. (2003) Outcomes of Parent Child Interaction Therapy: Mother's Report of Maintenance Three to Six Years after Treatment. *Journal of Clinical Child and Adolescence Psychology*, **32**, 419-429. http://dx.doi.org/10.1207/S15374424JCCP3203_10

[87] Love, J.M., Kisker, E.E., Ross, C., Raikes, H., Constantine, J., Boller, K. and Vogel, C. (2005) The Effectiveness of Early Head Start for 3-Year-Old Children and Their Parents: Lessons for Policy and Programs. *Developmental Psychology*, **41**, 885-901. http://dx.doi.org/10.1037/0012-1649.41.6.885

[88] U.S. Department of Health and Human Services, Administration for Children and Families (1995) Early Head Start Program Grant Availability: Notice. *Federal Register*, **60**, 14548-14578.

[89] Administration for Children and Families (2002) Pathways to Quality and Full Implementation in Early Head Start Programs. Department of Health and Human Services, Washington DC.

[90] Chazan-Cohen, R., Ayoub, C., Pan, B.A., Roggman, L., Raikes, H., Mckelvey, L., Whiteside-Mansell, L. and Hart, A. (2007) It Takes Time: Impacts of Early Head Start That Lead to Reductions in Maternal Depression Two Years Later. *Infant Mental Health Journal*, **28**, 151-170. http://dx.doi.org/10.1002/imhj.20127

19

Double Incomplete Pyloromyotomy (A. Ezzat Technique): A New Technique for Infantile Hypertrophic Pyloric Stenosis: Preliminary Study

Ahmed Ezzat Rozeik[1*], Radi Elsherbini[2], Hamdi Almaramhy[3]

[1]Pediatric Surgery Unit, Zagazig University, Al Sharqia Governorate, Egypt
[2]Pediatric Surgery Unit, Mansoura University, Mansoura, Egypt
[3]Faculty of Medicine, Taibah University, Medina, KSA
Email: *Ahmedezzat147@yahoo.com

Abstract

***Background-Purpose*: The study aimed to see the outcome of Double Incomplete Pyloromyotomy as new technique for surgical management of infantile hypertrophic pyloric stenosis (IHPS). *Methods*: This study was conducted in pediatric surgery unite, Zagazig University Hospital, Egypt. Fifteen patients were included in this study (11 male and 4 female) with IHPS from January 2012 to January 2013. Under general anesthesia, two longitudinal separated incisions at different planes as pyloromyotomy. *Results*: Postoperative vomiting and weight gain were recorded. Follow up period was 3 months. Vomiting improved within first 48 hours then stopped after that. Weight gain significantly increased after the operation when compared preoperatively. *Conclusion*: Double Incomplete Pyloromyotomy is a new, safe and effective procedure for treatment of infantile hypertrophic pyloric stenosis.**

Keywords

Hypertrophic Pyloric Stenosis, Double Incomplete Pyloromyotomy

1. Introduction

Infantile hypertrophic pyloric stenosis (IHPS) continues to be a common pediatric surgical condition, with an

*Corresponding author.

incidence reported of 1 to 8 per 1000 live births [1] [2]. Projectile non bilious vomiting and its complications are common presentations [3] [4]. Diagnosis mainly depends on abdominal ultrsonography [5] [6].

Ramstedt's pyloromyotomy remains the standard surgical treatment with an excellent outcome [7]-[10]. An alternative technique like a double-Y pyloromyotomy offers good results for management of this condition [11].

The aim of the present study was to see the outcome of surgical management of IHPS by Double Incomplete Pyloromyotomy.

2. Patients and Methods

A prospective study was planned between January 2102 and January 2103; fifteen patients were included in this study with diagnosis of IHPS by abdominal ultrasonography. These patients were managed by DIP technique. Patients with gross congenital anomalies were excluded from this study. All patients were fully prepared preoperatively regarding hydration and acid base and electrolytes balance.

3. Technique

Under general anesthesia, right upper quadrant incision was done. Delivery of pyloric mass into the wound. Two longitudinal incisions was performed: one incision started in one side of the mass from its upper end till middle of it, another incision started in other side of the mass from its lower end till the middle of it as **Figure 1** separation of pyloric muscle in both incisions till mucosa appear. After adequate hemostasis and checking of intact mucosa; abdominal closure in layers was done (A. Ezzat technique).

Oral feeding started 6 - 8 hours after surgery by dextrose water proceeding to half-strength milk then full feeds within the first 24 h postoperatively. Information on patient's demographics, postoperative vomiting and weight gain were collected. Patients were followed up for a period of 3 months.

4. Results

In this study of 15 patients; 11 were male while 4 were female. Mean age at presentation was 22 days (ranged from 16 days to 32 days). Projactile non bilious vomiting and acid-base disturbance were the main presentation in addition to weight loss and constipation. No mucosal perforation during operation or manifestations suggested it postoperatively. Vomiting improved then stopped within first 24 - 72 h after operation in all patients. We noted that weight gain observed in all patients from first week and proceeded till the end of follow up period. Mean preoperative weight was 2750 gms and the mean postoperative (after 3 months) was 5550 gms. No recurrence of vomiting or long-term complications and No need of re-do pyloromyotomy.

5. Discussion

Surgical management of infantile hypertrophic pyloric stenosis was described by Ramstedt in 1912. Till now it is the most popular procedure for IHPS [7]-[10]. Some modifications as Double-Y pyloromyotomy depending on the same principle with nearly the same outcome [11]. These procedures split the pyloric muscle completely in the same plane. Long-term follow of the patients specially after Ramstdt's procedure showed some unfavorable complications as rapid gastric emptying and increased duodenal reflux which explain increased incidence

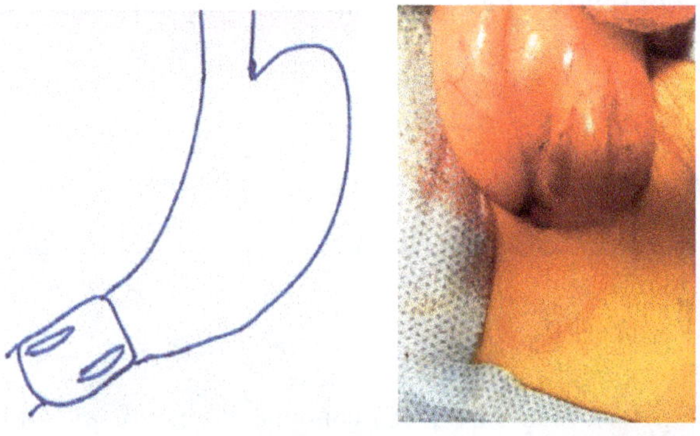

Figure 1. Incisions of Double Incomplete Pyloromyotomy.

of peptic ulcer in several series [12] [13]. Lasheen *et al.* [14] reported segmental internal sphincterotomy for treatment of chronic anal fissure by doing two incomplete incisions in different planes to decrease the incidence of fecal incontinence.

Depending on the same idea we applied double incomplete pyloromyotomy for surgical treatment of IHPS by doing two incomplete incisions in different planes of the pylorus. This new procedure has nearly the same outcome of Ramstedt's procedure with stopping of vomiting and significant weight gain along the follow up period. We suggest that the new technique decrease the incidence of rapid gastric emptying and duodenal reflux after Ramsted's procedure because of our technique did-not split the pyloric muscle in the same plane. In Ramstedt's procedure, the pyloric mucosa bulges after pyloromyotomy, leading to formation of a gutter inside the pylorus with stasis of food and susceptibility of gastritis and ulcer. In our technique the mucosa did-not bulge due to incomplete incisions and subsequently decreased the incidence of the complications.

Double Incomplete Pyloromyotomy offers the same results of Ramstedt's procedure regarding stopping vomiting, weight gain and low incidence of complications. This new technique needs longer follow up with studying of gastric emptying and pyloric sphincter function.

6. Conclusion

Double Incomplete Pyloromyotomy is a new, safe and effective technique for treatment Infantile Hypertrophic Pyloric Stenosis. It has the same results of stander Ramstedt's procedure but needs longer follow up and further studies.

References

[1] Panteli, C. (2009) New Insights into Pathogenesis of Infantile Pyloric Stenosis. *Pediatric Surgery International*, **25**, 1043-1052. http://dx.doi.org/10.1007/s00383-009-2484-x

[2] Gotly, L., Bland, A., Kimble, R., *et al.* (2009) Pyloric Stenosis: A Retrospective Study of an Australian Population. *Emergency Medicine Australasia*, **21**, 407-413.

[3] Chan, S.M., Chan, E.R., Chu, W.C., Cheung, S.T., Tam, Y.H. and Lee, K.H. (2011) Hypertrophic Pyloric Stenosis in a New Born: A Diagnostic Dilemma. *Hong Kong Medical Journal*, **17**, 245-247.

[4] Mahalik, S., Prasad, A., Sinha, A. and Kulshrestha, R. (2010) Delayed Presentation of Hypertrophic Pyloric Stenosis: A Rare Case. *Journal of Pediatric Surgery*, **45**, 9-11. http://dx.doi.org/10.1016/j.jpedsurg.2009.11.012

[5] Huang, Y.L., Lee, H.C., Yeung, C.Y., Chen, W.T., Jiang, C.B., Shew, J.C. and Wang, N.L. (2009) Sonogram before and after Pyloromyotomy: The Pyloric Ratio in Infantile Hypertrophic Stenosis. *Pediatrics & Neonatology*, **50**, 117-120. http://dx.doi.org/10.1016/S1875-9572(09)60046-2

[6] Muramori, K., Nagasaki, Y. and Kawanami, T. (2002) Ultrasonographic Serial Measurement of Morphologic Resolution of the Pylorus after Ramstedt's Pyloromyotomy for Infantile Hypertrophic Pyloric Stenosis. *Journal of Ultrasound in Medicine*, **26**, 1681-1687.

[7] Aspelund, G. and Langer, J.C. (2007) Current Management of Hypertrophic Pyloric Stenosis. *Seminars in Pediatric Surgery*, **16**, 27-33. http://dx.doi.org/10.1053/j.sempedsurg.2006.10.004

[8] Karen, W., Robert, H., Andrew, J.A., Caroline, K. and Nadia, B. (2010) Early Development Outcome of Infants with Infantile Hypertrophic Pyloric Stenosis. *Journal of Pediatric Surgery*, **45**, 2369-2372. http://dx.doi.org/10.1053/j.sempedsurg.2006.10.004

[9] Esmaeel, T., John, B., Sherif, E., Sebastien, D., Pramod, P., Helen, F. and Jean, M. (2007) Evaluation of Surgical Approaches to Pyloromyotomy: A Single-Center Experience. *Journal of Pediatric Surgery*, **42**, 865-868. http://dx.doi.org/10.1053/j.sempedsurg.2006.10.004

[10] Yagmurlu, A., Chalmer, J., Yoyngson, G., *et al.* (2004) Comparison of the Incidence of Complications in Open and Laparoscopic Pyloromyotomy: A Concurrent Single Institution Series. *Journal of Pediatric Surgery*, **39**, 292-296. http://dx.doi.org/10.1016/j.jpedsurg.2003.11.047

[11] Alalayet, Y.F., Miserez, M., Mansoor, K. and Khan, A.M. (2009) Double-Y Pyloromyotomy: A New Technique for Surgical Management of Infantile Hypertrophic Pyloric Stenosis. *European Journal of Pediatrics*, **19**, 17-20. http://dx.doi.org/10.1055/s-2008-1039025

[12] Tam, P.K., Saing, H., Koo, J., *et al.* (1985) Pyloric Function Five to Eleven Years after Ramstedt's Pyloromyotomy. *Journal of Pediatric Surgery*, **20**, 236-239.

[13] Sun, W.M., Doran, S.M., Jones, K.L., Davidson, G., Dent, J. and Horowitz, M. (2000) Long-Term Effect of Pyloro-

myotomy on Motility and Gastric Emptying. *The American Journal of Gastroenterology*, **95**, 92-100. http://dx.doi.org/10.1111/j.1572-0241.2000.01705.x

[14] Lasheen, A.E., Morsy, M.M. and Fiad, A.A. (2011) Segmental Internal Sphincterotomy: A New Technique for Treatment of Chronic Anal Fissure. *Journal of Gastrointestinal Surgery*, **15**, 2271-2274. http://dx.doi.org/10.1007/s11605-011-1689-1

20

Spectrum of Upper GI Endoscopy in Pediatric Population at a Tertiary Care Centre in Pakistan

Muhammad Rehan Khan[1], Shakeel Ahmed[1,2*], Syed Rehan Ali[1], Prem Kumar Maheshwari[1], Muhammad Saad Jamal[1]

[1]Department of Pediatrics and Child Health, The Aga Khan University Hospital, Karachi, Pakistan
[2]Department of Paediatrics, Medical & Dental College, Bahria University, Islamabad, Pakistan
Email: [*]shakeel.ahmed@aku.edu

Abstract

Although upper GI endoscopy is considered to be a gold standard in diagnosis of many pediatric gastrointestinal disorders, there is limited data about its utility from developing countries. We carried out this retrospective study at Aga khan University Hospital, Karachi, Pakistan from 2008-2012. During the study period, a total of 200 procedures were performed. Mean age of patients was 8.5 years. 66% of patients received general anesthesia for the procedure. Failure to thrive with suspected coeliac disease was the most common indication for the procedure, seen in 31% of patients. Gastritis was the most common abnormal endoscopic finding, seen in 14.5% of patients. Gastritis was the most common histopathological finding on biopsy, seen in 31% of the patients (n = 62). Findings were consistent with coeliac disease in 18% (n = 36), duodenitis, 10.5% (n = 21) and esophagitis, 4% (n = 8) of patients. No immediate post procedure complication was noted in our study.

Keywords

Upper GI Endoscopy, Children, Indications

1. Introduction

Gastrointestinal diseases are an important healthcare problem worldwide, especially in pediatric age group [1]. Bozzini is considered to be the pioneer of modern gastroenterology, who used candle-powered lichtleiter for the first time in medical history in 1805 [2]. After the introduction of flexible endoscopy by Hirschowitz in 1950's, use of upper GI endoscopy also started in pediatrics [3]. This led to inception of field of pediatric gastroenterol-

[*]Corresponding author.

ogy in 1960's in developed countries [4]. Later on, fiberoptic endoscopies for children were developed mainly in 1970's and upper GI endoscopy became a standard of care in diagnosis of many gastrointestinal problems in children [5]-[7]. Since then, pediatric gastroenterology is growing rapidly and has emerged as one the most diverse medical-surgical sub-specialty in modern medicine in the developed world [8].

Despite the high diagnostic yield, upper GI endoscopy is still an under-utilized tool and information regarding its efficacy is scanty in most of the developing countries [9]. This is mainly due to lack of awareness about the role of this important diagnostic modality in children which prevents referrals of these children to a center where this facility is available. On the other hand, factors like lack of trained pediatric gastroenterologists or lack of well-equipped pediatric endoscopic suites in resource-limited countries may also play an important role. Furthermore, there is lack of data from nonwestern countries regarding the appropriate indications of endoscopy in children or while referring a child for endoscopy [8]. Therefore, we carried out this hospital-based study to report the common indications, endoscopic/histopathological findings and complications of pediatric upper GI endoscopy in our setup to increase awareness amongst pediatricians.

2. Materials & Methods

The study was carried out in the Department of Paediatrics and Child Health at Aga Khan University Hospital, Karachi, Pakistan. Our hospital is a tertiary care referral center with well-equipped and advanced endoscopy suite. The medical records of all patients under the age of 15 years, who underwent upper GI endoscopy, from January 2008 to December 2012, were reviewed retrospectively using the electronic database system of our hospital. All of the pediatric patients in which upper GI endoscopy was performed during the study period were included in the study. The need for endoscopy was decided by general pediatricians. All pediatric upper GI endoscopies were performed by trained pediatric gastroenterologists/hepatologists. Informed consent was taken from parents/patients for the procedure after careful explanation of procedure details and potential complications. Mode of anesthesia was decided by gastroenterologists depending upon patient age, level of cooperation and physicians comfort level. Endoscopic findings were documented for each patient and biopsy materials for histopathology were taken. Patients were kept in recovery room to look for immediate post procedure complications related to procedure. Patients' demographic data including age, sex, and length of hospital stay were recorded. For the purpose of analysis, patients were divided into three age groups. Indications for upper GI endoscopy were recorded for each patient. Patients having height/weight below 5th percentile with suspected coeliac disease were labeled as failure to thrive. Mode of anesthesia, complications of procedure and histopathological findings of biopsied materials were recorded. Wherever available, findings of serologic tests were also analyzed to see their correlation with the histopathological findings. The collected data was entered into the SPSS (statistical package for social science) Version 18.0 and analyzed through its statistical program. The frequencies of various indications, endoscopic findings, and histopathological findings for upper GI endoscopy were calculated.

3. Results

During the study period, a total of 200 patients underwent upper GI endoscopy and biopsy. Mean age of patients was 8.5 years with range of 2 months to 15 years. Older children (aged 10 - 15 years) had highest frequency of upper GI endoscopy, *i.e.* 40% (n = 80), followed by youngest children (0 - 5 years of age), in which frequency of endoscopy was 32% (n = 63). The frequency of endoscopy in children between 5 - 10 years of age was 28% (n = 56). Around two thirds of the children (66%) were given general anesthesia for the procedure while in remaining only sedation was required. No immediate post procedure complications were noted in any of the patients during the file review. Failure to thrive with suspected coeliac disease was the most common indication for the procedure, seen in 31% patients (n = 62). **Table 1** describes the frequency of various indications for upper GI endoscopy in our study. In almost half of the patients (46%, n = 92), the endoscopic findings were normal and about one third of the patients (n = 61) had nonspecific endoscopic findings. Gastritis was the most common abnormal endoscopic finding, seen in 14.5% (n = 29) of patients. **Table 2** describes the details of endoscopic findings in study. Gastritis was the most common histopathological finding on biopsy, seen 31% (n = 62). Findings were consistent with coeliac disease in 18% (n = 36), duodenitis, 10.5% (n = 21) and esophagitis, 4% (n = 8) of patients. Around 7.5% (n = 15) of patients had nonspecific findings and 15.5% (n = 31) had normal histopathological findings. No biopsy/histopathology was done in 27 patients. Serological tests for coeliac disease were found positive in 37 patients before endoscopy. Out of these, 78% (n = 29) had pathological confirmation of disease on biopsy.

Table 1. Indications of upper GI endoscopy in children.

Indication	Number	% age
Failure to Thrive (Suspected Coeliac Disease)	62	31
Recurrent Abdominal Pain	37	18.5
Upper GI Bleeding	30	15
Chronic Vomiting	24	12
Chronic Diarrhea	20	10
Dysphagia	12	6
Hepatosplenomegaly	12	6

Table 2. Endoscopic findings.

Finding	Number	% age
Normal	92	46
Non-Specific Findings	61	30.5
Gastritis	29	14.5
Esophageal Varices	10	5
Esophagitis	5	2.5
Gastroduodenal Ulcer	3	1.5

4. Discussion

Upper GI endoscopy is one of the most specific, quick and cost effective diagnostic tool for a wide variety of gastrointestinal disorders in children, especially under the circumstances when other investigations are not conclusive. In addition to its diagnostic use, upper GI endoscopy also has an established therapeutic role and various disorders like upper GI bleeding, Mallory Weiss tear; gastric erosions can be effectively treated by endoscopy [10] [11]. Therefore, despite changing indications over a period of time, the disorders requiring upper GI endoscopy for diagnostic or therapeutic purposes in children have shown a rising trend [12].

In literature from most of the developing countries, recurrent abdominal pain has been reported as the commonest indication of upper GI endoscopy. In various reports, this frequency of abdominal pain is reported to be ranging from 8% to 43% [13]-[15]. In our study, the frequency of abdominal pain as an indication of upper GI endoscopy was 18.5%. So our results are comparable to other reports from developing countries. However, the most common indication of upper GI endoscopy in our study was failure to thrive (suspected coeliac disease), seen in 31% of children. No such finding is reported in literature from other developing countries. However, in a study from France, Jantchou *et al*, have reported a similar trend, where failure to thrive was the highest indication for performing upper GI endoscopy [16].

Similarly, almost half of the children (46%) who underwent upper GI endoscopy in our study had normal endoscopic findings while about one third (30.5%) of the patients had non-specific findings. Thus, endoscopic diagnosis was established in only one quarter of patients. Similar trends have been noted in other studies as well, where almost half of the endoscopies were normal [13] [14] [17]. Gastritis was the most common endoscopic finding in our study, seen in 14.5% of children. Similar reports have been shown in other studies as well.

Although, this procedure is safe and can be performed even without sedation or anesthesia in adult patients, there are no specific guidelines for pediatric age group in this regard. Even in latest consensus guidelines developed by Canadian association of gastroenterology, the concerns have been raised regarding sedation/anesthesia in children [18]. Although un-sedated procedure can be cost effective and time saving [19], in our study about 2/3 of the endoscopies were performed under general anesthesia. Approximately 60% of the upper GI related complications are secondary to sedatives/analgesic agents which can lead to cardiopulmonary compromise [20]. No immediate post procedure complications were noted in our study. However, there is need to develop guidelines for sedation in children not only to save resources but also to prevent unnecessary exposure to sedative/anesthetic agents which can be hazardous for children.

5. Conclusion

Upper GI endoscopy is a safe procedure in children. The awareness about its diagnostic and therapeutic role should be raised amongst pediatricians in developing countries. There is also a need to develop training programs of pediatric gastroenterology and pediatric endoscopic suites in developing countries so that children may benefit from this state of the art diagnostic modality.

Competing Interest

None.

Funding

None.

References

[1] El-Mouzan, M.I., Abdullah, A.M., Al-Sanie, A.M., *et al.* (2001) Pattern of Gastro Esophageal Reflux in Children. *Saudi Medical Journal*, **22**, 419-422.

[2] Sircus, W. (2003) Milestones in the Evolution of Endoscopy: A Short History. *Journal of the Royal College of Physicians of Edinburgh*, **33**, 124-134.

[3] Haight, M. and Thomas, D.W. (1995) Pediatric Gastrointestinal Endoscopy. *Gastroenterologist*, **3**, 181-186.

[4] Franciosi, J.P., Fiorino, K., Ruchelli, E., *et al.* (2010) Changing Indications for Upper Endoscopy in Children during a 20-Year Period. *Journal of Pediatric Gastroenterology & Nutrition*, **51**, 443-447. http://dx.doi.org/10.1097/MPG.0b013e3181d67bee

[5] Papp, J.P. (1973) Endoscopic Experience in 100 Consecutive Cases with the Olympus GIG Endoscope. *The American Journal of Gastroenterology*, **60**, 466-472.

[6] Gleason, W.A., Tedesco, F.J., Keating, J.P., *et al.* (1974) Fiber Optic Gastrointestinal Endoscopy in Infants and Children. *The Journal of Pediatrics*, **85**, 810-813. http://dx.doi.org/10.1016/S0022-3476(74)80347-1

[7] Graham, D.Y., Klish, W.J., Ferry, G.D., *et al.* (1978) Value of Fiber Optic Gastrointestinal Endoscopy in Infants and Children. *Saudi Medical Journal*, **71**, 558-560. http://dx.doi.org/10.1097/00007611-197805000-00022

[8] Ginger, M.A. (2001) Gastroenterologic Endoscopy in Children: Past, Present and Future. *Current Opinion in Pediatric*, **13**, 429-434. http://dx.doi.org/10.1097/00008480-200110000-00008

[9] Okello, T.R. (2006) Upper Gastrointestinal Endoscopic Findings in Adolescents at Lacor Hospital, Uganda. *African Health Sciences*, **6**, 39-42.

[10] El-Mouzan, M.I., Al-Mofleh, I.A., Abdullah, A.M., *et al.* (2004) Indications and Yield of Upper Gastrointestinal Endoscopy in Children. *Saudi Medical Journal*, **25**, 1223-1225.

[11] Aduful, H., Naaeder, S., Darko, R., *et al.* (2007) Upper Gastrointestinal Endoscopy at the Korle Bu Teaching Hospital, Accra, Ghana. *Ghana Medical Journal*, **41**, 12-16.

[12] Murray, J.A., Van Dyke, C., Plevak, M.F., *et al.* (2003) Trends in the Identification and Clinical Features of Celiac Disease in a North American Community, 1950-2001. *Clinical Gastroenterology and Hepatology*, **1**, 19-27. http://dx.doi.org/10.1053/jcgh.2003.50004

[13] Joshi, M.R., Sharma, S.K. and Baral, M.R. (2005) Upper GI Endoscopy in Children- in an Adult Suite. *Kathmandu University Medical Journal* (*KUMJ*), **3**, 111-114.

[14] Mudawi, H.M., El Tahir, M.A., Suleiman, S.H., *et al.* (2009) Paediatric Gastrointestinal Endoscopy: Experience in a Sudanese University Hospital. *Eastern Mediterranean Health Journal*, **15**, 1027-1031.

[15] Hafeez, A., Ali, S. and Hassan, M. (2000) An Audit of Pediatric Upper Gastrointestinal Endoscopies. *Journal of the College of Physicians and Surgeons Pakistan*, **10**, 13-15.

[16] Jantchou, P., Schirrer, J. and Bocquet, A. (2007) Appropriateness of Upper Gastrointestinal Endoscopy in Children: A Retrospective Study. *Journal of Pediatric Gastroenterology and Nutrition*, **44**, 440-445. http://dx.doi.org/10.1097/MPG.0b013e31802c6847

[17] Quine, M.A., Bell, G.D., McCloy, R.F., *et al.* (1994) Appropriate Use of Upper Gastrointestinal Endoscopy—A Prospective Audit. Steering Group of the Upper Gastrointestinal Endoscopy Audit Committee. *Gut*, **35**, 1209-1214.

http://dx.doi.org/10.1136/gut.35.9.1209

[18] Bishop, P.R., Nowicki, M.J., May, W.L., *et al.* (2002) Unsedated Upper Endoscopy in Children. *Gastrointestinal Endoscopy*, **55**, 624-630. http://dx.doi.org/10.1067/mge.2002.123417

[19] Armstrong, D., Barkun, A., Bridges, R., *et al.* (2012) Canadian Association of Gastroenterology Consensus Guidelines on Safety and Quality Indicators in Endoscopy. *Canadian Journal of Gastroenterology*, **26**, 17-31.

[20] ASGE Standards of Practice Committee, Ben-Menachem, T., Decker, G.A., *et al.* (2012) Adverse Events of Upper GI Endoscopy. *Gastrointestinal Endoscopy*, **76**, 707-718. http://dx.doi.org/10.1016/j.gie.2012.03.252

21

Cholelithiasis in Children with Sickle Cell Disease in Ouagadougou Pediatric Hospital

Fla Kouéta[1,2*], Sonia Kaboret[1,2], Caroline Yonaba[1,3], Aïssata Kaboré[1,2], Lassina Dao[1,2], Sak-Wend-Tongo Daïla[2], Hamidou Savadogo[2], Emile Bandré[1,4], Diarra Yé[1,2]

[1]Training and Research Unit of Health Sciences, University of Ouagadougou, Ouagadougou, Burkina Faso
[2]Service of Medical Pediatrics, Charles de Gaulle Pediatric University Teaching Hospital, Ouagadougou, Burkina Faso
[3]Department of Pediatrics, Yalgado University Teaching Hospital, Ouagadougou, Burkina Faso
[4]Pediatric Surgery Service, Charles de Gaulle Pediatric University Teaching Hospital, Ouagadougou, Burkina Faso
Email: *kouetafla@yahoo.com

Abstract

Introduction: Sickle cell disease (SCD) causes chronic hemolysis which is a risk factor for cholelithiasis. Its development may lead to severe and life-threatening complications. Objective: Determine the prevalence of cholelithiasis, the conditions of diagnosis and related factors. Materials and Method: We retrospectively reviewed records of 110 patients with sickle cell disease followed up in Charles de Gaulle University Pediatric Hospital from January 2003 to December 2013, including 103 patients who had abdominal ultrasonography. Results: Cholelithiasis prevalence was 24.3%. The mean age of patients was 10.8 years, (range 3 to 15 years). Sex ratio was 2.1. In 88% cases, cholelithiasis was diagnosed based on the characteristic symptoms of right hypocondrial pain, fever and icterus. Most factors associated with cholelithiasis were as follows: age above 10 years (OR = 4), occurrence of at least three (03) vaso-occlusive crises per year (OR = 7.6), history of blood transfusion (OR = 8), right hypochondrial pain (OR = 4.5) and icterus (OR = 15). Only 20% of patients suffering from a symptomatic cholelithiasis underwent laparoscopic cholecystectomy and results were conclusive. Conclusion: Patients with sickle cell disease, especially those aged above 10, should be routinely tested for cholelithiasis using abdominal ultrasonography at least once a year. Because of the difficulties in managing evolutive complications in case of an emergency in our context, we advocate laparoscopic cholecystectomy of any cholelithiasisas soon as it is diagnosed in children with sickle cell disease.

*Corresponding author.

Keywords

Cholelithiasis, Sickle Cell Disease, Children

1. Introduction

Cholelithiasis is a frequent complication of chronic hemolysis due to sickle cell disease (SCD) [1]. It is sometimes revealed by digestive symptoms difficult to distinguish from painful abdominal vaso-occlusive crises (recurrent abdominal pain sometimes similar to biliary colic, nausea, vomiting). However, cholelithiasis is often asymptomatic and can lead to serious complications (cholecystitis, cholangitis, pancreatitis, septicemia starting in the bile) which can jeopardize patients' lives [2] [3]. If excessive bilirubin excretion related to chronic hemolysis is a major risk factor for gallstones formation, other conducive factors which have not been identified yet could intervene [1] [4]. Many studies show that the prevalence of cholelithiasis in patients with sickle cell disease increases with age and affects 6% of patients before 15 years of age and more than 50% of young adults [1] [5] [6]. Gallstones treatment is equivocal but most of studies recommend cholecystectomy in the symptomatic cases and regular ultrasonography in the other cases [3] [7]. In Charles de Gaulle University Pediatric Hospital of Ouagadougou, children with SCD have been followed up since 2002 but patients have to bear the fees [8]. Ultrasonography is not always accessible due to its cost. The diagnosis of cholelithiasis is often based on clinical signs and the risk of developing complications is high. It is in this context that we found it appropriate to carry out this study to determine the prevalence of cholelithiasis, the conditions of diagnosis, the factors associated with its occurrence and the treatment adapted to our context of limited resources.

2. Patients and Methods

We carried out a retrospective study to describe and review the records of all patients with SCD followed up in Charles de Gaulle University Pediatric Hospital (CHUP-CDG) between January 1st, 2003 and December 31st, 2013. During the period of study, 110 patients with SCD were followed up every 3 months and had at least one biological checkup every 6 months based on full blood count far away from any complication. Annual abdominal ultrasonography was routinely proposed to all patients. It was also performed in case of abdominal pain or in the occurrence of clinical signs of symptomatic cholelithiasis. Thus, one hundred and three (103) patients had had abdominal ultrasonography during the period of study, either routinely or with the occurrence of warning signs and these were all included in the study. For each patient, we collected data on clinical monitoring and/or hospitalization records and on epidemiological aspects (age, sex, parents' socioeconomic status), clinical data (pathological history, motives for consultation, physical examination data), paraclinical data (hemoglobin electrophoresis, full blood count, abdominal ultrasonography, biochemical checkup: serum transaminase, bilirubinemia), data on medical and surgical treatment and on the course of the disease. Parents' socioeconomic status was arbitrarily classified according to the father's occupation and divided into two (02) categories: average socioeconomic level (civil servants, liberal professions, traders, the military and paramilitary); low socioeconomic level (farmers, breeders, informal sector, the unemployed, pupils, students).

To identify epidemiological, clinical and biological factors likely to be associated with the occurrence of cholelithiasis, we compared patients suffering from cholelithiasis (Group I) with the other patients whose abdominal ultrasonography was normal (Group II). Data were collected and analyzed on microcomputer with Epi-Info software, Version 3.5.1. Group I (cases) and group II (witnesses) were compared using the Chi-squared test at a significance level of 5% and calculation of Odds ratio with their confidence intervals (IC) at 95%. Factors in which the confidence interval did not include the value 1 were deemed to be high risk factors for cholelithiasis occurrence.

3. Results

3.1. Epidemiological Data

3.1.1. Prevalence of Cholelithiasis

Out of 103 patients with SCD who had had an abdominal ultrasonography, 25 suffered from cholelithiasis, hence a prevalence of 24.3%. Hemoglobin electrophoresis revealed 14 SC patients (56%) and 11 SS patients (44%) among patients suffering from cholelithiasis.

3.1.2. Distribution of Cholelithiasis Cases by Age and Sex

Patients' mean age during cholelithiasis diagnosis was 10.8 years (range—3 to 15 years). The age group from 10 to 15 years was the most affected with 16 cases (64%) (see **Table 1**). We registered 17 boys (68%) and 8 girls (32%). Sex-ratio was 2.1.

3.1.3. Socioeconomic Level

The socioeconomic level was deemed average in 17 parents (68%) and low in 8 parents (32%).

3.2. Clinical Data

3.2.1. Frequency of Vaso-Occlusive Crises

Out of 25 patients, 23 had a history of vaso-occlusive crises including 20 who experienced more than 3 vaso-occlusive crises per year, representing 80% of cases.

3.2.2. History of Transfusion

Ten (10) patients had already had at least one blood transfusion, representing 40%.

3.2.3. Conditions of Diagnosis

Right hypocondrial pain (68%), fever (60%) and icterus (56%) were the main conditions for diagnosing cholelithiasis, as shown in **Table 2**. Only 3 cases of cholelithiasis were routinely detected.

3.2.4. Physical Signs

On examination, some general signs were observed: a mucocutaneous paleness in 12 patients (48%) and icterus in the other14 patients (56%). Physically, 14 patients (56%) felt a pain at deep palpation of right hypocondrium and 03 patients (12%) presented with persistent pain in the same hypocondrium. Hepatomegaly and splenomegaly were observed in 6 (24%) and 2 cases (8%), respectively. For 8 patients (32%), physical examination was normal.

3.3. Paraclinical Data

3.3.1. Results of Abdominal Ultrasonography

Abdominal ultrasonography objectived a gall bladder containing gallstones in 24 cases and "Sludge" in 01 case. In 05 cases, gallstones size ranged from 10 to 27 mm in diameter with a mean size of 14.60 mm. In 19 patients, we observed "multi-microlithiases" with gallstones measuring less than 5 mm in diameter and in 1 case, a "small lithiasis" measuring between 5 and 10 mm. Moreover, all patients had normal sonographic patterns of liver and common bile duct. Ultrasonography revealed complications such an acute cholecystitis in 07 patients, representing 28% of cases.

3.3.2. Results of Biological Examinations

Full blood count revealed hemoglobin level below 6 g/dl in 6 patients (24%) and ranging from 06 to 10 g/dl in the other 19 patients (76%). A hyperleucocytosis above 15,000 white blood cells/mm^3 was observed in 16 cases

Table 1. Distribution of the 25 cholelithiasis patients by age and sex.

Range of age (years)	Sex		Total n (%)
	Female n (%)	Male n (%)	
<5	1 (4)	3 (12)	4 (16)
6 - 10	1 (4)	4 (16)	5 (20)
11 - 15	6 (24)	10 (40)	16 (64)
Total	8 (32)	17 (68)	25 (100)

Table 2. Conditions of diagnosis of the 25 cases of cholelithiasis.

Conditionof diagnosis	Number	(%)
Right hypocondrial pain	17	68
Fever	15	60
Icterus/subicterus	14	56
Diffuse abdominal pain	04	16
Nausea/vomiting	03	12
Dark urines	02	8
Routine diagnosis	03	12

(64%) with predominant neutrophils.

Other lab tests revealed high serum transaminase in 46% of patients and high total bilirubin in 60% of cases. Moreover, creatinemia and blood sugar turned normal in all our patients.

3.4. Therapeutic Aspects

Out of 25 cases of cholelithiasis, 19 were hospitalized and the other 6 were followed up as outpatients. Patients were initially admitted in pediatric care unit, then, 9 patients were transferred to surgical care unit in the same hospital. Medical treatment often consisted in healing clinical and biological disorders observed and it was associated with a symptomatic treatment made up of analgesic, anti-inflammatory and antispasmodic medicines. In surgical care unit, 5 patients underwent a cold laparoscopic cholecystectomy within a mean time of 17.4 days after cholelithiasis was diagnosed through abdominal ultrasonography (range—04 to 34 days).No major surgery aftermath was reported in all cases. The mean hospital stay was 7.4 days (range—01 to 19 days) with on average 9 days in pediatric care unit and 5 days in pediatric surgery.

After hospital stay, patients were proposed a monthly, 3 months and then half-yearly follow-up as well as abdominal ultrasonography. Most of patients failed to have abdominal ultrasonography. After one year's follow-up, 14 patients who were not operated became asymptomatic under medical treatment and 4 patients were lost to follow up.

3.5. Factors Associated with Cholelithiasis

Table 3 shows epidemiological and clinical factors likely to be associated with the occurrence of cholelithiasis in our patients. Age above 10 years (OR = 4), occurrence of at least 3 vaso-occlusive crises per year (OR = 7.6), history of blood transfusion (OR = 8), right hypocondrial pain (OR = 4.5) and icterus (OR = 15) were mainly associated with cholelithiasis.

4. Discussion

Sickle cell disease is a genetic disease that causes anemia as well as acute and chronic tissue injuries in many organs [1]. Providing better care in our unit has increased the life expectancy of children with SCD [8]. Yet, its development can lead to chronic complications such as cholelithiasis which should be known and managed. Despite the retrospective nature of our study, which could introduce bias in the estimation of the prevalence of gallstones and especially symptomatic forms, we have achieved significant results and conducted the following discussion.

4.1. Prevalence of Cholelithiais

Prevalence of cholelithiasis in children with SCD varies according to studies. We observed a prevalence of 24.3% in our series. Our results are similar to those of Athanassiou-Metaxa and al in Greece [9] who reported a frequency of 27.1%. Other authors as Silva in Greece and Itoua in Nigeria [10] [11] reported a prevalence greatly superior to ours, 40.9% and 31.30% respectively. However, many other African studies reported lower prevalence: 9.3% in Côte d'Ivoire, 9.4% in Senegal and 11.5% in Sudan [1] [2] [12]. Differences observed

Table 3. Factors associated with cholelithiasis.

Factors	Group I (n = 25)	Group II (n = 78)	OR (IC95%)	p
Type of hemoglobin				
SC	14	41	1 (0.4 - 3)	0.7
SS	11	37	1.0	
Age				
>10 years	16	20	5 (1.8 - 15.2)	0.0004
≤10 years	9	58	1.0	
Sex				
male	17	45	1.6 (0.7 - 4.5)	0.3
female	8	33	1.0	
Socioeconomic level				
low	8	36	0.6 (0.2 - 1.6)	0.2
average	17	42	1.0	
Vaso-occlusive crises ≥ 3/an				
yes	20	27	7.6 (2.3 - 26.1)	0.00007
no	5	51	1.0	
History of blood transfusion				
Yes	10	06	8 (2.2 - 29.9)	0.001
no	15	72	1.0	
Right hypocondrial pain				
Yes	17	30	4.5 (1.6 - 13.3)	0.001
no	8	48	1.0	
Icterus				
yes	14	06	15 (4.3 - 57.4)	$<10^{-6}$
no	11	72	1.0	

between prevalences could be related to patients' age in the series, their mode of selection or clinical signs. In our study, the relatively high prevalence of cholelithiasis can be explained inter alia by better care provision to patients with SCD and increased access to ultrasonography, which is an essential tool in the diagnosis of this pathology. Diagne and al in Senegal [2] reported that cholethiais on the whole occurred less frequently in patients of West Africa than in those of Central Africa. This would be related to the fact that in case of SCD, the Bantu haplotype which is more frequent in Central Africa experiences more severe symptoms with chronic and more important hemolysis whereas the Senegal and Benin haplotype which is the majority in West Africa presents with less severe symptoms. The intermingling of populations could progressively reduce the scope of this observation.

4.2. Conditions of Diagnosis

Conditions under which cholelithiasis is diagnosed in children with SCD vary according to series. In our study as in Sarnaik and al [13] and Bond and al [14], cholelithiasis was, from the onset, diagnosed in case of symptoms evocative of bile ducts disorders (right hypocondrial pain, icterus and fever) in 88%, 60% and 56% of cases, respectively. On the other hand, in the work of Attala [1] and Parez [3], cholelithiasis was initially detected through a routine ultrasonography. The diagnosis of cholelithiasis with clinical signs is a late diagnosis. This situation is prejudicial to patients due to high risk of death if complications occur [2]. Recurrent high temperature (60%) and cholecystitis in 28% of cases reveal in our series major complications in children with SCD. Annual abdominal ultrasonography required for the follow-up of our patients should therefore be done routinely and free of charge for parents who are unable to bear fees.

4.3. Factors Associated with the Occurrence of Cholelithiasis

Factors that lead to gallstones formation in case of chronic hemolysis such as sickle cell disease have not been fully understood [15]. In our study, age above 10 years, occurrence of at least 3 vaso-occlusives crises per year, history of blood transfusion, right hypocondrial pain and icterus were reported. These observations are similar to those of literature in which the prevalence of cholelithiasis in patients with SCD always increases with age and seriousness of disease [1] [2] [3] [7]. However, if an increased bilirubin excretion related to chronic or recurrent hemolysis remains a significant factor for cholelithiaisis occurrence, all patients who experience an important hemolysis do not develop cholelithiasis. Other contributory factors play therefore a complementary role. According to Everson *et al.* [4], some defects of biliary function and the metabolism of bile acids may contribute. Moreover, some authors reported the role of food factors (fatty food and diet low in fiber) in patients living in Europe and USA [16] [17]. Factors leading to cholelithiasis are numerous, equivocal and depend on age. It is therefore possible that early care while reducing the exposure to factors aggravating chronic hemolysis, reduces the risk of cholelithiasis.

4.4. Therapeutic Aspects

In our series, only 20% of patients with symptomatic cholelithiasis underwent laparoscopic cholecystectomy. Despite the equivocal treatment attitude towards cholelithiasis, most of studies agree on cholecystectomy in symptomatic forms [1]-[3]. In asymptomatic forms, two attitudes are opposed. Some authors advocate abstention and follow-up [7] [18] whereas other authors recommend cold cholecystectomy before the onset of any complication [19] [20]. In our context, the second attitude seems more reasonable because of fear of complications in case of emergency. But this attitude is faced with financial difficulties and sometimes the reluctance of parents who fear the aftermath of surgery which was simple in all our operated patients.

Laparoscopic cholecystectomy is the treatment of choice of cholelithiasis in children with SCD, because of its effectiveness and harmlessness in comparison with laparotomy which is a classical surgery [21]. This technique is used recently though uncommon in our health center. Considering challenges for obtaining regular ultrasonography during follow-up of patients and difficulties in the management of complications in case of emergency, we recommend as Parez and al in Paris and Diagne and al in Dakar [2] [3], the routine laparoscopic cholecystectomy in any patient with SCD showing or not a symptomatic cholelithiasis.

5. Conclusion

Cholelithiasis is frequent in children with SCD in Burkina Faso. It should be routinely screened using ultrasonography in any patient with SCD, especially those above 10 years of age. Because of the difficulties in managing evolutive complications in case of an emergency in our context, we advocate laparoscopic cholecystectomy way of all gallstones since its discovery in sickle cell children. The implementation of a national programme of sickle cell disease, the introduction of a routine neonatal screening and a regular follow-up could contribute to reduce morbidity and mortality in children with SCD in our country.

Conflict of Interest

No.

References

[1] Attalla, B.A.I., Karrar, Z.A., Ibnouf, G., Mohamed, A.O., Abdelwahab, O., Nasir, E.M., *et al.* (2013) Outcome of cholelithiasis in Sudanese children with Sickle Cell Anaemia (SCA) after 13 Years Follow-Up. *African Health Sciences*, **13**, 154-159. http://dx.doi.org/10.4314/ahs.v13i1.21

[2] Diagne, I., Badiane, M., Moreira, C., Signaté-Sy, H., Ndiaye, O., Lopez-Sail, P., *et al.* (1999) Lithiase biliaire et drépanocytose homozygote en pédiatrie à Dakar (Sénégal). *Archives de Pédiatrie*, **6**, 1286-1292.

http://dx.doi.org/10.1016/S0929-693X(00)88890-9

[3] Parez, N., Quinet, B., Batut, S., Grimprel, E., Larroquet, M., Audry, G., *et al.* (2001) Lithiase biliaire chez l'enfant drépanocytaire: Expérience d'un hôpital pédiatrique parisien. *Archives de Pédiatrie*, **8**, 1045-1049. http://dx.doi.org/10.1016/S0929-693X(01)00581-4

[4] Everson, G.T., Nemeth, A., Kourourian, S., Zogy, D., Leff, N.B., Dixon D., *et al.* (1989) Gallbladder Function Is Altered in Sickle Haemoglobinopathy. *Gastroenterology*, **96**, 1307-1316.

[5] Akinyanju, O. and Ladapo, F. (1979) Cholelithiasis and Biliary Tract Disease in Sickle Cell Disease in Nigerians. *Postgraduate Medical Journal*, **55**, 400-402. http://dx.doi.org/10.1136/pgmj.55.644.400

[6] Dos Santos, G.A.P., Bellomo-Brandão, M.A. and Da Costa-Pinto, E.A.L. (2008) Gallstones in Children with Sickle Cell Disease Followed up at a Brazilian Hematology Center. *Arquivos de Gastroenterologia*, **45**, 313-318. http://dx.doi.org/10.1590/S0004-28032008000400010

[7] Serjeant, B.R. and Serjeant, B.E. (1993) Management of Sickle Cell Disease; Lessons of Jamaïcan Cohort Study. *Blood Reviews*, **7**, 137-145. http://dx.doi.org/10.1016/0268-960X(93)90001-K

[8] Yé, D., Kouéta F., Dao, L., Kaboret, S. and Sawadogo, A. (2008) Prise en charge de la drépanocytose en milieu pédiatrique: Expérience du centre hospitalier universitaire pédiatrique Charles-de-Gaulle de Ouagadougou (Burkina Faso). *Santé*, **18**, 70-75.

[9] Athanassiou-Metaxa, M., Tsatra, I. and Koussi, A. (2002) Lithiase biliaire chez les patients drépanocytaires: L'expérience grecque. *Archives de Pédiatrie*, **8**, 878. http://dx.doi.org/10.1016/S0929-693X(02)00014-3

[10] Silva, I.V., Reis, A.F., Palare, M.J., Ferrao, A., Rodrigues, T. and Morais, A. (2015) Sickle Cell Disease in Children: Chronic Complications and Search of Predictive Factors for Adverse Outcomes. *European Journal of Haematology*, **94**, 157-161. http://dx.doi.org/10.1111/ejh.12411

[11] Itoua-Ngaporo, A., Ngoma, K. and Paris, J.C. (1987) La prevalence de la lithiase biliaire dans la drépanocytose homozygote. *Médecine et Chirurgie Digestives*, **16**, 479-482.

[12] Abby, C.B., Sangaré, A., Bougouma, A., Méité, M., Kéita, A., Djédjé, A.T., *et al.* (1996) Lithiase biliaire et drépanocytose. *Rev Méd Côte-d'Ivoire*, **78**, 27-31.

[13] Sarnaik, S., Slovis, T.L., Corbett, D.P., Emami, A. and Whitten, C.F. (1980) Incidence of Cholelithiasis in Sickle Cell Anemia Using the Ultrasonic Gray-Scale Technique. *The Journal of Pediatrics*, **96**, 1005-1008. http://dx.doi.org/10.1016/S0022-3476(80)80626-3

[14] Bond, L.R., Hatty, S.R., Horn, M.E.C., Dick, M., Meire, H.B. and Bellingham, A.J.G. (1987) Stones in Sickle Cell Disease in the United Kingdom. *BMJ*, **295**, 234-236. http://dx.doi.org/10.1136/bmj.295.6592.234

[15] Bogue, C.O., Murphy, A.J., Gerstle, J.T., Moineddin, R. and Daneman, A. (2010) Risk Factors, Complications, and Outcomes of Gallstones in Children: A Singlecenter Review. *Journal of Pediatric Gastroenterology & Nutrition*, **50**, 303-308. http://dx.doi.org/10.1097/MPG.0b013e3181b99c72

[16] Nzeh, D.A. and Adedoyin, M.A. (1989) Sonographic Pattern of Gallbladder Disease in Children with Sickle Cell Anaemia. *Pediatric Radiology*, **19**, 290-292. http://dx.doi.org/10.1007/BF02467294

[17] Werlin, S.L. and Scott, J.P. (1996) Is Biliary Sludge a Stone-in-Waiting? *The Journal of Pediatrics*, **129**, 321-322. http://dx.doi.org/10.1016/S0022-3476(96)70061-6

[18] Durosinmi, M.A., Ogunseyinde, A.O., Olatunji, P.O. and Esnas, J.F. (1989) Prevalence of Cholelithiasis in Nigerians with Sickle-Cell Disease. *African Journal of Medical Sciences*, **18**, 223-227.

[19] Stephens, C.G. and Scott, R.B. (1980) Cholelithiasis in Sickle Cell Anaemia: Surgical or Medical Management. *Archives of Internal Medicine*, **140**, 648-651. http://dx.doi.org/10.1001/archinte.1980.00330170064026

[20] Malone, B.S. and Werlin, S.L. (1988) Cholecystectomy and Cholelithiasis in Sickle Cell Anaemia. *American Journal of Diseases of Children*, **142**, 799-800.

[21] Diop, N., Diao-Bah, M., Ndiaye-Pape, L., Diouf, E., Kane, O., Bèye, M., *et al.* (2008) Priseen charge peri-operatoire de la cholecystectomie par voielaparoscopique chez l'enfantdrépanocytaire homozygote. *Archives de Pédiatrie*, **15**, 1393-1397. http://dx.doi.org/10.1016/j.arcped.2008.06.012

22

Transient Macroamylasemia in a Severely Multiple-Handicapped Child Following the Development of Acute Bronchitis

Yoshihiko Sakurai

Department of Pediatrics, Matsubara Tokushukai Hospital, Matsubara, Japan
Email: ysakurai-th@umin.ac.jp

Abstract

Macroamylasemia is a condition of elevated serum amylase levels in which normal serum amylase form a complex with high molecular weight proteins such as immunoglobulins. This is a case report on a patient with macroamylasemia following acute asthmatic bronchitis. A 5-year-old male with cerebral palsy and developmental retardation was admitted to our hospital because of high fever and severe cough. Treatment of the respiratory symptoms provided symptomatic improvement, but the serum amylase levels became suddenly elevated. Although acute pancreatitis associated with respiratory infection was initially suspected, a predominant salivary isoamylase, normal serum lipase level, low urine amylase level, and low amylase-creatinine clearance ratio (ACCR) (0.58%) indicated macroamylasemia. The serum amylase level decreased, and the ACCR increased within normal range 2 weeks after discharge. Both of these indicators have been within normal range over the past year. Transient macroamylasemia can be misdiagnosed as acute pancreatitis, especially in a severely multiple-handicapped child who is unable to complain. The ACCR is useful in the diagnosis of macroamylasemia.

Keywords

Acute Respiratory Infections, Amylase-Creatinine Clearance Ratio (ACCR), Macroamylasemia, Multiple-Handicapped Child

1. Introduction

Macroamylasemia is a condition in which normal serum amylase form a complex with high molecular weight proteins such as immunoglobulin A and rarely immunoglobulin G [1]. In 1964, Wilding *et al.* firstly described the presence in circulating blood of an enzymatically active macromolecular amylase-immunoglobulin complex as a cause of persistent hyperamylasemia [2]. In 1967, Berk *et al.* referred to this condition as macroamylasemia [3]. Macroamylase undergoes a slower renal clearance rate due to its high molecular mass over a wide range (molecular weight, 150,000 - 2,000,000 Da) [4]. A decrease in the urinary excretion of amylase results in retention in blood and an elevation in the serum amylase levels. Macroamylasemia reportedly occurs in 2.5% of all hyperamylasemic patients, and in 1% of apparently healthy adults with normal amylase levels [1]. It has been associated with various diseases such as celiac disease, lymphoma, the human immunodeficiency virus infection, monoclonal gammopathy, rheumatoid arthritis, and ulcerative colitis. The exact prevalence of macroamylasemia in children remains unknown, and there have only been a few reports on pediatric cases with celiac disease [5], lymphoma in Wiskott-Aldrich syndrome [6], Crohn disease [7], and appendicitis [8]. In the present case, a severely multiple-handicapped boy had a significantly elevated plasma amylase level while in the hospital for acute asthmatic bronchitis.

2. Case Presentation

A 5-year-old male was admitted to our hospital with complaints of high fever and severe cough. He had hypoxic-ischemic encephalopathy in addition to severe perinatal asphyxia, epilepsy, developmental disorder, esophageal hiatal hernia, gastroesophageal reflux, and food allergy to eggs and peanuts. The patient had been managed at another hospital with eperisone, tizanidine, and chlordiazepoxide for intractable myotonia. An elemental diet had been administered through a nasogastric tube. His family history was unremarkable, and his past history showed frequent hospitalization because of recurrent lower respiratory tract infection.

One month before admission, he underwent gastrostomy successfully at another hospital for nutritional support, because nasogastric tube feeding did not fully protect against aspiration or ensure an adequate nutrition intake. Fervescence and cough developed 3 days before admission and persisted. A physical examination on admission showed marked emaciation (height, 100 cm; body weight, 9.8 kg) with a high temperature (38.9°C) and tachypnea (respiratory rate, 52/min). The saturation of peripheral oxygen with a pulse oximeter was 88%. Chest auscultation revealed bilateral fine inspiratory crackles and end expiratory wheeze. Laboratory investigations demonstrated a white blood cell count of 4800/μL with normal differential. C-reactive protein (CRP) was markedly increased at 14.71 mg/dL, and procalcitonin was 2.42 ng/mL. No other significant abnormality was found in the blood biochemical tests, including the amylase level. Rapid diagnostic tests for the RS virus, adenovirus, and mycoplasma were all negative. Chest radiograph revealed an infiltrative shadow in the right hilar region and lower lung field. Although a low white blood cell count that is still within normal range may result from an overwhelming infection that exhausts white blood cells faster than they can be produced, hepatic dysfunction, renal dysfunction, and coagulopathy that are frequently observed in such a severe infection were not evident. Based on these findings, he was diagnosed with acute asthmatic bronchitis. Short-acting bronchodilators, inhaled corticosteroids, and intravenous antibiotics were commenced. He also received intravenous fluids to prevent dehydration. A congested nose developed and the creatine kinase levels increased probably due to hypertonia; these symptoms and aberrant values were transiently observed after admission. However, his respiratory status was gradually improved, and he became lively and active on hospital day 9. On hospital day 10, the CRP level was decreased to 0.14 mg/dL within normal range, but only a modest increase in amylase was observed (189 IU/L). Dysfunction of the liver and kidney was not evident. A change in facial expression was unclear when the parotid gland and submaxillary gland were palpated. No swelling of the glands was observed. On the assumption that the mild elevation of amylase was transient, he stayed out overnight at his home on a trial basis. He returned to the hospital without any incident on the following day (12). In anticipation of discharge, blood examination was conducted, which revealed an unexpected further elevation in amylase (443 IU/L). Abdominal tenderness was unclear. Suspecting acute pancreatitis associated with acute infection, abdominal ultrasound imaging was performed, but it could not depict the pancreas very clearly. Since oozing blood from the puncture site was persistent, clotting function tests were performed but revealed normal clotting ability except for a mild prolongation of prothrombin time (PT): PT (13.4 sec), activated partial thromboplastin time (APTT, 29.0 sec), fibrinogen (332 mg/dL), fibrin and fibrinogen degradation product (FDP, <2.5 μg/mL), and D-dimer (<0.5 μg/mL). Blood chemistry revealed that the serum lipase level was within normal range (16 U/L). Amylase isoenzyme analysis revealed that the pancreatic amylase was 6%, while the salivary amylase was 94%. Furthermore, urine amylase was below the lower limit of normal (73 IU/L), and the amylase-creatinine clearance ratio (ACCR) was calculated to be 0.58%. Based on these findings, the patient was diagnosed with macroamylasemia, and he was discharged on hospital day 17 after observing the clinical course. Two weeks after discharge, the amylase level was decreased within normal range (59 IU/L), and the ACCR was increased to more than 1% (1.12%). The serum amylase level and ACCR have been within normal range over the past year.

3. Discussion

In the present case, the serum amylase levels were elevated during the convalescent phase of acute asthmatic bronchitis. Since tenderness and swelling of the salivary glands were not evident, mumps was likely negative and acute pancreatitis was suspected. Pancreatitis is a rare condition in children. The predominant causes for developing pancreatitis in children include trauma; congenital pancreaticobiliary malformations; drugs such as anticonvulsant valproate; toxins; viral infections; hereditary disorders; and metabolic disorders [9]. In the present case, acute pancreatitis associated with respiratory infection or drugs was initially suspected. However, on the basis of the laboratory findings, including the normal level of serum lipase, lower level of urine amylase, and reduced ACCR, macroamylasemia was diagnosed. Serum lipase is a useful backup test to confirm pancreatic insufficiency [10], while serum amylase is a sensitive marker. In macroamylasemia, amylase levels increase in blood and decrease in urine, resulting in the reduction of ACCR. It is well accepted that ACCR is very useful for diagnosing macroamylasemia [11] [12]. ACCR shows 1% - 5% in normal individuals. ACCR decrease to less than 1% in macroamylasemia, whereas significant elevation is observed in acute pancreatitis [13]. It was difficult to interpret physical findings in the current patient; however, a decrease in the ACCR aided in the differential diagnosis.

In the present case, as the amylase level elevated on hospital day 12 in the convalescent phase of acute respiratory infection, immunoglobulins exhibiting a cross reactivity with amylase might emerge with an increase in immunoglobulins against a pathogenic organism. This might cause macroamylasemia to develop.

To our knowledge, there have been few reports on acute respiratory infections-associated macroamylasemia.

4. Conclusion

Our case indicates the possible development of transient macroamylasemia in pediatric patients with acute respiratory infections. When encountering a patient with hyperamylasemia, the possibility of macroamylasemia should be considered in the differential diagnosis. In addition, the ACCR is helpful in differentiating between acute pancreatitis and macroamylasemia.

References

[1] Klonoff, D.C. (1980) Macroamylasemia and Other Immunoglobulin-Complexed Enzyme Disorders. *Western Journal of Medicine*, **133**, 392-407.

[2] Wilding, P., Cooke, W. and Nicholson, G. (1964) Globulin-Bound Amylase: A Cause of Persistently Elevated Levels in Serum. *Annals of Internal Medicine*, **60**, 1053-1059. http://dx.doi.org/10.7326/0003-4819-60-6-1053

[3] Berk, J.E., Kizu, H., Wilding, P. and Searcy, R.L. (1967) Macroamylasemia: A Newly Recognized Cause for Elevated Serum Amylase Activity. *The New England Journal of Medicine*, **277**, 941-946. http://dx.doi.org/10.1056/NEJM196711022771801

[4] Levitt, M.D., Duane, W.C., and Cooperband, S.R. (1972) Study of Macroamylase Complexes. *The Journal of Laboratory and Clinical Medicine*, **80**, 414-422.

[5] Barera, G., Bazzigaluppi, E., Viscardi, M., Renzetti, F., Bianchi, C., Chiumello, G. and Bosi, E. (2001) Macroamylasemia Attributable to Gluten-Related Amylase Autoantibodies: A Case Report. *Pediatrics*, **107**, E93. http://dx.doi.org/10.1542/peds.107.6.e93

[6] Yoshida, K., Minegishi, Y., Okawa, H., Yata, J., Tokoi, S., Kitagawa, T. and Utagawa, T. (1997) Epstein-Barr virus-Associated Malignant Lymphoma with Macroamylasemia and Monoclonal Gammopathy in a Patient with Wiskott-Aldrich Syndrome. *Pediatric Hematology and Oncology*, **14**, 85-89. http://dx.doi.org/10.3109/08880019709030889

[7] Venkataraman, D., Howarth, L., Beattie, R.M. and Afzal, N.A. (2012) A Very High Amylase Can Be Benign in Paediatric Crohn's Disease. *BMJ Case Reports*, 2012. http://dx.doi.org/10.1136/bcr.02.2012.5917

[8] Ko, J. and Lee, D. (2009) Macroamylasemia in a 4-Year-Old Girl with Abdominal Pain. *Korean Journal of Pediatrics*, **52**, 1283-1285. http://dx.doi.org/10.3345/kjp.2009.52.11.1283

[9] Li, H., Qian, Z., Liu, Z., Liu, X., Han, X. and Kang, H. (2010) Risk Factors and Outcome of Acute Renal Failure in Patients with Severe Acute Pancreatitis. *The Journal of Critical Care*, **25**, 225-229. http://dx.doi.org/10.1016/j.jcrc.2009.07.009

[10] Winslet, M., Hall, C., London, N.J. and Neoptolemos, J.P. (1992) Relation of Diagnostic Serum Amylase Levels to Aetiology and Severity of Acute Pancreatitis. *Gut*, **33**, 982-986. http://dx.doi.org/10.1136/gut.33.7.982

[11] Levitt, M.D., Rapoport, M. and Cooperband, S.R. (1969) The Renal Clearance of Amylase in Renal Insufficiency, Acute Pancreatitis, and Macroamylasemia. *Annals of Internal Medicine*, **71**, 919-925. http://dx.doi.org/10.7326/0003-4819-71-5-919

[12] Kazmierczak, S.C., Van Lente, F., McHugh, A.M. and Katzin, W.E. (1988) Macroamylasemia with a Markedly Increased Amylase Clearance Ratio in a Patient with Renal Cell Carcinoma. *Clinical Chemistry*, **34**, 435-438.

[13] Murray, W.R. and Mackay, C. (1977) The Amylase Creatinine Clearance Ratio in Acute Pancreatitis. *British Journal of Surgery*, **64**, 189-191. http://dx.doi.org/10.1002/bjs.1800640311

23

Etiologies and Outcome of Children with Purulent Meningitis at the Yaounde Gyneco-Obstetric and Pediatric Hospital (Cameroon)

Séraphin Nguefack[1,2*], Andréas Chiabi[1,2], Jacob Enoh[1,3], El Hadji Djouberou[2], Evelyn Mah[1,2], Karen Kengne Kamga[1], Sandra Tatah[2], Elie Mbonda[1,2]

[1]Departement of Pediatric Neurology, Yaounde Gynaeco-Obstetric and Pediatric Hospital, Yaounde, Cameroon
[2]Faculty of Medicine and Biomedical Sciences, University of Yaounde I, Yaounde, Cameroon
[3]Departement of Pediatric, University of Cocody-Abidjan, Abidjan, Côte d'Ivoire
Email: [*]seraphin_nguefack@yahoo.fr

Academic Editor: Carl E. Hunt, George Washington University School of Medicine and Health Sciences, USA

Abstract

Background: Bacterial meningitis is one of the most severe infections in infants and children. It is associated with high mortality and neurological sequelae. In order to improve the prognosis of infants and children with purulent meningitis, we decided to conduct this study whose main objective was to identify the main pathogens responsible and describe the outcome in infants and children aged 2 months to 15 years admitted for purulent meningitis at the Yaounde Gyneco-Obstetric and Pediatric Hospital (YGOPH). Method: This was a cross-sectional study with retrospective data collection and consecutive sampling. Our study was conducted from 1 January 2009 to 31 December 2013. The patients included in the study were infants and children aged from 2 months to 15 years who were admitted for bacterial meningitis at the YGOPH, confirmed by bacteriological examination of cerebrospinal fluid (CSF) with identification of the pathogen by culture or soluble antigen. The data was analyzed using SPSS Version 18.0 and Excel 2007. The Chi-square test was used to determine the association of various variables. The significance threshold was set as P < 0.05. Results: We selected 171 cases of purulent meningitis who represented 1.54% of admitted patients. The sex ratio was 1.2. We noted that 45% of our patients were aged 2 months to 1 year. The main presenting complaints were fever (98.8%), seizures (44.4%) and vomiting (28.7%). *Haemophilus influenzae* was found in 67 children (39.2%), followed by *Streptococcus pneumoniae*

[*]Corresponding author.

in 54 children (31.6%) and *Neisseria meningitidis* in 17 children (9.9%). Acute complications (status epilepticus, coma) were seen in 33% of patients. The statistically significant (P < 0.05) factors for poor prognosis were aged from 2 months to 1 year (P = 0.0004), coma (P = 0.32), intracranial hypertension (P = 0.0001), the pathogen (P = 0.0032 *Pneumococcus*), a delay of more than three days between the onset of the disease and the treatment (P = 0.0134) and brain abscess (P = 0.0001). We identified 32 deaths (18.7%) and 17 cases (9.9%) with neurological sequelae before discharge. Conclusion: The incidence of acute bacterial meningitis remains high in our context. The main causes were *Haemophilus influenzae, Streptococcus pneumoniae* and *Neisseria meningitis.* The mortality rate was high with poor prognosis factors such as age less than 12 months, delayed care, pneumococcal meningitis, coma, brain abscess, and intracranial hypertension. Focus should be placed on strengthening the routine immunization on vaccine-preventable diseases of infants and children against *Haemophilus influenzae, Pneumococcus* and *Meningococcus.*

Keywords

Bacterial Meningitis, Etiologies, Outcome, Children, Cameroon

1. Introduction

Meningitis is one of the most severe infections in infants and children with an incidence of 25 per 100,000 children in Africa [1]. This infection is associated with high rates of acute complications, death and the risk of long-term morbidity. Its outcome was generally fatal before the advent of antibiotics whose discovery, along with those of vaccines, improved on the incidence and prognosis of the disease [2] [3].

Although morbidity, mortality and occurrence of sequelae have diminished, these continue to be important in the pediatric population of developing countries, and their severity is highest in infants and children [3]. In 2012, in the course of the surveillance of meningitis in Africa the World Health Organization (WHO) [4] identified 22,000 meningitis cases in 14 countries in the meningitis belt. In Cameroon, several studies have been done on this subject [5]-[8]. Case fatality rates ranging from 8% to 27.44% and rates of appearance of sequelae ranging from 4% - 20% have been reported in studies conducted in different parts of the country [5]-[8]. In order to improve the prognosis of bacterial meningitis in infants and children in our environment, we decided to conduct this study whose aim was to determine the etiology and describe the prognosis in infants and children aged 2 months to 15 years who had been admitted for purulent meningitis at the Yaounde Gyneco-obstetric and Pediatric Hospital.

2. Method

This was a descriptive cross-sectional study, with retrospective data collection for the period from 1 January 2009 to 31 December 2013. Sampling was consecutive. All patients aged 2 months to 15 years admitted in the pediatric unit with the diagnosis of bacterial meningitis based on the clinical and bacteriological criteria, through identification of the pathogen in CSF culture or soluble antigen in the CSF. We excluded patients in whom the diagnosis of meningitis was established but the pathogen was not identified. We selected all patients with meningitis who fulfilled our inclusion criteria through the registers of the pediatric unit. Data collected included: gender, age, weight of the child, the clinical signs of the child at the time of admission, the findings of the physical examination, the results of the cytology and bacteriology CSF analysis, CSF soluble antigen test, acute complications (death, altered state of consciousness, status epilepticus), sequelae at the time of discharge (psychomotor regression, motor deficit, hydrocephalus). The results were analyzed using SPSS 18.0 and Microsoft Office Excel 2007. The statistical test Chi-square was used to determine associations between variables. The significance threshold was set as P < 0.05.

3. Results

3.1. Study Population

We included 171 patients aged 2 months to 15 years seen between 1 January 2009 and 31 December 2013, with purulent meningitis, in whom a pathogen had been identified. During the same period we had 11035 patients aged 2 months to 15 years admitted in the unit, thus patients with purulent meningitis represented 1.54% of admitted patients. We noted a peak incidence in the age group of 2 to 12-month (45%, **Figure 1**). The average age was 39.4 ± 32.1 months and age range 2 months to 15 years. The sex ratio was 1.2.

3.2. Presenting Complaints

The main presenting complaints were fever (98.8%), seizures (44.4%) and vomiting (28.7%) (**Table 1**).

3.3. Etiologies

Haemophilus influenzae was the most common pathogen (**Table 2**). It constituted 39.2% of organisms that caused purulent meningitis, followed by *Streptococcus pneumoniae* with 31.6% of the cases. In the age group from 2 months to 2 years *Haemophilus influenzae* was most incriminated.

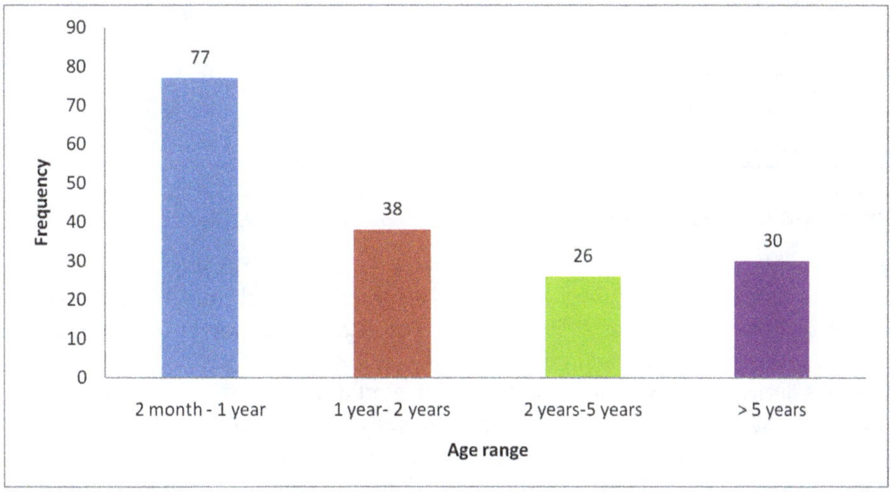

Figure 1. Distribution of patients according to age groups.

Table 1. Distribution of patients according to the chief complaint.

Symptoms	Number	Percentage (%)
Fever	169	(98.8)
Seizures	76	(44.4)
Vomiting	49	(28.7)
Coma	30	(17.5)
Irritability	28	(16.4)
Head ache	20	(11.7)
Agitation	19	(11.1)
Grunting	8	(4.7)
Excessive crying	7	(4.1)
Somnolence	6	(3.5)
Constipation	4	(2.3)
Photophobia	2	(1.2)
Refuse to breast feed	2	(1.2)
Purpura fulminans	2	(1.2)

Table 2. Distribution of pathogens according to age.

Germs	2 month - 1 yr	1 yr - 2 yr	2 yr - 5 yr	>5 yr	Total
H .influenzae	43	13	2	9	67
S. pneumoniae	19	9	15	11	54
N. meningitidis	2	3	8	5	18
Group B Streptococcus	6	5	0	0	11
Group C Streptococcus	1	0	0	5	6
Salmonella	2	2	0	0	4
E. coli	0	2	0	0	2
Klebsiella pneumoniae	2	0	0	0	2
Pasteurella sp	1	1	0	0	2
Staphylococcus aureus	0	2	0	0	2
Citrobacter sp	0	1	0	0	1
Pseudomonas aeruginosa	0	0	1	0	1
Other streptococcus sp	1	0	0	0	1
Total	**77**	**38**	**26**	**30**	**171**

3.4. Outcome and Sequelae

The average number of days of hospitalization was 15.35 days ± 8.851 days, ranging from 1 day to 41 days. The period of time between onset of fever and that of antibiotics ranged from 1 to 23 days giving an average of 4.8 days ± 4 days. Fifty-seven patients (33.3%) had complications during hospitalization (**Table 3**). Note that the same patient may have had several complications simultaneously. Status epilepticus and coma were the main complications during hospitalization (**Table 3**). The mortality rate observed in our study was 18.7% (32 deaths); 122 patients (71.3%) recovered without immediate sequelae and 9.9% had recovered with immediate sequelae (**Table 4**). We found a statistically significant association ($P < 0.05$) between alteration of consciousness, intracranial hypertension, cerebral abscess and progression to neurological sequelae and death. We equally found a statistically significant association ($P < 0.05$) between *Streptococcus pneumoniae*, *Haemophilus influenzae* and poor clinical outcome. We recorded 17 deaths (53.1%), and 44.4% of the sequelae were due pneumococcal infection, thus making it the most virulent pathogen. Other poor prognostic factors ($P < 0.05$) were age less than 12 months and the delayed care above 3 days after onset of symptoms.

4. Discussion

The incidence of bacterial meningitis in our study remained high with 1.54% of admissions. This figure could be underestimated because we excluded patients in whom the pathogen was not identified. The sex ratio of 1.2 was close to Faye [9] in Ivory Coast who found a sex ratio of 1.3 in 2003. Meanwhile Sile [6] in northern Cameroon found a sex ratio of 1.6 in 1999. We did not find an explanation for this male predominance. The average age of our patients was 32.1 months with a standard deviation of 39.4, close to the average age of most authors [5] [10] [11]. Clinically, the study noted that the major symptoms to suggest meningitis in infants and children were fever, seizures and vomiting in respectively 98.8%, 44.4% and 28.7% of patients (**Table 1**).

In our study, *Haemophilus influenzae* was the most common pathogen, found in 39.2% of the patients, followed by *Streptococcus pneumoniae* and *Neisseria meningitidis* with respectively 31.6 and 10.5% of the patients (**Table 2**). In a study done in the same unit between 2004 and 2009 *Haemophilus influenzae* was the most commonly identified pathogen followed by *Streptococcus pneumoniae* and *Neisseria meningitidis*, respectively, in 40.3%, 34.2% and 5.4% [5]. Our results are also similar to those reported in Senegal by Cisse [12] who found *Haemophilus influenzae* (42.3%) followed by *Streptococcus pneumoniae* (31.9%) and *Neisseria meningitidis* (11.2%). Almuneef [13] in Saudi Arabia also identified *Haemophilus influenzae* as the first pathogen in bacterial meningitis in persons younger than 5 years followed by *pneumococcus* and *meningococcus*. Other authors [14] [15] in Mozambique and Angola also had, with some variation at the relative frequencies, globally the same results as our study with *Haemophilus influenzae* as the first cause of meningitis before the age of 15 years. How-

Table 3. Complications found during hospitalization.

Complications	Number	Percentage (%)
Status epilepticus	40	54.7
Coma	18	24.6
Motor deficits	9	12.3
Cerebral abscess	4	5.4
ICHT*	1	1.3
Digestive haemorrhage	1	1.3
Total	73	100

*Intracranial hypertension.

Table 4. Distribution of patients according to sequelae at time of hospital discharge.

Sequelae	Number	Percentage (%)
Psychomotor Regression	5	2.9
Deafness	4	2.4
Hemiparesis	4	2.4
Hydrocephaly	3	1.8
Tetra paresis	2	1.2
Facial paralysis	1	0.6
Total	17	9.9

ever other studies [7] [8] [16] done locally in Cameroon and other African studies [1] [17] [18] reported, with some variation in the relative frequencies, a predominance of *Streptococcus pneumoniae*, followed by *Haemophilus influenzae* and *Neisseria meningitis*. Massenet [19] in a study in the northern part of Cameroon found a high prevalence of *Neisseria meningitidis* with 70.2%, followed by 19.5% with *Streptococcus pneumoniae* and *Haemophilus influenzae* with 10.3%. This predominance of *Neisseria meningitidis* in the study of Massenet is explained by the fact that the study was conducted in the northern part of the country which lies in the African meningitis belt. The predominance of *Haemophilus* in our study may be related to selection bias because we have included only the patients who had a positive culture or positive soluble antigen. However the high incidence of meningitis caused by *Haemophilus influenzae* may also be related to the lack of vaccination in most of these patients, because since the vaccine was introduced in 2008, a decrease in the incidence of *Haemophilus influenzae* meningitis was expected. This is unlike the study of Wall [17] in Malawi that showed a significant decline in *Haemophilus influenzae* meningitis after the introduction of the vaccine.

The mortality rate observed in our study was 18.5%. This rate is close to the mortality rate of 21.8% presented by Gervaix [8] in Cameroon in 2012 and the 20.3% of deaths found by Gomes [20]. It is less than the mortality rate reported in other studies [7] [10] in Cameroon which were respectively 27.4% and 29.8%. This mortality rate is also lower than the 24% found by Roca [14] in Mozambique. The most vulnerable age group is that of two months to one year, which represented 43.7% of deaths and 38.8% of sequelae. The vulnerability of children under one year was also found by other authors [7] [8].

Streptococcus pneumoniae was the pathogen responsible for most of the deaths and sequelae in our study as confirmed by several other studies [7] [8] [21]-[23]. Seventeen patients had at least one sequela at the time of discharge representing of 9.9%. This rate is similar to that found by Moufdi [24] who reported 10.2% of sequelae at time of discharge. This frequency of sequelae is probably underestimated because of the absence of an evaluation long after the acute episode. In evaluating these patients later, these sequelae would certainly be more severe.

The poor prognostic factors were age < 12 months, pneumococcal infection, delayed care > 3 days, the presence of a coma, and signs of intracranial hypertension. Pelkonen [15] in Angola found as poor prognostic factors coma and delayed care, while Gervaix [8] found as poor prognostic factors: age < 2 years and pneumococcal infection. Farag [25] found age < 12 months, and Kirimi [26] in Turkey had coma as a factor of poor prognosis.

5. Conclusion

The incidence of acute bacterial meningitis remains high in our context. The main causative pathogens are *Haemophilus influenzae, Streptococcus pneumoniae* and *Neisseria meningitidis*. The mortality and acute sequelae remain high with poor prognostic factors such as age less than 12 months, delays in care, pneumococcal meningitis, coma, brain abscess, and intracranial hypertension. A focus should be placed on strengthening the routine immunization on vaccine-preventable diseases of infants and children against *Haemophilus influenzae, pneumococcus* and *meningococcus*.

References

[1] Peltola, H. (2001) Burden of Meningitis and Order Severe Infection of Children in Africa: Implications for Prevention. *Clinical Infetious Diseases*, **31**, 64-75. http://dx.doi.org/10.1086/317534

[2] Chavez-Bueno, S. and McCracken, G.H. (2005) Bacterial Meningitis in Children. *Pediatric Clinics of North America*, **52**, 795-810. http://dx.doi.org/10.1016/j.pcl.2005.02.011

[3] Koko, J., Dufillot, D. and Gahouma, D. (1996) Mortalité hospitalière dans le service de pédiatrie générale de L'Hôpital pédiatrique d'Owando (Libreville-Gabon): Aspects caractéristiques. *Annales de Pédiatrie*, **43**, 624-630.

[4] Organisation Mondiale de la santé (2012) Rapport sur les statistiques de santé dans le monde disponible sur le site. http://who.int/gho/publication/world-health-statistics/full.pdf

[5] Tiodoung, T.A. (2008) Aspects cliniques, bactériologiques, thérapeutiques et évolutifs des méningites bactériennes du nourrisson et de l'enfant à propos de 149 cas à l'HGOPY. Université des Montagnes, Cameroon.

[6] Sile, M.H., Sile, H., Mbonda, E., Feuzeu, R. and Fonkoua, M.C. (1999) Les méningites purulentes de l'enfant au Nord Cameroun: aspects cliniques, bactériologiques et thérapeutiques. *Médecine d'Afrique Noire*, **46**, 16-20.

[7] Bernard-Bonin, A.C. and Tetanye, E. (1985) Les méningites purulentes de l'enfant à Yaoundé: Aspects épidémiologiques et pronostiques. *Annales de la Société Belge de Médecine Tropicale*, **65**, 59-68.

[8] Gervaix, A., Taguebue, J., Bescher, B.N., *et al.* (2012) Bacterial Meningitis and Pneumococcal Serotype Distribution in Children in Cameroon. *The Pediatric Infectious Diseases Journal*, **31**, 1084-1087.

[9] Faye, K., Doukou, E.S., Boni, C., Akoua-Koffi, C. and Diallo-Touré, K. (2003) Agents des méningites purulentes communautaires de l'enfant: Tendance épidémiologique à Abidjan, Cote d'Ivoire, de 1999 à l'an 2000. *Bulletin de la Société de Patholologie Exotique*, **96**, 313-316.

[10] Ntapli, A. (1993) Etude des séquelles neurologiques des méningites bactériennes chez le nourrisson et l'enfant à l'hôpital central de Yaoundé. Thèse de Médecine. Université de Yaoundé I.

[11] Bingen, E.C., Lévy, F., De la Rocque, M., Boucherat, Y. and Aujard, R.C. (2005) Méningites à pneumocoque de l'enfant en France : Age de survenue et facteurs de risque médicaux. *Archives de Pédiatrie*, **12**, 1187-1189. http://dx.doi.org/10.1016/j.arcped.2005.04.076

[12] Cisse, E., Sow, H.D., Ouangre, A.R., Gaye, A., Sow, A.I., Samb, A. and Fall, M. (1989) Méningites bactériennes dans un hôpital pédiatrique en zone tropicale. *Médecine Tropicale*, **49**, 265-269.

[13] Almuneef, M., Memish, Z., Khan, Y., Kagallwala, A. and Alshaalan, M. (1998) Childhood Bacterial Meningitis in Saudia Arabia. *Journal of Infection*, **36**,157-160. http://dx.doi.org/10.1016/S0163-4453(98)80005-4

[14] Roca, A., Bassat, Q., Morais, L., Machevo, S., Sigaúque, B., O'Callaghan, C., *et al.* (2009) Surveillance of Acute Bacterial Meningitis among Children Admitted to a District Hospital in Rural Mozambique. *Clinical Infectious Diseases*, **48**, S172-S180. http://dx.doi.org/10.1086/596497

[15] Pelkonen, T., Roine, I., Monteiro, L., Correia, M., Pitkäranta, A., Bernardino, L. and Peltola, H. (2009) Risks Factors for Death and Severe Neurological Sequelae in Childhood Bacterial Meningitis in Sub-Saharan Africa. *Clinical Infectious Diseases*, **48**, 1107-1110. http://dx.doi.org/10.1086/597463

[16] Fonkoua, M.C., Cunin, P., Sorlin, P., Musi, J. and Martin, M.V. (2001) Les méningites d'étiologie bactérienne à Yaoundé (Cameroun) en 1999-2000. *Bulletin de la Société de Pathologie Exotique*, **94**, 300-303.

[17] Wall, E.C., Everett, D.B., Mukaka, M., Bar-Zeev, N., Feasey, N., Jahn, A., *et al.* (2014) Bacterial Meningitis in Malawian Adults, Adolescents, and Children during the Era of Antiretroviral Scale-Up and *Haemophilus influenza* Type b Vaccination, 2000-2012. *Clinical Infectious Diseases*, **58**, 137-145. http://dx.doi.org/10.1093/cid/ciu057

[18] Kisakye, A., Mukambi, I., Nansera, D., Lewis, R., Braka, F., Wobudeya, E., *et al.* (2009) Surveillance for *Streptoccus pneumoniae* Méningitis in Children Aged < 5 Years: Implication for Immunization in Uganda. *Clinical Infectious Diseases*, **48**, S153-S161. http://dx.doi.org/10.1086/596495

[19] Massenet, D., Birguel, J., Azowe, F., Ebong, C., Gake, B., Lombart, J.-P. and Boisier, P. (2013) Epidemiologic Pattern of Meningococcal Meningitis in Northern Cameroon in 2007-2010: Contribution of PCR-Enhanced Surveillance. *Pathogens and Global Health*, **107**, 15-20. http://dx.doi.org/10.1179/2047773212Y.0000000070

[20] Gomes, I., Melo, A., Lucena, R., Cunha-Nascimento, M.H., Ferreira, A., Góes, J., *et al.* (1996) Prognosis of Bacterial Meningitis in Children. *Arquivos de Neuro-Psiquiatria*, **53**, 407-411. http://dx.doi.org/10.1590/S0004-282X1996000300008

[21] Yaro, S., Lourd, M., Traore, Y., Njanpop-Lafourcade, B.-M., Sawadogo, A., Sangare, L., *et al.* (2006) Epidemiological and Molecular Characteristics of Highly Lethal Pneuococcal Meningitis Epidemic in Burkina Faso. *Clinical Infectious Diseases*, **43**, 693-700. http://dx.doi.org/10.1086/506940

[22] Tetanye, E., Yondo, D., Bernard-Bonnin, A.C., Tchokoteu, P.F., Kago, I., Ndayo, M. and Mbede, J. (1990) Initial Treatment of Bacterial Meningitis in Yaounde, Cameroon: Theoretical Benefits of Ampicilline-Chloramphenicol Combination versus Chloramphenicol Alone. *Annals of Tropical Paediatrics*, **10**, 285-291.

[23] Thabet, F., Tilouche, S., Tabarki, B., Amrib, F., Guedichec, M.-N., Sfar, M.-T., *et al.* (2007) Mortalité par méningites à pneumocoque chez l'enfant. Facteurs pronostiques à propos d'une série de 73 observations. *Archives de Pédiatrie*, **14**, 334-337. http://dx.doi.org/10.1016/j.arcped.2006.11.012

[24] Moufdi, A. (2007) Les méningites purulentes du nourrisson et de l'enfant. Thèse de Médecine, Université Mohamed V-Souissi de Rabat, Rabat.

[25] Farag, H.F., Abdel-Fattah, M.M. and Youssri, A.M. (2005) Epidemiological, Clinical and Prognostic Profile of Acute Bacterial Meningitis among Children in Alexandria, Egypt. *Indian Journal of Medical Microbiology*, **23**, 95-101. http://dx.doi.org/10.4103/0255-0857.16047

[26] Kirimi, E., Tuncer, O., Arslan, S., Ataş, B., Caksen, H., Uner, A. and Oner, A.F. (2003) Prognostic Factors in Children with Purulent Meningitis in Turkey. *Acta Medica Okayama*, **57**, 39-44.

24

Fever among Children with Sickle-Cell Disease: Findings from the General Pediatric Ward of the Owendo Pediatric Hospital in Libreville, Gabon

Jean Koko[1,3*], Daniel Gahouma[1,3], Simon Ategbo[3], Cathérine Seilhan[2], Armelle Pambou[1], André Moussavou[3]

[1]General Pediatrics Service, Owendo Peditric Hospital (OPH), Libreville, Gabon
[2]Laboratory of Medical Biology, Owendo Pediatric Hospital (OPH), Libreville, Gabon
[3]Pediatrics Department, Faculty of Medicine, Health Sciences University (USS), Libreville, Gabon
Email: *jeankoko06@yahoo.fr

Academic Editor: Carl E. Hunt, George Washington University School of Medicine and Health Sciences, USA

Abstract

Sickle-cell disease (SCD) represents a substantial public health problem in Gabon. Fever is one of the principal reasons for the hospitalization of children afflicted by major sickle-cell disorder, since it can be a clinical reflection of severe infections that have the potential to become life threatening. Objectives: Identification of the main causes of fever in children with SCD in our clinical setting, with the aim of optimizing treatments. Patients and Methods: This is a retrospective study of all the medical files for children with SCD that were admitted to our ward, over a two year period, due to fever (>38.5°C) lasting more than 24 hours. Only those files that contained at least the following five fundamental medical examinations were retained for further evaluation: Complete Blood Count (CBC), blood smear, blood culture, urine culture and chest X-ray. Out of a total of 118 admissions (103 patients), 87 (73.7%) were due to the incidence of fever. The medical files of 11 patients were deemed to be unusable. Seventy-six episodes of fever were observed among 69 children, of which 42 were male and 27 female (sex ratio of 1.5). Among these, seven (10%) were admitted twice. Results: The age groups that were most affected included 12 - 18 year-olds (30 cases: 43.5%) and 6 - 12 year-olds (26 cases: 37.7%). The most common accompanying symptoms were bone and joint pain (43.4%), asthenia (22.4%), cough (19.7%), vomiting (17%) and headache (15.8%). The specific cause of the fever could not be pinpointed in 29 cases (38.1%). Aside from these cases, the main causes of fever were malaria (30.3%) and bronchopulmonary infections (22.4%). The white blood cell count was >20,000/mm^3 in 47% of respiratory infections, 43.5% of the cases involving malaria and 55.2% of cases of fever with unknown cause. Hemoglobin levels

*Corresponding author.

were <5g/dl for 52.2% of the cases involving malaria and 22.6% for those of unknown origin. For four patients, all less than 10 years of age, the disease was fatal. Conclusion: For the majority of fever episodes, the underlying cause could not be determined. Nonetheless, malaria was identified as one of the principal identifiable causes of fever among children with SDC in Libreville. Treatment for malaria upon admission, and the promotion of preventative measures, therefore seems to be appropriate for our clinical setting. In light of the large number of unresolved cases, systematic prescription of broad-spectrum antibiotics may also be called for.

Keywords

Sickle-Cell Disease, Fever, Malaria, Acute Lower Respiratory Infections (ALRI), Gabon

1. Introduction

Sickle cell disease (SCD) is the most widespread and most serious form of hemoglobin disorders [1]. Sub-Saharan Africa is the most affected area, with an incidence of sickle cell trait ranging from 2 to 30%, depending on the specific region [1]-[4]. According to recent estimates, close to 275,000 afflicted children are born worldwide each year, of which 80% are in Africa [1]. In Gabon, SCD is a major public health problem, with 24% of the population carriers of hemoglobin S (HbS) and a 2% - 3% level of SS (HbSS) homozygous [5] [6]. Infectious complications are responsible for high rates of morbidity and mortality in SCD patients [4] [7]-[12]. In developed countries, the initiation of effective preventive measures (newborn screening, oral penicillin prophylaxis, pneumococcal and Haemophilus type b immunization) has resulted in the dramatic reduction in these rates [7] [12] [13]. This preventive strategy remains not easily accessible in sub-Saharan Africa, except for some pilot projects [14] [15]. Fever may be the expression of these infections, as shown by several authors [16]-[20], but to our knowledge no similar studies have been conducted to date in Gabon. Also in case of occurrence of fever, the physician is confronted with the haunting of a serious infection requiring prompt and aggressive treatment. The aim of this study was to determine the main causes of fever in children with sickle cell disease in our context, in order to optimize therapeutic management.

2. Patients and Methods

Records of children with sickle cell disease, hospitalized in our department for fever (axillary temperature > 38.5˚C) evolving for more than 24 hours over a period of 24 months, were retrospectively analyzed. They were known sickle cell patients, the diagnosis having been made previously, most often during the development of acute complications. The hospital receives patients unselected, brought directly to the emergency room by the parents, or sent by other health facilities instead. No specific monitoring is organized there. Children are hospitalized alone without escorts. We selected only those files containing at least the following five tests: Complete Blood Count (CBC), blood smear (BS) to detect malaria parasites, urine culture, blood culture (≥1), and chest X-ray. A lumbar puncture was performed in cases of meningeal syndrome or other signs that indicated neurological issues. Out of a total of 118 admissions (103 patients), 87 (73.7%) were due to the incidence of fever. From the latter group, records from eleven patients were deemed to be unusable (incomplete files). Seventy-six episodes of fever were observed among 69 children (seven children were admitted twice or more). There were 42 boys and 27 girls, resulting in a gender ratio of 1.5. All of the patients were homozygous SS. None were receiving regular health checks and there was no documentable evidence of specific preventative measures (e.g. oral penicillin, pneumococcal and *Haemophilus influenzae* type b vaccination). The protocol of care in emergency included a dual probabilistic antibiotic treatment cefotaxime + gentamicin in addition to quinine salt perfusion. Transfusion of packed red blood cells was performed in all patients with hemoglobin < 5 g/dl. Ethical approval for the study was obtained from the research and ethics committee of the Faculty of Medicine of the Health Sciences University, Libreville, Gabon. Statistical analyses were performed using the Chi-squared distribution and Fisher's exact test for measures < 3. A p-value of <0.05 was considered to be significant.

3. Results

The most represented age groups were 12 - 18 year-olds (30 cases: 43.5%) and 6 - 12 year-olds (26 cases: 37.7%)

(**Figure 1**). The most common associated symptoms (**Table 1**) were bone and joint pain (43.4%), weakness (22.4%) and cough (19.7%). **Table 2** lists the causes of the fever. Three patients (3.9%) had urinary tract infection; the isolated microbes being *Escherichia Coli* (two cases) and *Klebsiella pneumoniae* (one case). The cause of the fever could only be clearly established for 29 of the cases (38.1%). The blood cultures were positive six times (8.7%); *Streptococcus pneumoniae* (two cases) and *Haemophilus influenzae* (two cases) were all associated with pulmonary impairment. *Klebsiella pneumoniae* (one case) and *Salmonella* spp (one case) were the other organisms that were detected. Lumbar punctures, which were carried out 8 times (11.6%), were normal: for one child undergoing convulsions, five children between the ages of 6 and 12 who had headaches and back pain, and two children of three and four years of age, respectively, who experienced vomiting and weakness. Analysis of symptoms associated with the fever (**Table 1**) indicated a significant difference (p = 0.002) between respiratory tract infections and malaria in terms of coughing fits. White blood cell counts were >20,000/mm^3 for 47% of the cases involving respiratory infections, 43.5% of the malaria cases and 55.25% of the cases of fever with unknown origin (**Table 3**); and there was no significant difference between these values. Four fatalities were documented (5.8%): two cases of acute anemia involving malaria in a two year old girl and a seven year old boy, one case of *Salmonella* spp septicemia for a four year old boy, and one case of a boy, aged 5, who was undergoing convulsions and for whom the cause could not be determined.

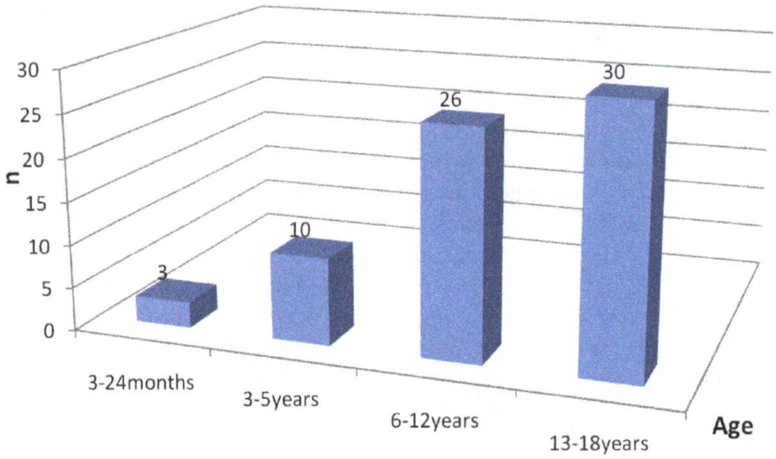

Figure 1. Age distribution of the 69 sickle cell disease patients.

Table 1. Functional signs depending on the cause of fever in the 69 children with sickle cell disease admitted to the Owendo Pediatric Hospital (HPO).

Causes symptoms	Malaria n = 23 (%)	Bronchopulmonary infection n = 17 (%)	Undetermined causes n = 29 (%)	Urinary tract infection n = 3 (%)	Osteomyelitis n = 2 (%)	Total (%)	p-value
Weakness	8 (34.8)*	2 (11.8)	4 (13.8)*	1 (33.3)	2 (100)	17 (22.4)	0.07
Headache	4 (17.4)	2 (11.8)	5 (17.2)	1 (33.3)	0 (0.0)	12 (15.8)	
Abdominal pain	5 (21.7)	2 (11.8)	3 (10.3)	0 (0.0)	0 (0.0)	10 (13.1)	
Bone and joint pain	7 (30.4)*	7 (41.2)	15 (51.7)*	2 (66.7)	2 (100)	33 (43.4)	0.12
Back pain	0 (0.0)	0 (0.0)	4 (13.8)	1 (33.3)	0 (0.0)	5 (6.6)	
Chest pain	0 (0.0)	2 (11.8)	3 (10.3)	1 (33.3)	0 (0.0)	6 (7.9)	
Cough	4 (17.4)*	11 (64.7)*	0 (0.0)	0 (0.0)	0 (0.0)	15 (19.7)	0.002
Vomiting	5 (21.7)	2 (11.8)	5 (17.2)	1 (33.3)	0 (0.0)	13 (17.1)	
Vertigo	2 (8.7)	0 (0.0)	0 (0.0)	0 (0.0)	0 (0.0)	2 (2.9)	
Convulsions	0 (0.0)	0 (0.0)	1 (3.4)	0 (0.0)	0 (0.0)	0 (0.0)	

*Compared values.

Table 2. Causes of fever among the 69 children with SCD who were admitted to the OPH.

Causes	n	%
Bronchopulmonary infections	17	22.4
-Bronchopneumonia	11	14.5
-Pneumonia	6	7.9
Malaria	23	30.3
Bone and joint infections	2	2.6
Urinary tract infections	3	3.9
Bacteremia	6	8.7
-Salmonella spp	1	1.3
-Streptococcus pneumoniae	2	2.6
-Haemophilus influenzae	2	2.6
-Klebsiella pneumoniae	1	1.3
Hepatitis B	1	1.3
Undetermined causes	29	38.1
Total	**76**	**100**

Table 3. Levels of white blood cells and hemoglobin according to the principal causes of fever among the 69 children with SCD admitted to the Owendo Pediatrics Hospital.

Causes	Respiratory infections n = 17 (%)	Malaria n = 23 (%)	Undetemined causes n = 29 (%)	Urinary tract infection n = 3 (%)	Bone and joint infections n = 2 (%)	p-value
Leukocytes						
<10000/mm³	1 (5.9)	3 (13)	0 (0.0)	0 (0.0)	0 (0.0)	0.63
10000 - 20000/mm³	8 (47)*	10 (43.5)*	13 (44.8)	1 (33.3)	1 (50)	
>20000/mm³	8 (47)*	10 (43.5)*	16 (55.2)	2 (66.6)	1 (50)	
Hemoglobin						
≤5 g/dl	4 (23.5)	12 (52.2)*	8 (27.6)*	1 (33.3)	1 (50)	
>5 g/dl	13 (76.5)	11 (47.8)*	21 (72.4)*	2 (66.6)	1 (50)	0.07

*Compared values.

4. Discussion

The limitations of this study are inherent to its retrospective nature: no inclusion of patients seen in outpatient, many incomplete records and many cases of undetermined cause. A prospective study would refine our results that nevertheless provide valuable information.

Bacterial infections represent the main complication associated with SCD, resulting in elevated morbidity and mortality rates [4] [7]-[12]. Therefore, in case of fever, most protocols of care as well as international recommendations advocate routine prescription of broad-spectrum antibiotics [7] [10]-[12] [16]-[20]. It is however difficult to implement such treatment in Africa since these drugs are expensive and are not always readily available in the health facilities. The objective of this study was to assess the causes of fever in Libreville, with the aim of optimizing the administration of antibiotics. In light of the large number of cases of unknown origin (38.1%) and the frequency of respiratory and other infections (22.4%), it seems clear that systematic administration of antibiotics is advisable for patients in Gabon with SCD. Malaria remains, however, the main cause of fever that can be definitively associated with SCD, since it occurred in 30.3% of our patient cohort. This rate is higher than that observed by Rahimy *et al.* at Cotonou (6.7%) [14], but this involved a cohort of monitored children who were receiving anti-malarial prophylaxis [13]. On the other hand, Gabon is situated in an area where malaria is holo-endemic. Transmission of the parasite is hence stable and continuous throughout the year, and this may explain these rates. While it is generally accepted that the hemoglobin S trait has a protective role against severe forms of malaria [2] [21] [22], it is also known that the latter exacerbates the anemia due to hyperhemolysis and presents a trigger for vaso-occlusion crisis (VOC) [7] [21]. Therefore, 12 of the 23 patients (52.2%) afflicted by malaria had severe anemia (Hb < 5g/dl), hence requiring a transfusion (**Table 3**). A similar frequency (54.4%) was found by Ntetani Aloni *et al.* in Kinshasa [23]. Among these, we encountered two deaths, which confirm the observations made by McAuley *et al.* in Kenya [24]. Since the abandonment of the anti-malarial chemoprophylaxis in Gabon because of high levels of chloroquine resistance, the insecticide treated bed net is now the only effective preventive measure recommended.

Bronchopulmonary infections were the second cause of fever in our study (22.4%). These typically are major determinants of morbidity and mortality in sickle cell disease [7]. They accounted for 42.8% of infections we observed in a previous report [8] and 40.4% of cases in Libreville as reported by Thuillez *et al.* [6]. In a study by Wierenga *et al.*, acute chest syndrome (ACS) was the second leading cause of fever with 21.8% and was the only pulmonary involvement [17]. The ACS is conventionally defined as the association of chest pain with shortness of breath and a recent radiological abnormalities (infiltrate), all against a backdrop of fever [7] [17]. This frequently requires treatment in the intensive care unit. Although the distinction between a beginning ACS and a simple pneumonia is often difficult, we took the diagnosis of pneumonia and bronchopneumonia given the absence of dyspnea in our patients and the favorable outcome with conventional treatment. *Streptococcus pneumoniae* and *Haemophilus influenzae* type b are the most frequently implicated pathogens, and to a lesser degree atypical bacteria such as *Mycoplasma pneumonia.* As we will see later, many studies note the effectiveness of antibiotic prophylaxis with oral penicillin and vaccination in the prevention of these diseases [7] [12] [14] [25] [26]. The infection can also be caused by viruses, which does not diminish its potential severity in which it can trigger a vaso-occlusive crisis through fever, hypoxia and dehydration, all three factors of sickling [7].

Urinary tract infections constitute another frequent cause of fever in children with SCD. We only found three cases, or 3.9%. This is similar to the 2.4% incidence observed by Wierenga *et al.* in Jamaica [17], but considerable lower than the 26% noted by Mava *et al.* in Nigeria [27]. In a previous investigation undertaken at our ward, 42.8% of the observed bacterial infections were urinary tract infections [8].

Bacteremia represents the main threat to children with SCD. We detected six cases (8.7%) of which one was septicemia, compared to 6.1% for Wierenga *et al.* in Jamaica [17], 6.6% for Williams *et al.* in Kenya [25] or 0.8% for Baskin *et al.* in Boston [26]. This low incidence that we observed is probably due to the self-administration of antibiotics, which is a common practice in Libreville that is often not revealed by parents for fear of being reprimanded by the health care staff. In our Hospital, on the other hand, since children are admitted on their own, their mothers often prefer other forms of health care. It is also possible that, due to lack of parental knowledge, fever in some young children goes undiagnosed, causing them to perish without even being admitted to Hospital. All of these reasons can explain the low proportion of children less than 5 years old in our study. In addition to being the most commonly encountered, *Streptococcus pneumonia, Haemophilus influenzae* type b and *Salmonella* spp are also the most dreaded bacteria [7] [11] [25]. Thanks to the combined effects of oral penicillin and a range of vaccines, a discrete decline in invasive infections has been observed in recent years in the developed world [7] [12] [13] [26]-[28]. In Gabon, as elsewhere in sub-Saharan Africa, this preventative strategy does not exist due to inefficiencies in the health care system and due to the cost of the antibiotics and vaccines. In keeping with opinions expressed by other authors [13] [27]-[29], we believe that a preventative approach remains attainable in Africa, provided that proactive measures are taken to ensure systematic neonatal screening and to provide ready access to vaccines and oral penicillin, similar to what has been done successfully at Cotonou in Benin [14]. In the meantime, despite the availability of only minimal resources, it is nonetheless entirely possible to implement medical care that will improve the outcome for youngsters in Gabon who are afflicted with SCD.

In keeping with the low incidence of bacteremia, only two cases (2.6%) of bone and joint infections were detected, and none case involved meninges. Our previous investigations [8] [9] had already demonstrated that these locations were affected relative infrequently among individuals in Gabon with SCD. These observations were substantiated by Thuillez *et al.* in a cohort of nearly 300 patients [6].

For more than one-third of the cases (38.1%), none cause could be identified. This differs from the 16.7% reported in Benin [14]. Nearly half of these patients experienced severe bone and joint pain (**Table 1**). Analysis of white blood cells and the level of hemoglobin failed to provide significant clues regarding the disease etiology (**Table 3**). Bégué *et al.* [7] reported that the elevated fever did not always correspond to an underlying infection. Rather, it was associated with complications such as pulmonary thrombosis and multiple bone infarcts. For the patient cohort in Jamaica [17], these painful bouts occurred in 27.3% of cases, and they were deemed to be the sole cause of the fever in 12.1% of the cases. It is now known that the occurrence of a bone infarct induces inflammatory cytokine production and other pyrogenic products that are responsible for elevated body temperatures [7] [17]. In the other cases (aside from VOCs), like Wierenga *et al.* [17] we believe that these high fevers involve infections of viral origin or atypical microbes that are not included in our hospital's diagnostic screening protocol.

5. Conclusion

Fever remains a common reason for consultation in sickle cell child. It can be an expression of a serious infection requiring emergency care. In Africa more than elsewhere, the risk of infection is an ongoing concern for medical staff. The highlight of our study is that none etiology was found in the vast majority of cases. However, bronchopulmonary infections and malaria occupy a significant place in Libreville. Given that definitive exclusion of a bacterial infection is not possible, we believe that the prescription of broad-spectrum antibiotics by parenteral route remains a wise precaution, despite the high cost of this therapeutic strategy.

Conflict of Interest

None.

References

[1] Modell, B. and Darlison, M. (2008) Global Epidemiology of Haemoglobin Disorders and Derived Service Indicators. *Bulletin of the World Health Organization*, **86**, 480-487. http://dx.doi.org/10.2471/BLT.06.036673

[2] Labie, D. and Elion, J. (2010) La drépanocytose: Problème de l'Afrique. *Médecine Tropicale*, **70**, 449-453.

[3] Diagne, I., Diagne-Gueye, N.D.R., Signate-Sy, H., *et al.* (2003) Prise en charge de la drépanocytose chez l'enfant en Afrique: expérience de la cohorte de l'hôpital d'enfants Albert Royer de Dakar. *Médecine Tropicale*, **63**, 513-520.

[4] Grosse, S.D., Odame, I., Atrash, H.K., Amendah, D.D., Piel, F.B. and Williams, T.N. (2011) Sickle Cell Disease in Africa. A Neglected Cause of Early Childhood Mortality. *American Journal of Preventive Medicine*, **41**, S398-S405.

[5] Gendrel, D., Nardou, M. and Gendrel, C. (1991) Le poids de la drépanocytose dans un service de pédiatrie africain. In: Galactéros, F. and Dormont, S., Eds., *Drépanocytose et santé publique*, Inserm/Centre international de l'enfance, Paris, 153-154.

[6] Thuillez, V., Ditsambou, V., Mba, J.R. Mba Meyo, S. and Kitengue, J. (1996) Aspects actuels de la drépanocytose chez l'enfant au Gabon. *Archives de Pédiatrie*, **3**, 668-674. http://dx.doi.org/10.1016/0929-693X(96)87087-4

[7] Bégué, P. and Castello-Herbreteau, B. (2001) Infections graves chez l'enfant drépanocytaire: Aspects cliniques et prévention. *Archives de Pédiatrie*, **8**, 732S-741S. http://dx.doi.org/10.1016/S0929-693X(01)80189-5

[8] Koko, J., Kani, F., Reymond-Yéni, A., Onewin-Andjanga, G., Moussavou, A. and Gahouma, D. (1999) Infections bactériennes chez l'enfant drépanocytaire à Libreville. *Archives de Pédiatrie*, **6**, 1131-1132. http://dx.doi.org/10.1016/S0929-693X(00)86994-8

[9] Koko, J., Dufillot, D., M'ba-Meyo, J., Gahouma, D. and Kani, F. (1998) Mortalité des enfants drépanocytaires dans un service de pédiatrie en Afrique Centrale. *Archives de Pédiatrie*, **5**, 965-969. http://dx.doi.org/10.1016/S0929-693X(98)80003-1

[10] Wethers, D.L. (2000) Sickle Cell Disease in Childhood: Part II. Diagnosis and Treatment of Major Complications and Recent Advances in Treatment. *American Family Physician*, **62**, 1309-1314.

[11] Ramakrishnan, M., Moïsi, J.C., Klugman, K.P., Iglesias, J.M., Grant, L.R., Mpoudi-Etame, M. and Levine, O.S. (2010) Increased Risk of Invasive Bacterial Infections in African People with Sickle-Cell Disease: A Systematic Review and Meta-Analysis. *Lancet Infectious Diseases*, **10**, 329-337. http://dx.doi.org/10.1016/S1473-3099(10)70055-4

[12] Di Nuzzo, D.V.P. and Fonseca, S.F. (2004) Sickle Cell Disease and Infection. *Jornal de Pediatria* (*Rio de Janeiro*), **80**, 347-354. http://dx.doi.org/10.2223/JPED.1218

[13] Chakravorty, S. and Williams, T.N. (2014) Sickle Cell Disease: A Neglected Chronic Disease of Increasing Global

Health Importance. *Archives of Disease in Childhood*, Published Online.

[14] Rahimy, M.C., Gangbo, A., Ahouignan, G., Anagonou, S., Boco, V. and Alihonou, E. (1999) Outpatient Management of Fever in Children with Sickle Cell Disease (SCD) in an African Setting. *American Journal of Hematology*, **62**, 1-6. http://dx.doi.org/10.1002/(SICI)1096-8652(199909)62:1<1::AID-AJH1>3.0.CO;2-C

[15] Tshilolo, L., Aissi, L.M., Lukusa, D., Kinsiama, C., Wembonyama, S., Gulbis, B. and Vertongen, F. (2009) Neonatal Screening for Sickle Cell Anaemia in the Democratic Republic of the Congo: Experience from a Pioneer Project on 31 204 Newborns. *Journal of Clinical Pathology*, **62**, 35-38. http://dx.doi.org/10.1136/jcp.2008.058958

[16] McIntosh, S., Rooks, Y., Ritchey, A.K. and Pearson, H.A. (1980) Fever in Young Children with Sickle Cell Disease. *The Journal of Pediatrics*, **96**, 199-204. http://dx.doi.org/10.1016/S0022-3476(80)80802-X

[17] Wierenga, K.J.J., Hambleton, I.R., Wilson, R.M., Alexander, H., Serjeant, B.E. and Serjeant, G.R. (2001) Significance of Fever in Jamaican Patients with Homozygous Sickle Cell Disease. *Archives of Disease in Childhood*, **84**, 156-159. http://dx.doi.org/10.1136/adc.84.2.156

[18] Narang, S., Fernandez, I.D., Chin, N., Lerner, N. and Weinberger, G.A. (2012) Bacteremia in Children with Sickle Hemoglobinopathies. *Journal of Pediatric Hematology/Oncology*, **34**, 13-16. http://dx.doi.org/10.1097/MPH.0b013e318240d50d

[19] Bansil, N.H., Kim, T.Y., Tieu, L. and Barcega, B. (2013) Incidence of Serious Bacterial Infections in Febrile Children with Sickle Cell Disease. *Clinical Pediatrics* (*Philadelphia*), **52**, 661-666. http://dx.doi.org/10.1177/0009922813488645

[20] Shihabuddin, B.S. and Scarfi, C.A. (2014) Fever in Children with Sickle Cell Disease: Are All Fevers Equal? *Journal of Emergency Medicine*, **47**, 395-400. http://dx.doi.org/10.1016/j.jemermed.2014.06.025

[21] Gendrel, D., Kombila, M., Nardou, M., Gendrel, C., Djouba, F. and Richard-Lenoble, D. (1991) Protection against *Plasmodium falciparum* Infection in Children with Hemoglobin S. *The Pediatric Infectious Disease Journal*, **10**, 620-621. http://dx.doi.org/10.1097/00006454-199108000-00013

[22] Williams, T.N., Mwangi, T.W., Wambua, S., Alexander, N.D., Kortok, M., Snow, R.W. and Marsh, K. (2005) Sickle Cell Trait and the Risk of *Plasmodium falciparum* Malaria and Other Childhood Diseases. *The Journal of Infectious Diseases*, **192**, 178-186. http://dx.doi.org/10.1086/430744

[23] Aloni, M.N., Tshimanga, B.K., Ekulu, P.M., Ehungu, J.L.G. and Ngiyulu, R.M. (2013) Malaria, Clinical Features and Acute Crisis in Children Suffering from Sickle Cell Disease in Resource-Limited Settings: A Retrospective Description of 90 Cases. *Pathogens and Global Health*, **107**, 198-201. http://dx.doi.org/10.1179/2047773213Y.0000000089

[24] McAuley, C.F., Webb, C., Makani, J., Macharia, A., Uyoga, S., Opi, D.H., *et al.* (2010) High Mortality from *Plasmodium falciparum* Malaria in Children Living with Sickle Cell Anemia on the Coast of Kenya. *Blood*, **116**, 1663-1668. http://dx.doi.org/10.1182/blood-2010-01-265249

[25] Williams, T.N., Uyoga, S., Macharia, A., Ndila, C., McAuley, C.F., Opi, D.H., *et al.* (2009) Bacteraemia in Kenyan Children with Sickle-Cell Anaemia: A Retrospective Cohort and Case-Control Study. *The Lancet*, **374**, 1364-1370. http://dx.doi.org/10.1016/S0140-6736(09)61374-X

[26] Baskin, M.N., Goh, X.L., Heeney, M.M. and Harper, M.B. (2013) Bacteremia Risk and Outpatient Management of Febrile Patients with Sickle Cell Disease. *Pediatrics*, **131**, 1035-1041. http://dx.doi.org/10.1542/peds.2012-2139

[27] De Montalembert, M. and Tshilolo, L. (2007) Les progrès thérapeutiques dans la prise en charge de la drépanocytose sont-ils applicables en Afrique subsaharienne? *Médecine Tropicale*, **67**, 612-616.

[28] Quinn, C.T., Rogers, Z.R. and Buchanan, G.R. (2004) Survival of Children with Sickle Cell Disease. *Blood*, **103**, 4023-4027. http://dx.doi.org/10.1182/blood-2003-11-3758

[29] Ware, R.E. (2013) Is Sickle Cell Anemia a Neglected Tropical Disease? *PloS Neglected Tropical Diseases*, **7**, e2120. http://dx.doi.org/10.1371/journal.pntd.0002120

25

Vacuum Assisted Closure (VAC) and Platelet-Rich Plasma (PRP): A Successful Combination in a Challenging Case of Gastroschisis

Vincenzo Domenichelli*, **Simona Straziuso, Maria Domenica Sabatino, Silvana Federici**

Pediatric Surgical Unit, "Infermi" Hospital, AUSL Romagna, Rimini, Italy
Email: *zodott@me.com

Abstract

Giant gastroschisis could be a surgical challenge concerning the abdominal wall reconstruction. Many techniques have been described for both primary or staged closure but sometimes neither of them is succesful in all patients. We are presenting the combined use of Vacuum Assisted Closure (VAC) and Platelet-Rich Plasma (PRP) to improve the result in this difficult case. The use of VAC device is a well known procedure in the treatment of adult difficult wounds closure. It consists of a sponge applied directly on the abdominal wall defect, covered with a transparent dressing and connected to a controlled continuous negative pressure system [1]. Platelet-rich plasma (PRP) is an autologous concentration of human platelets in a small volume of plasma. Due to this combination it provides multiple growth and healing factors actively secreted by platelets which have been shown to begin and accelerate wound healing [2] [3]. The association between VAC and PRP was effective in the shrinkage and reduction of the abdominal defect. Fifteen months after the removal of the VAC device the fascia appears competent with a cutaneus scar that will need a plastic correction in the future. The VAC should be considered as a helpful and effective device in case of complicated giant gastroschisis or omphalocele when traditional treatment is not sufficient.

Keywords

Vacuum Assisted Closure, Gastroschisis, Platelet-Rich Plasma, Abdominal Wall Defect

1. Introduction

Gastroschisis is a relatively common congenital malformation of the abdominal wall.

*Corresponding author.

In the last decade the treatment of choice has been the primary closure. After the description of Bianchi's technique many of these patients have been treated in NICU with a manual reduction of the bowel into the abdominal cavity [4].

Whenever this approach cannot be applied the traditional silo bag for staged reduction is used.

We are describing a case in which all the possible ways have been used to reach the closure of the abdominal defect but due to the underdevelopment of the abdominal cavity and the presence of thickened intestinal wall the reduction was not possible using traditional techniques.

2. Case Report

F. M., female, was born via vaginal delivery at 34th week of gestational age with a very huge gastroschisis which was diagnosed during a late prenatal ultrasound. At birth the Apgar scores were 9/10 and the infant weight was 2500 grams.

The patient was in good clinical condition and then transferred to the neonatal intensive care unit (NICU) of our hospital. The majority of the intestinal loops were outside the abdominal wall and were immediately covered by a sterile plastic bag. At a first examination a "mesenterium commune" and a plastic peritonitis of the outer loops were seen.

After an unsuccesful attempt of manual reduction [4], a surgical procedure with partial reduction of the bowels into the abdominal cavity, appendectomy and resection of an ileal atresia was performed in the operating room. An Alexis® wound retractor was then used as a Silo bag to contain the remaining extra-abdominal loops for a later stage reduction (**Figure 1**).

In the immediate postoperative period the patient had stable vital signs with a moderate dyspnea.

Further investigations in the NICU didn't show any associated congenital abnormality. The child was managed with antibiotic therapy and total parenteral nutrition.

During the following days several progressive reductions were attempted and in 9th postoperative day a Gore-Tex® patch was placed to close the abdominal wall defect.

On the 19th day of life the baby girl passed normal stools.

Eleven days after the positioning of the patch, an inflammatory infiltration of the wound occurred with an almost complete dehiscence, presenting the underneath Gore-Tex on the surface.

We then planned to start a VAC treatment (ActiVAC®, KCI System). The black sponge (KCI VAC® Granufoam™) was applied on the Gore-Tex mesh which was partially detached (**Figure 2**). We applied the VAC with a negative pressure, ranging from 50 to 75 mmHg which kept the wound clean, lowering the risk of infections and helping the closure of the wound itself.

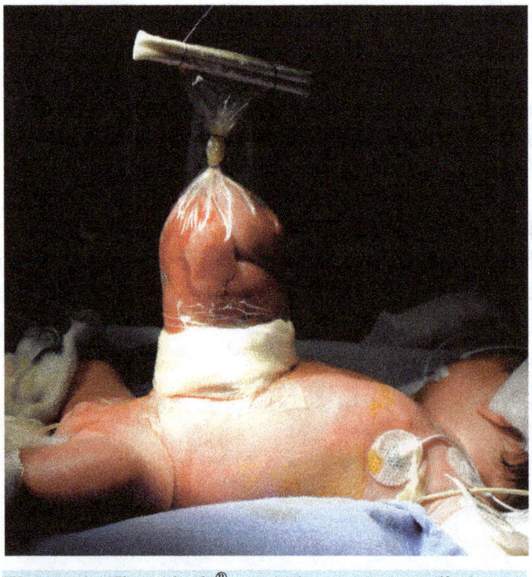

Figure 1. The Alexis® wound retractor applied as a Silo bag.

The VAC was applied for 33 days and changed every 48/72 hours. Granulation tissue was discovered under the patch which at this point was completely removed and therefore we decided to start a PRP treatment to further support the healing process. The PRP was continued for 7 days [5]. VAC treatment was continued for other 14 days. The patient was sent home at 2 months of life and the VAC set changed every 72/96 hrs on an outpatient basis without sedation. Towards the end of the treatment the device was changed at longer intervals. Subsequently the wound was covered with hydrocolloidal adhesive medication until its complete recovery.

The initial abdominal wall defect was 6 × 2.5 cm and decreased throughout the period of treatment (**Figure 3**).

During the treatment no infections occurred. We observed a complete wound closure; the abdominal wall appears competent without ventral hernia with acceptable skin scar which, of course, will need further plastic surgery (**Figure 4**).

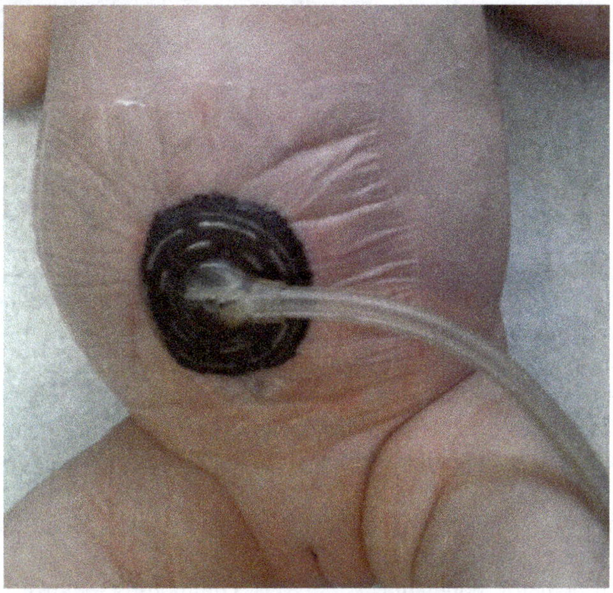

Figure 2. The VAC device during negative pressure.

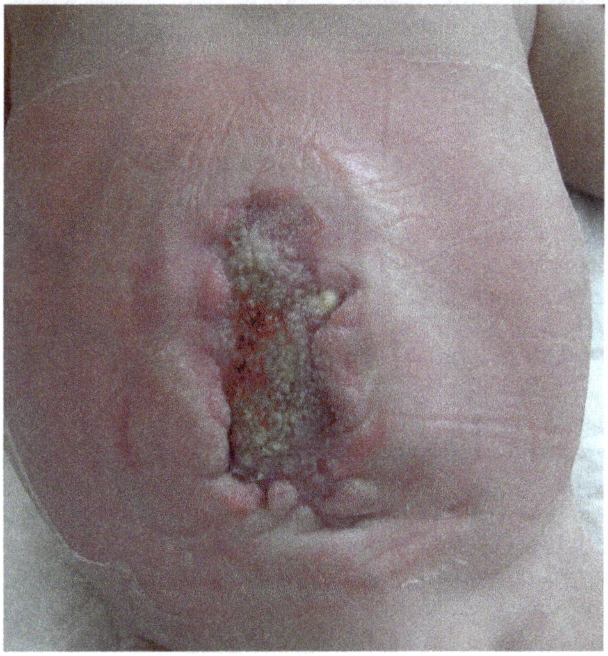

Figure 3. The abdominal wall defect after the PRP treatment.

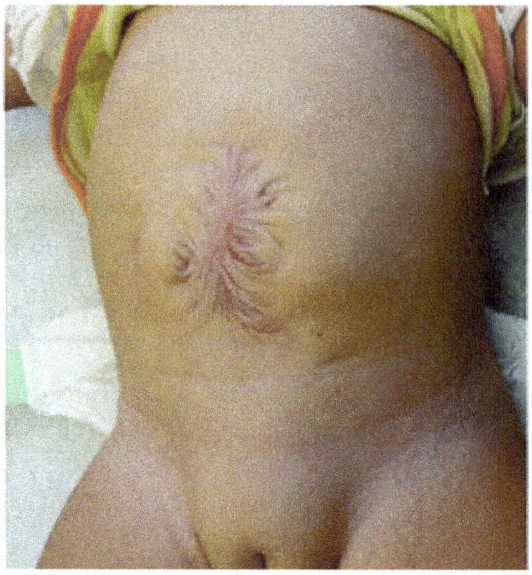

Figure 4. The final scar at complete healing.

3. Discussion

The VAC therapy has been reported as a successful alternative also in treating difficult cases of abdominal wall defects in children and newborns in NICU [1] [6] [7].

Vacuum-assisted closure appears to increase microcirculation, granulation tissue coverage and contraction rate and to decrease wound edema and infections [8]-[10]. Its use helped the reduction of abdominal wall defects in a short period of time keeping the abdominal cavity dry and lowering the risk of wound infections.

It is simple to apply and to use at the bedside or on an outpatient basis. It is well tolerated in the pediatric age [11].

Topical treatment using platelet derived factors has increasingly been described as being capable of accelerating wound healing and tissue repair [12].

The use of prp in pediatric population is not very common—as shown by the little international literature available [3] [13]—but we believe that in some selected cases could be of great help for its peculiar properties.

Therefore VAC devices and PRP together, should be considered as a helpful and effective alternative in complicated giant gastroschisis or omphalocele when traditional treatments are not sufficient.

References

[1] Kilbride, K.E., Cooney, D.R. and Custer, M.D. (2006) Vacuum-Assisted Closure: A New Method for Treating Patients with Giant Omphalocele. *Journal of Pediatric Surgery*, **41**, 212-215. http://dx.doi.org/10.1016/j.jpedsurg.2005.10.003

[2] Marx, R.E. (2004) Platelet-Rich Plasma: Evidence to Support Its Use. *Journal of Oral and Maxillofacial Surgery*, **62**, 489-496. http://dx.doi.org/10.1016/j.joms.2003.12.003

[3] Sidman, J.D., Lander, T.A., *et al.* (2008) Platelet-Rich Plasma for Pediatric Tonsillectomy Patients. *Laryngoscope*, **118**, 1765-1767. http://dx.doi.org/10.1097/MLG.0b013e31817f18e7

[4] Bianchi, A. and Dickson, A.P. (1998) Elective Delayed Reduction and No Anesthesia: "Minimal Intervention Management" for Gastrochisis. *Journal of Pediatric Surgery*, **33**, 1338-1340. http://dx.doi.org/10.1016/S0022-3468(98)90002-1

[5] Baird, R., Gholoum, S., Laberge, J.M., *et al.* (2010) Management of a Giant Omphalocele with an External Skin Closure System. *Journal of Pediatric Surgery*, **45**, 17-20. http://dx.doi.org/10.1016/j.jpedsurg.2010.05.004

[6] Gabriel, A. and Gollin, G. (2006) Management of Complicated Gastroschisis with Porcine Small Intestinal Submucosa and Negative Pressure Wound Therapy. *Journal of Pediatric Surgery*, **41**, 1836-1840. http://dx.doi.org/10.1016/j.jpedsurg.2006.06.050

[7] Fenton, S.J., Dodgion, C.M., Meyer, R.L., *et al.* (2007) Temporary Abdominal Vacuum-Packing Closure in the Neonatal Intensive Care Unit. *Journal of Pediatric Surgery*, **42**, 957-961. http://dx.doi.org/10.1016/j.jpedsurg.2007.01.029

[8] McCord, S.S., Naik-Mathuria, B.J., Murphy, K.M., *et al.* (2007) Negative Pressure Therapy Is Effective to Manage a Variety of Wounds in Infants and Children. *Wound Repair and Regeneration*, **15**, 296-301.

http://dx.doi.org/10.1111/j.1524-475X.2007.00229.x

[9] Miller, P.R., Meredith, J.W., Johnson, J.C., *et al.* (2004) Prospective Evaluation of Vacuum-Assisted Fascial Closure after Open Abdomen. *Annals of Surgery*, **239**, 608-616. http://dx.doi.org/10.1097/01.sla.0000124291.09032.bf

[10] Fleck, T., Simon, P., Burda, G., *et al.* (2006) Vacuum Assisted Closure Therapy for the Treatment of Sternal Wound Infections in Neonates and Small Infants. *Interactive CardioVasc Thoracic Surgery*, **5**, 285-288. http://dx.doi.org/10.1510/icvts.2005.122424

[11] Butter, A., Emran, M., Al-Jazaeri, A., *et al.* (2006) Vacuum-Assisted Closure for Wound Management in the Pediatric Population. *Journal of Pediatric Surgery*, **41**, 940-942. http://dx.doi.org/10.1016/j.jpedsurg.2006.01.061

[12] Mazzucco, L., Borzini, P. and Gope, R. (2010) Platelet-Derived Factors Involved in Tissue Repair from Signal to Function. *Transfusion Medicine Reviews*, **24**, 218-234. http://dx.doi.org/10.1016/j.tmrv.2010.03.004

[13] Nagaveni, N.B., Praveen, R.B., Umashankar, K.V., *et al.* (2010) Efficacy of Platelet-Rich Plasma (PRP) in Bone Regeneration after Cyst Enucleation in Pediatric Patients—A Clinical Study. *Journal of Clinical Pediatric Dentistry*, **35**, 81-87. http://dx.doi.org/10.17796/jcpd.35.1.q69168v5268234k9

26

Measurement of Transcutaneous Bilirubin with Bilicheck as a Jaundice Screening Method in Neonates in Pediatric Emergency Departments

Concepción Míguez*, Mercedes Fariñas Salto, Rafael Marañón

Pediatric Emergency Department, Hospital General Universitario Gregorio Marañón, Madrid, Spain
Email: *c.miguez09@gmail.com

Abstract

Objectives: To study the reliability of a transcutaneous bilirubinometer (Bilicheck) to determine bilirubin levels in neonates consulting for jaundice in a Paediatric Emergency Department (ED), and to evaluate its usefulness as a screening method. Methods: Prospective observational study realized between June of 2005 and December of 2005 in neonates consulting at a paediatric emergency department for jaundice, in whom we realized both transcutaneous and total serum bilirubin measurements (TcB and TSB). We collected demographic variables, analytical variables (serum and transcutaneous bilirubin levels), length of stay in the ED, and need for treatment. Results: 66 children were included aged 2 to 31 days (81% of the sample were 2 to 7 days old). There was a close and statistically significant correlation between TcB and TSB ($r = 0.81$, $p < 0.001$). The area under the ROC curve was of 0.90, allowing detecting newborns with jaundice susceptible of treatment with TcB levels ≥ 13 mg/dL (sensitivity 92%, specificity 63, 5%, a positive predictive value 39% and a negative predictive value 97%). The number of venous punctures could be reduced in 50%. The medium stay in the ED was of 2 hours when performing serum measurements. Conclusions: A linear correlation exists between TcB-TSB. TcB measurement cannot replace that of TsB, however it could be used as a screening method in an ED to determine which neonates need confirmation by TsB measurement. The use of transcutaneous bilirubinometer would reduce both the number of painful interventions in neonates and the medium length of stay in ED, consequently reducing iatrogenesis.

Keywords

Jaundice, Bilirubinometer, Screening, Transcutaneous Bilirubin, Seric Bilirubin

*Corresponding author.

1. Introduction

The yellowish coloration of skin and mucosa (jaundice) is a frequent diagnosis in neonates. This coloration can be observed when serum bilirubin levels are higher than 5 mg/dL. Two thirds of all newborn infants are estimated to present a certain degree of jaundice during their first weeks of life. In a percentage of cases, bilirubin levels can exceed neurotoxic levels, with the subsequent risk of producing kernicterus [1]-[3].

Causes of jaundice in neonates are diverse, ranging from physiological jaundice which usually requires no treatment, to septic shock which requires hospitalization in intensive care units.

Evaluation of jaundice in a paediatric emergency department requires a precise medical history, physical examination and at times, laboratory tests.

Although intensity and localization of jaundice is commonly used as an indicator of bilirubin blood concentration, the correlation between visual estimation and actual bilirubin concentration is poor [4] [5].

In 2004, the American Academy of Paediatrics published clinical practice guidelines on management of neonatal hyperbilirubinemia, affirming that visual estimation of the degree of jaundice can lead to errors, therefore bilirubin levels should be determined by measurement of total serum bilirubin (TSB) or by transcutaneous bilirubin (TcB), and interpreted according to the age (in hours) of the newborn infant [1] [2].

Previous studies have demonstrated that TcB determinations represent good estimations of the TSB levels in term and late preterm neonates in their first days of life; however, they tend to underestimate TSB at high levels. Recent studies indicate that the TcB determination is more accurate than visual estimation methods [4] [6].

The principle objective of our study was to evaluate the reliability of a transcutaneous bilirubinometer (Bili Chek®) and to determine its usefulness in an emergency department as a screening method in newborn infants susceptible to treatment. Secondary objectives were to find out whether the use of a transcutaneous bilirubinometer could reduce the number of venous punctures (without however affecting the percentage of admissions), as well as the average length of stay in the emergency department.

2. Materials and Methods

We performed a prospective observational study from June 2005 through December 2005 amongst neonates that consulted for jaundice in the Emergency Department. The study took place in the emergency service of the Hospital General Universitario Gregorio Marañón in Madrid, which usually attends to 60,000 children aged 2 days to 16 years.

The study meets the Helsinki Declaration standards and has been approved by our hospital's clinical investtigation and ethics committee.

The population we studied consisted of all children aged 2 to 30 days (both included) which consulted the emergency department for jaundice. We excluded preterm babies, infants aged more than 30 days, infants who had previously received phototherapy and neonates with clinical signs of dehydration or toxic aspect.

The variables collected in the study are shown in **Table 1**.

In all children included in the study, we measured both transcutaneous and serum bilirubin levels.

TSB measurement was made in our hospital's biochemistry laboratory by spectrophotometry.

TcB measurement was made with a transcutaneous bilirubinometer (Bilicheck, by Philips brand). The determination of TcB with the bilirubinometer was done by 5 skin measurements in the forehead, upper third of the thorax, areas free of hair or skin blemishes. The equipment then calculated the average of all 5 determinations in mg/dL.

Table 1. Variables collected in the study.

- Demographic variables: age, sex, race.
- Personal history: group incompatibility, birth weight, gestational age, Apgar score at birth.
- Medical history variables: feeding (breast, formula, breast and formula).
- Physical examination variables: weight, presence or absence of cephalohematoma or broken clavicle.
- Laboratory variables: transcutaneous bilirubin levels and serum bilirubin.
- Income: yes/no
- Length of stay in emergency department.

We considered infants older than 48 hours of life with bilirubin levels ≥ 18 mg/dl as being susceptible to treatment (we did not consider preterm, low weight at birth, nor group incompatibility).

For the administration of treatment the American Academic of Paediatrics guideline in management of hyperbilirubinemic in the newborn infant 35 or more weeks of gestation were followed.

The data was introduced in Access 2003 database and was then treated statistically with SPSS program version 14.

We performed a correlation, regression and variance analysis. With the use of a ROC curve we determined the sensitivity and specificity of transcutaneous bilirubin measurement, as well as the optimal cut-off point performing a checkout with serum bilirrubin in neonates with jaundice.

3. Results

66 children were included in the study (82% of those who consulted for jaundice and met the inclusion criteria at the time of the study). The patients were aged 2 to 30 days of life. 81% of the samples were in their first week of life.

The demographic characteristics of the children in the study are shown in **Table 2**.

We compared TSB and TcB determinations in all patients, finding a statistically significant linear correlation between both measurements ($r = 0.81$, $r^2 = 0.66$, $p < 0.001$), as shown in **Figure 1**. The maximum and minimum difference found between the bilirubin numbers determined with both methods was of −10 mg/dL and −0.4 mg/dL, suggesting that Bilicheck underestimates TSB levels.

Using variance analysis, we analysed whether demographic characteristics such as race, weight, presence or not of group incompatibility had an influence on the precision of TcB measurement. No influence was found.

With the use of a ROC curve we determined the sensitivity and specificity of transcutaneous bilirubin levels, as well as the optimal cut-off point for detecting jaundice requiring treatment. The area under the ROC curve was of 0.90 (95% confidence interval [0.82 - 0.98]) (**Figure 2**).

In the coordinates table transcutaneous bilirubin levels (**Table 3**).

By analyzing the ROC curves optimal cutoff of the bilirrubin transcunateous with increased sensitivity, specificity and negative predictive value was detected in those neonates that they should perform serum bilirrubin to be eligible for treatment.

This optimal cutoff was 13 mg/dl transcuataneous bilirrubin corresponding to a 18 mg/dl serum bilirrubin (value close to the levels of phototherapy depending on the weight, age, gestational age, and days of life).

TcB levels of 13 mg/dL seems to be the optimal cut-off point for detecting need of treatment, with 92.9% sensitivity, 62.1% specificity, a positive predictive value of 39% and a negative predictive value of 97% (**Table 4**).

Half of our patients presented TcB levels <13 mg/dL, and were therefore not susceptible for treatment and did not need further confirmation with TSB determination. This leads to suppose that 50% of the neonates included

Table 2. The demographic characteristics of the children in the study.

Characteristics	Range or percentage (n)
Gestational age	37 - 41 sem
Birth weight	2190 - 3920 gr
Breastfeeding	71% (47)
Breast and formula feeding	19.6% (13)
formula feed	9% (6)
Caucasian race	74.2% (49)
Others races	25.6% (17)
Blood group incompatibility	13.6% (9)
Cephalohematoma	3% (2)
Clavicle fracture	3% (2)
Apgar score at birth <7	1.5% (1)

Table 3. Coordinates table transcutaneous bilirubin levels: optimal cut-off point for detecting need of treatment.

Transcutaneous bilirubin levels (mg/dl)	Sensitivity	1-Specificity
3.5	1.0	1.0
5	1.0	0.98
9.5	1.0	0.90
10	1.0	0.86
11	1.0	0.71
12	1.0	0.5
13	**0.93**	**0.38**
14	0.85	0.173
15	0.57	0.077

Table 4. Sensitivity, specificity, positive predictive value and negative predictive value of transcutaneous bilirubin level (13 mg/dl) for detection of jaundice phototerapy susceptible.

	Sensitivity	Specificity	Positive predictive value	Negative predictive value
Transcutaneous bilirrubin level = 13 mg/dl	93%	62%	39%	97%

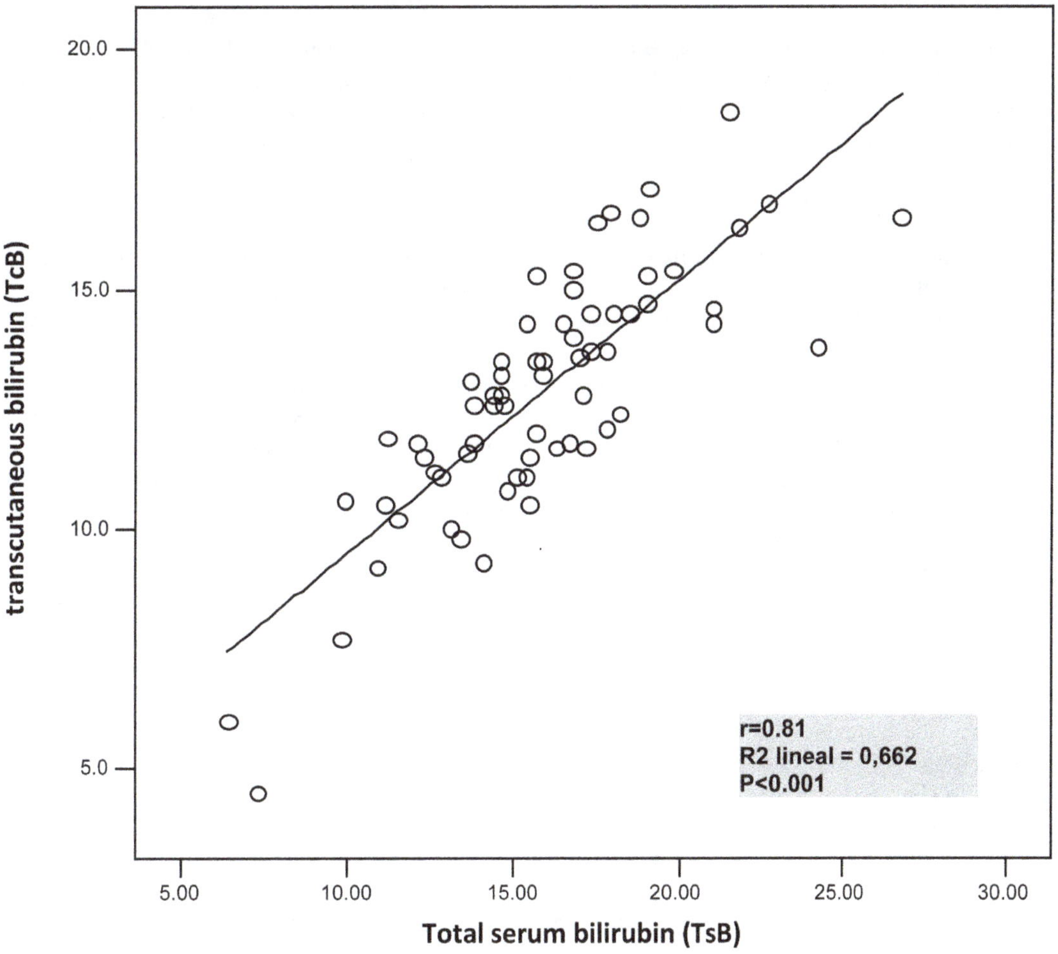

Figure 1. Comparison of total serum bilirrubin and transcutaenous bilirubin determinations (r = 0.81; p < 0.001).

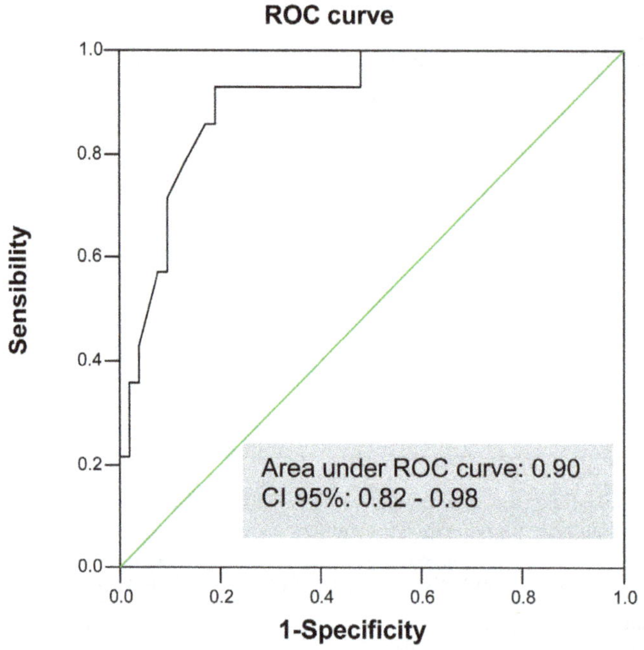

Figure 2. ROC curve for transcutaneous bilirubin levels.

in this study didn't actually need a venous puncture to determine serum bilirubin level.

In 61 of all 66 patients, we noted the time of entrance and time of exit of the Emergency Department, observing a mean time of stay of 2 hours when performing venous puncture for the determination of TSB (minimum 50 minutes, maximum 4 hours).

4. Discussion

The evaluation of the efficacy of non invasive methods for the determination of hyperbilirubinemia in the jaundice neonate is of great importance in daily clinical practice.

Non-invasive bilirubin measurement methods include visual estimation of hyperbilirubinemia and TcB determination with a bilirubinometer.

The visual estimation of hyperbilirubinemia has shown to correlate to TSB in various studies [4] [6], however it has limitations such as the difficulty in indentifying jaundice in dark-skinned babies [5]. Recent studies have shown that TcB determination has a better correlation than visual estimation methods [4] [6].

As in previous studies, we have found a statistically significant linear correlation between TSB and TcB determination with Bilicheck. However, this correlation decreases as serum bilirubin levels increase, which seems to affect Bilicheck's precision.

In our study, a sub estimation in bilirubin levels is observed when using Bilicheck, as in previous studies [7]-[9]. The cut-off point obtained was of 13 mg/dL. Higher levels obtained with our bilirubinometer determined a higher probability of having TSB levels susceptible to treatment. In these cases, a serum bilirubin determination should be performed to confirm TcB results.

In the last few years, different systems have been designed to measure bilirubin levels transcutaneous. Those that have been the most studied (Minolta/Hill-Room Air Shields Transcutaneous Jaundice Meter-103 and Bilicheck) have shown a good correlation with serum levels of bilirubin and have proven to be useful screening methods [10]-[14].

The impossibility to measure bilirubin fractions (direct, indirect), and the fact that it cannot be used if the patient has previously received treatment with phototherapy are some of the limitations linked to the use of bilirubinometers.

According to the AAP guidelines, serum bilirubin should be measured in case of high TcB levels, toxic or septic aspect, infants older than 3 weeks old, or if a direct bilirubin determination is needed [1]-[3].

The bilirubinometer used in our study (Bilicheck) measures TcB using full-spectrum light (380 to 760 nm) reflected by the skin. The use of a multiple-spectrum wavelength allows to distinguish different optical densities due to bilirubin and other possible confusion factors such as haemoglobin, melanin, skin depth. This method allows thus to quantify tissue and capillary bilirubin omitting confusion factors. This measurement is therefore theoretically independent of ethnic origin, age and weight of the newborn [10]-[13].

High resolution liquid chromatography is the reference technique for measuring TSB. Bilicheck uses it as a standard reference. This technique is scarcely used in laboratories due to its technical difficulties and complicated use on a daily basis. The use of different laboratory techniques might explain the different correlations between TcB and TSB in different studies. In our hospital for example, our laboratory uses direct spectrophotometry for the measurement of TSB, with which we have correlated Bilicheck findings in our study.

In our sample, as well as in a study published by Maria Das Graças da Cunha Leite *et al.*, the correlation between bilirubin levels measured with Bilicheck and serum bilirubin was not affected by race, age or weight at birth [15] [16].

In the case of premature babies, various studies have demonstrated the efficacy of transcutaneous bilirubinometer in this subgroup [17] [18]. However a few studies refer that race and skin colour might affect the measurement of TcB in this subgroup [19]-[22].

The use of a transcutaneous bilirubinometer as a screening method decreases the number of venous and capillary punctures in neonates with jaundice [7] [16].

In our study if the bilirubinometer had been used to determine the need for a serum bilirubin determination in infants with TcB 13 mg/dL or higher, the number of blood tests would have been reduced in 50% and only one patient actually needing phototherapy would have been lost. In a study published by Samanta *et al.* [7] where TcB cut-off point was 14 mg/dL, the number of venous punctures was reduced in 55%.

Reducing venous and capillary punctures in these children would reduce pain and iatrogenesis and would increase the personnel and parents' satisfaction.

In our study, we recorded the time of admission and discharge for each child, to evaluate the average time of stay needed for the measurement of TSB in infants with jaundice. The average stay was of 2 hours (minimum 50 minutes, maximum 4 hours). This time would have been reduced if the need for a serum determination had been checked beforehand with Bilicheck.

In some studies, the reduction in the length of stay in the emergency department has proven to be one of the utilities of the transcutaneous bilirubinometer in the emergency ward [23] [24].

This reduction in the length of stay allows a better flow of patients amongst an emergency department, and reduces the risk of transmission of infectious diseases.

5. Limitations

Although Bilicheck was used in all cases to determine TcB, measurements were obtained by different operators, which could have led to errors.

6. Conclusions

Although Bilicheck cannot replace the measurement of serum bilirubin as a reference test, the correlation found between these two methods shows that it could be an interesting tool to discriminate neonates in need of a blood test to evaluate jaundice.

The use of TcB as a screening method in neonates that consult in an emergency department would reduce the use of invasive methods, iatrogenesis, and length of stay in the department and would allow starting treatments more promptly. In this case, TSB measurement should be performed if TcB is higher that 13 mg/dL, in children who have been treated previously with phototherapy or if a toxic aspect is detected.

Acknowledgements

The authors would like to thank Dr. Julie Cayrol. M. D. Pediatric Emergency Department. Hospital General Universitario Gregorio Marañón. Madrid who translation of the text into English.

Declaration

No sponsorship or conflicts of interest were declared by the authors.

Conflicts of Interest

The authors declare that they have no conflicts of interest.

References

[1] American Academy of Pediatrics, Subcommittee on Hyperbilirubinemia (2004) Management of Hyperbilirubinemia in the Newborn Infant 35 or More Weeks of Gestation [Published Correction Appears in Pediatrics. 2004, **114**, 1138]. *Pediatrics*, **114**, 297-316. http://dx.doi.org/10.1542/peds.114.1.297

[2] Canadian Paediatric Society, Fetus and Newborn Committee (2007) Guidelines for Detection, Management and Prevention of Hyperbilirubinemia in Term and Late Preterm Newborn Infants (35 or More Weeks' Gestation). *Paediatr Child Health*, **12**, 401-407.

[3] Maisels, M.J., Bhutani, V.K., Bogen, D., *et al.* (2009) Hyperbilirubinemia in the Newborn Infant 9 or = 35 Weeks' Gestation: An Update with Clarifications. *Pediatrics*, **124**, 1193-1198. http://dx.doi.org/10.1542/peds.2009-0329

[4] Keren, R., Tremont, K., Luan, X. and Cnaan, A. (2009) Visual Assessment of Jaundice in Term and Late Preterm Infants. *Archives of Disease in Childhood—Fetal and Neonatal Edition*, **94**, F317-F322. http://dx.doi.org/10.1136/adc.2008.150714

[5] Kaplan, M., Shchors, I., Algur, N., *et al.* (2008) Visual Screening versus Transcutaneous Bilirubinometry for Predischarge Jaundice Assessment. *Acta Paediatrica*, **97**, 759-763. http://dx.doi.org/10.1111/j.1651-2227.2008.00807.x

[6] Moyer, V.A., Ahn, C. and Sneed, S. (2000) Accuracy of Clinical Judgment in Neonatal Jaundice. *Archives of Pediatrics and Adolescent Medicine*, **154**, 391-394.

[7] Samanta, S., Tan, M., Kissack, C., *et al.* (2004) The Value of Bilicheck as Screening Tool for Neonatal Jaundice in Term and Near-Term Babies. *Acta Paediatrica*, **93**, 1486-1490. http://dx.doi.org/10.1111/j.1651-2227.2004.tb02634.x

[8] Nanjundaswamy, S., Petrova, A., Mehta, R., Bernstein, W. and Hegyi, T. (2004) The Accuracy of Transcutaneous Bilirubin Measurements in Neonates: A Correlation Study. *Biology of the Neonate*, **85**, 21-25. http://dx.doi.org/10.1159/000074953

[9] Wong, C.M., van Dijk, P.J.E. and Laing, I.A. (2002) A Comparison of Transcutaneous Bilirubinometers: SpectRx BiliCheck versus Minolta AirShields. *Archives of Disease in Childhood—Fetal and Neonatal Edition*, **87**, 137-140. http://dx.doi.org/10.1136/fn.87.2.F137

[10] Bhutani, V.K., Gourley, G.R., Adler, S., Kreamer, B., Dalin, C. and Johnson, L.H. (2000) Noninvasive Measurement of Total Serum Bilirubin in a Multiracial Predischarge Newborn Population to Assess the Risk of Severe Hyperbilirubinemia. *Pediatrics*, **106**, E17. http://dx.doi.org/10.1542/peds.106.2.e17

[11] Maisels, M.J. (2006) Transcutaneous Bilirubinometry. *Neoreviews*, **7**, e217-e225. http://dx.doi.org/10.1542/neo.7-5-e217

[12] Samanta, S., Tan, M., Kissack, C., Nayak, S., *et al.* (2004) The Value of Bilicheck as a Screening Tool for Neonatal Jaundice in Term an Near-Term Babies. *Acta Paediatrica*, **93**, 1486-1490. http://dx.doi.org/10.1111/j.1651-2227.2004.tb02634.x

[13] Rubaltelli, F., Gourley, G., Loskamp, N., *et al.* (2001) Transcutaneous Bilirrbin Measurement a Multicenter Evaluation of a New Device. *Pediatrics*, **107**, 1264-1271. http://dx.doi.org/10.1542/peds.107.6.1264

[14] Thayyil, S. and Marriott, L. (2005) Can Transcutaneous Bilirubinometry Reduce the Need for Serum Bilirubin Estimations in Term and near Term Infants? *Archives of Disease in Childhood*, **90**, 1311-1312. http://dx.doi.org/10.1136/adc.2004.070292

[15] Bertini, G. and Rubaltelli, F. (2002) Non-Invasive Bilirubinometry in Neonatal Jaundice. *Seminars in Neonatology*, **7**, 129-133. http://dx.doi.org/10.1053/siny.2002.0100

[16] da Cunha Leite, M. das G., de Araújo Granato, V., Facchini, F.P. and Marba, S.T.M. (2007) Comparison of Transcutaneous and Plasma Bilirubin Measurement. *Jornal de Pediatria*, **83**, 283-286. http://dx.doi.org/10.2223/JPED.1619

[17] Fouzas, S., Karatza, A.A., Skylogianni, E., Mantagou, L. and Varvarigou, A. (2010) Transcutaneous Bilirubin Levels in Late Preterm Neonates. *Journal of Pediatrics*, **157**, 762-766. http://dx.doi.org/10.1016/j.jpeds.2010.04.076

[18] Zecca, E., Barone, G., De Luca, D., Marra, R., Tiberi, E. and Romagnoli, C. (2009) Skin Bilirubin Measurement during Phototherapy in Preterm and Term Newborn Infants. *Early Human Development*, **85**, 537-540. http://dx.doi.org/10.1016/j.earlhumdev.2009.05.010

[19] Yu, Z.B., Dong, X.Y., Han, S.P., Chen, Y.L., Qiu, Y.F., Sha, L., *et al.* (2011) Transcutaneous Bilirubin Nomogram for Predicting Neonatal Hyperbilirubinemia in Healthy Term and Late-Preterm Chinese Infants. *European Journal of Pediatrics*, **170**, 185-191. http://dx.doi.org/10.1007/s00431-010-1281-9

[20] Mishra, S., Chawla, D., Agarwal, R., Deorari, A.K. and Paul, V.K. (2010) Transcutaneous Bilirubin Levels in Healthy

Term and Late Preterm Indian Neonates. *Indian Journal of Pediatrics*, **77**, 45-50. http://dx.doi.org/10.1007/s12098-010-0007-3

[21] Wainer, S., Rabi, Y., Parmar, S.M., Allegro, D. and Lyon, M. (2009) Impact of Skin Tone on the Performance of a Transcutaneous Jaundice Meter. *Acta Paediatrica*, **98**, 1909-1915. http://dx.doi.org/10.1111/j.1651-2227.2009.01497.x

[22] De Luca, D., Jackson, G.L., Tridente, A., Carnielli, V.P. and Engle, W.D. (2009) Transcutaneous Bilirubin Nomograms: A Systematic Review of Population Differences and Analysis of Bilirubin Kinetics. *Archives of Pediatrics & Adolescent Medicine*, **163**, 1054-1059. http://dx.doi.org/10.1001/archpediatrics.2009.187

[23] Lam, T.S., Tsui, K.L. and Kam, C.W. (2008) Evaluation of a Point of Care Transcutaneous Bilirubinometer in Chinese Neonates at an Accident and Emergency Department. *Hong Kong Medical Journal*, **14**, 356-360.

[24] Yamamoto, L.G., Killeen, J. and French, G.M. (2012) Transcutaneous Bilirubin Measurement Methods in Neonates and Its Utility for Emergency Department Use. *Pediatric Emergency Care*, **28**, 380-387. http://dx.doi.org/10.1097/PEC.0b013e31824dcb43

27

Renal Amyloidosis Following Chronic Osteomyelitis in a Patient with Congenital Insensitivity to Pain and Anhidrosis

Sevgi Yavuz*, Aydin Ece

Division of Pediatric Nephrology, Dicle University, Diyarbakir, Turkey
Email: *drsyavuz@gmail.com

Abstract

Congenital insensitivity to pain and anhidrosis (CIPA) is a rare form of hereditary sensory and autonomic neuropathy. It is characterized by impaired perception of pain and temperature, anhidrosis and intellectual disability. Self mutilating behaviors lead to accidental injuries. The limb lesions are often infected and frequently progress to chronic osteomyelitis. In pediatrics, amyloidosis usually occurs secondary to chronic inflammatory diseases. The coexistence of amyloidosis and CIPA has not previously been reported in literature. A CIPA case complicated with nephrotic syndrome and renal amyloidosis following chronic osteomyelitis is presented here. This report emphasizes the importance of close follow-up of patients by urine analysis for the risk of developing amyloidosis particularly in the presence of chronic infections.

Keywords

Pain Insensitivity, Anhidrosis, Osteomyelitis, Nephrotic Syndrome, Amyloidosis

1. Introduction

Congenital insensitivity to pain and anhidrosis (CIPA), also known as hereditary sensory and autonomic neuropathy type IV (HSAN IV), is an autosomal recessive disorder caused by mutations in neuropathic tyrosine kinase receptor type 1 (NTRK1) gene encoding the nerve growth factor receptor [1]. The failure in differentiation and migration of neural crest cells leads to the complete absence of small myelinated and unmyelinated nerve fibers, thereby resulting in impaired pain perception and autonomic dysfunction. The characteristic clinical features of CIPA include recurrent episodes of unexplained pyrexia, anhidrosis, mental retardation and insensitivity

*Corresponding author.

to pain with subsequent self-mutilation. Furthermore, patients often suffer from skin lacerations and fractures which are frequently complicated by persistent wound infections, septic arthritis and osteomyelitis [1] [2].

The amyloidosis is characterized by extracellular deposition of proteins in various tissues as insoluble fibrils. To date almost 25 different amyloid fibrils have been known to cause amyloidosis. In pediatrics, the most common form of amyloidosis is reactive AA amyloidosis secondary to chronic inflammatory diseases [3]-[5]. Here, we present a boy with CIPA who developed renal AA amyloidosis following chronic osteomyelitis.

2. Case Report

A 13-year-old boy was admitted with swelling throughout the body. He was the first child of consanguineous parents. The insensitivity to pain, self-mutilating behaviors, mental retardation, lack of sweating, unexplained fever and vomiting attacks were noticed during infancy. He experienced right femur fracture at 4 years old and consequently had several operations on his right leg. He frequently hospitalized for recurrent cellulitis and osteomyelitis for the last four years. Several courses of parenteral antibiotics and debridement of soft tissues had been performed. The orthopedists recommended right leg amputation, however this was not approved by his parents. He had a sister suffering from similar complaints. On physical examination, his weight and height were below the 3rd percentile. He had generalized edema with a warm and thick skin. Palms and soles were hyperkeratotic. There was prominent scarring and tissue loss upon lips and fingertips due to biting. His right thigh was edematous and erythematous. He had miscellaneous trophic ulcers and chronic destructive changes on his knees (**Figure 1**). Neurological examination revealed mild hypotonia with insensitivity to superficial and deep pain stimuli. Laboratory investigations showed anemia (hgb: 10.9 g/dl), nephrotic range proteinuria (urine protein/urine creatinine: 3 mg/mg), hypoalbuminemia (albumin: 0.5 g/dl) and hyperlipidemia (total cholesterol: 216, triglyceride: 200 mg/dl). Acute phase reactants were increased (erythrocyte sedimentation rate: 50 mm/h, C-reactive protein: 20 mg/L). Renal (urea: 22 mg/dl, serum creatinine: 0.4 mg/dl) and liver function tests (ALT: 20 mg/dl, AST: 16 mg/dl), serum complements (C_3: 98 mg/dl, C_4: 16 mg/dl)) and immunoglobulin levels were within normal limits. Both anti-nuclear antibody (ANA), anti-double stranded DNA (anti-DNA) and viral markers were negative. No mutation was detected on Familial Mediterranean Fever genetic analysis. Renal ultrasonography was normal. Electromyography (EMG) indicated polyneuropathy affecting motor and sensorial fibers. The patient showed no obvious pain with EMG needle insertion. The sural nerve biopsy showed degeneration in nerve fibers. A clinical diagnosis of CIPA was established. Genetic analysis was not made because of its unavailability in our country. Given the additional nephrotic syndrome, a renal biopsy was performed and the findings were consistent with renal amyloidosis (**Figure 2**). Immunosuppressive drugs were not given because of presence of chronic infection. Angiotensin converting enzyme inhibitor (ACEI) and lipid lowering agents were started. The patient required several parenteral antibiotics courses and albumin infusions. His parents persisted for not approving limb amputation. At the end of twelve months of follow-up, the patient progressed to

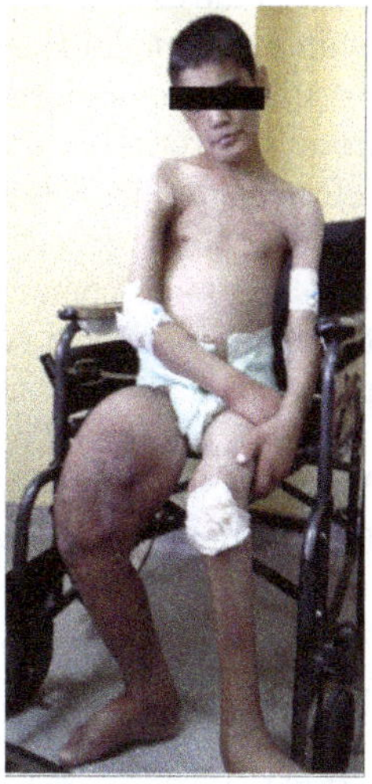

Figure 1. Photography of the patient showing generalized edema with edematous and erythematous right leg, miscellaneous trophic ulcers and chronic destructive changes on knees.

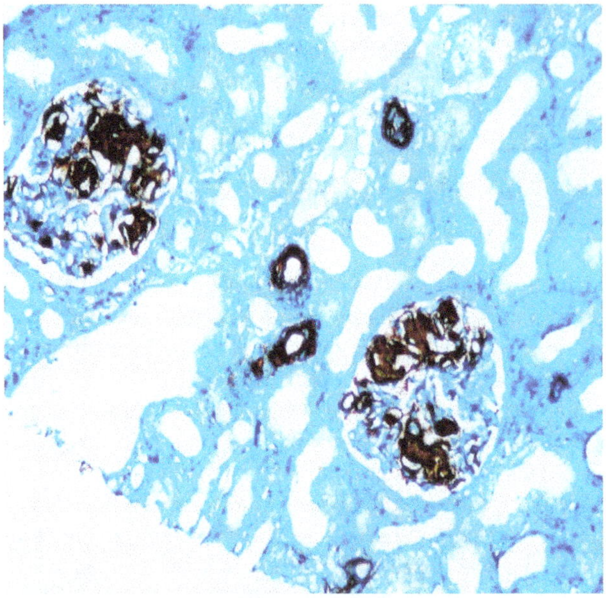

Figure 2. Positive immunoperoxidase staining for AA amyloid in glomerular mesangium and capillary walls (×200).

chronic kidney disease (CKD) and was died due to septic shock.

3. Discussion

CIPA is a very rare form of hereditary sensory and autonomic neuropathy. To date, a few hundred cases have been described. Patients have a clinical triad of impaired perception of pain and temperature, anhidrosis and intellectual disability. Their lifespan is usually short. Hyperprexia and sepsis account for the death in vast majority of the patients [6]. The present case exhibited typical clinical picture of CIPA despite the lack of confirmation by genetic analysis. The sibling with similar medical history supported our opinion.

Orthopedic problems are one of the most characteristic and serious complications of CIPA. The insensitivity to pain leads to multiple accidental injuries. The limb lesions are often infected and frequently progress to chronic osteomyelitis, at times requiring limb amputation [7] as we observed in our patient. On the other hand the close relationship between longstanding infections including osteomyelitis and amyloidosis has been well described in literature [8] [9]. However, amyloidosis has not previously been reported in CIPA. The current CIPA case is the first that is complicated with renal amyloidosis probably due to chronic osteomyelitis.

The kidney is a major target organ for systemic amyloidosis. Asymptomatic proteinuria is the most common initial presentation of renal disease. Nephrotic syndrome occurs in more than one fourth of patients at the time of diagnosis [5]. Similarly, our patient was referred after the onset of nephrotic syndrome. Furthermore, the amount of proteinuria and renal function vary according to the extent and/or site of amyloid deposition [3]. Uda *et al.* reported that glomerular amyloid depositions are more common and have a worse prognosis compared to vascular and tubular depositions in rheumatoid arthritis-related AA amyloidosis [10]. Likewise, glomerular accumulation was more prominent and progression to renal dysfunction was accelerated in the present case.

The prognosis of renal amyloidosis is generally poor and usually progress to ESRD if untreated. The major therapeutic strategy is to suppress the inflammatory activity by specific treatment of underlying disorder [1]-[3]. The medical approach in our patient was a dilemma. We were unable to eliminate chronic osteomyelitis since the parents disapproved limb amputation. Palliative treatment with ACEI and albumin infusions was administered until CKD has developed. Prevention and training programmes were applied since no specific treatment for CIPA has been available. The skin was kept clean and moisture. The parents were trained to minimize the injuries.

4. Conclusion

In conclusion, the present CIPA case is the first case that is complicated with renal amyloidosis due to chronic osteomyelitis. This report emphasizes that patients with CIPA should be closely followed up by urine analysis for the risk of developing amyloidosis particularly in the presence of chronic infections.

Conflict of Interest

None.

References

[1] Indo, Y., Tsurata, M., Hayashida, Y., *et al.* (1996) Mutations in TRKA/NGF Receptor Gene in Patients with Congenital Insensitivity to Pain with Anhidrosis. *Nature Genetics*, **13**, 485-488. http://dx.doi.org/10.1038/ng0896-485

[2] Sztriha, L., Lestringant, G.G., Hertecant, J., Frossard, P.M. and Masouyé, I. (2001) Congenital Insensitivity to Pain with Anhidrosis. *Pediatric Neurology*, **25**, 63-66. http://dx.doi.org/10.1016/S0887-8994(01)00278-8

[3] Bilginer, Y., Akpolat, T. and Ozen, S. (2011) Renal Amyloidosis in Children. *Pediatric Nephrology*, **26**, 1215-1227. http://dx.doi.org/10.1007/s00467-011-1797-x

[4] Dember, L.M. (2006) Amyloidosis-Associated Kidney Disease. *Journal of the American Society of Nephrology*, **17**, 3458-3471. http://dx.doi.org/10.1681/ASN.2006050460

[5] Nishi, S., Alchi, B., Imai, N. and Gejyo, F. (2008) New Advances in Renal Amyloidosis. *Clinical and Experimental Nephrology*, **12**, 93-101. http://dx.doi.org/10.1007/s10157-007-0008-3

[6] Bonkowsky, J.L., Johnson, J., Carey, J.C., Smith, A.G. and Swoboda, K.J. (2003) An Infant with Primary Tooth Loss and Palmar Hyperkeratosis: A Novel Mutation in the $NTRK_1$ Gene Causing Congenital Insensitivity to Pain with Anhidrosis. *Pediatrics*, **112**, 237-241. http://dx.doi.org/10.1542/peds.112.3.e237

[7] Shorer, Z., Shaco-Levy, R., Pinsk, V., Kachko, L. and Levy, J. (2013) Variation of Muscular Structure in Congenital Insensitivity to Pain with Anhidrosis. *Pediatric Neurology*, **48**, 311-313. http://dx.doi.org/10.1016/j.pediatrneurol.2012.12.015

[8] Odabas, A.R., Cetinkaya, R., Selcuk, Y., Erman, Z. and Bilen, H. (2002) Clinical and Biochemical Outcome of Renal Amyloidosis. *International Journal of Clinical Practice*, **56**, 342-344.

[9] Tuglular, S., Yalcinkaya, F.I., Paydas, S., *et al.* (2002) A retrospective Analysis of 287 Secondary Amyloidosis Cases in Turkey. *Nephrology Dialysis Transplantation*, **17**, 2003-2005. http://dx.doi.org/10.1093/ndt/17.11.2003

[10] Uda, H., Yokota, A., Kobayashi, K., *et al.* (2006) Two Distinct Clinical Courses of Renal Involvement in Rheumatoid Patients with AA Amyloidosis. *The Journal of Rheumatology*, **33**, 1482-1487.

28

Early-Stage Juvenile Fibromyalgia in a 12-Year-Old Girl

Yoshihiko Sakurai

Department of Pediatrics, Matsubara Tokushukai Hospital, Matsubara, Japan
Email: ysakurai-th@umin.ac.jp

Abstract

Juvenile fibromyalgia (JFM) is often diagnosed at a later stage. Therefore, little is known about its early phase. A 12-year-old girl with persistent lumbago without fever consulted an orthopedist, but imaging studies showed no abnormalities and analgesics were ineffective. She therefore visited our pediatric clinic. On digital palpation, she had pain in 13 of the 18 tender point sites of fibromyalgia. The blood test results were unremarkable. A medical interview revealed character tendencies often seen in patients with JFM; she was serious-minded, uncompromising, and showed excessive concern for others. Furthermore, psychological stress for the approaching annual sports day might have built up. All factors considered, early-stage JFM was the probable diagnosis. The patient accepted the diagnosis and understood that the disease may be psychogenic. Getting through the sports day cured her symptoms. This case highlights the importance of initial care, including a detailed explanation, in those with JFM.

Keywords

Juvenile Fibromyalgia, Early Stage, Character Tendency, Psychological Stress, Initial Care

1. Introduction

Fibromyalgia (FM) is a common chronic disease characterized by the presence of multiple symptoms such as widespread, constant pain throughout the body, sleeping disturbances, abnormal exhaustion, and cognitive problems, without chronic inflammation and no organic disorder in the etiology [1]. Although this condition occurs more commonly in women between the ages of 20 and 50, it can also affect men, teenagers, and children. Juvenile FM (JFM) is frequently overlooked, and often a long time is required to reach a correct diagnosis. As symptoms of JFM tend to be prolonged and may not resolve for longer period than previously thought [2], it is desirable to diagnose JFM as early as possible. However, the detailed symptoms and course of JFM in the early phase remain relatively less known. We herein report the case of a 12-year-old girl with early-stage JFM, in whom successful participation in a school event led to rapid resolution of symptoms. Informed consent was obtained from the patient and her parents for publication of this case report.

2. Case Presentation

A 12-year-old girl visited the orthopedic outpatient clinic at our hospital with complaints of a 1-month history of lumbago. Physical examination and computed tomography (CT) imaging revealed no abnormal findings. The finger-to-floor distance (FFD) was 0 cm. The prescribed topical ketoprofen patch was not effective. The 1-week administration of an analgesic (acetaminophen: 400 mg/day) did not reduce her pain; however, she did not develop a fever during this period. Furthermore, as cervical pain appeared, the patient and her mother were both very anxious regarding the unexplained, prolonged pain.

The patient was the only daughter of her parents. The family history was negative for rheumatic, autoimmune, or metabolic bone diseases. The patient's medical history was also negative. However, her backache, for which she had consulted an orthopedist, had been intermittent for several months, while she had had no fever since she noticed the lumbago. Furthermore, her pain was not localized to the lower back but was widespread, occurring at several sites. On physical examination, digital palpation yielded that she had pain in 13 of the 18 tender point sites (**Figure 1**). Tenderness was also evident over both thighs and the lateral sides of both feet. The other physical findings and neurologic findings were unremarkable. A complete blood count (CBC) showed a white blood cell count of 6,100 /μL (neutrophils 45.8%, lymphocytes 48.9%, monocytes 3.3%, basophils 0.7%, and eosinophils 1.3%). The erythrocyte sedimentation rate was 5.5 mm/h and C-reactive protein level was 0.01 mg/dL. The aspartate aminotransferase and alanine transaminase levels were 27 IU/mL and 23 IU/mL, respectively. Her immunoglobulin levels were within normal range (immunoglobulin (Ig)A 155 mg/dL, IgG 1328 mg/dL, and IgM 140 mg/dL). Levels of complement proteins were also within normal range (C3 103 mg/dL, C4 20.1 mg/dL, and total complement activity (CH50) 41 U/mL). The antinuclear antibody test was negative. Thus, organ dysfunction and inflammation were not evident. A history of present illness, medical history, physical findings, and laboratory findings ruled out the differential diagnoses of rheumatic, orthopedic, and neurologic diseases. When all these facts were considered, the early phase of JFM was suspected.

Through a medical interview, the patient's character and living environment were revealed. She usually slept late at night and sometimes had fearful dreams. Her mother said that she had been strict with the patient and thought that she had scolded the patient more often than other mothers with children of the same age would have done. The patient liked school, enjoyed her classes, and had many friends in school. She served as the class representative and often arbitrated quarrels between classmates, but would worry afterwards whether she had made the right decision. She was liable to take on problems by herself without discussing them with anyone. Her ho-

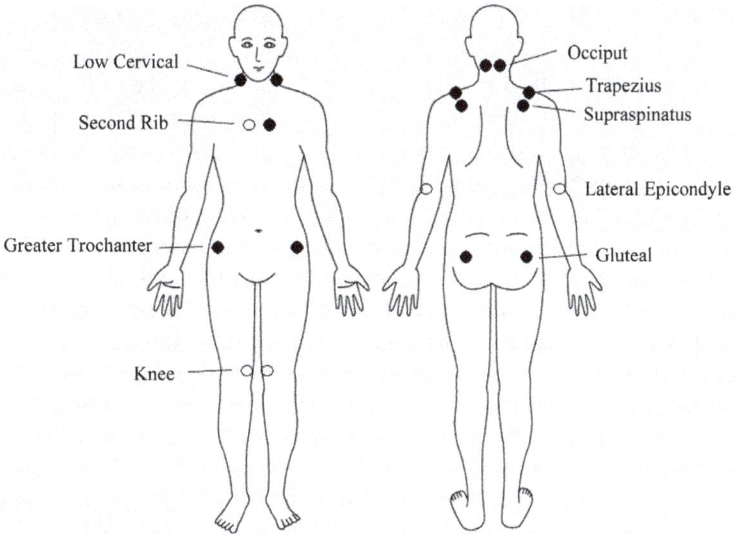

Figure 1. The 18 tender points associated with fibromyalgia. The closed circle indicates positive tender points, and the open circle represents points negative for tenderness. In this patient, 13 of 18 tender points were positive.

meroom teacher would often advise her to express herself more freely.

The annual sports day at the patient's school was to be held within 2 months of her initial visit. At previous annual sports days, she had been selected for the relay team for 3 successive years. She was very chagrined when she had lost a relay race at the sports day held the previous year. She really wanted to win this upcoming race as it was going to be her last race in the elementary school phase and she had been practicing to run faster. Unfortunately, she found it difficult to continue practicing due to varying intensity of pain; moreover, she was afraid that the foot pain might occur in the race and prevent her from winning. The patient was also selected for an event where she would have to climb on top of a human pyramid, a kind of coordinated group gymnastic event. She was chosen to be at the top because she was relatively small in stature, but she was afraid of heights and had not shared this fact with anyone. The upcoming school event (the sports day), as well as her strained relationship with her mother, were likely the important psychological factors affecting her condition.

The patient's parents, especially her mother, were strongly advised to change the way they treated the patient and asked to avoid interacting with her very strictly. Analgesic medication was prescribed in a single dose as needed for severe pain. After the first visit, the pain persisted, but the intensity was slightly reduced. She continued attending school, and her everyday life was not seriously affected. The patient was able to climb to the top of the human pyramid in a rehearsal 1 day prior to the actual sports day; she repeated the successful feat on the sports day. She was also able to complete the relay race successfully.

The patient's systemic pain ceased completely immediately after the sports day. She stated that it did not matter whether she won or lost, and she did not share the outcome of the relay race with her attending doctor. When her parents asked her about the state of her health, she claimed that she no longer had any pain or tenderness. At present, she has been pain-free for more than 1 year.

3. Discussion

Chronic pain is not necessarily rare in children. About 30% of children and adolescents have chronic pain that lasts for more than 3 months [3]-[5], which may include so-called growing pains and Osgood-Schlatter disease that develops in athletes. However, we seldom encounter a pediatric patient who has pain or tenderness at several points, which is specific to FM. In such cases, JFM as well as growing pains should be kept in mind in the differential diagnosis of chronic pains. Growing pains are more common in younger children than JFM and often appear in the night and resolve spontaneously [6], whereas JFM symptoms are chronic or last for months to years. Although the definitive diagnostic criteria of JFM are not yet established, several criteria have been proposed, in which the detection of tender points is of vital importance [7]-[10]. In our case, neither the American College of Rheumatology criteria [10] nor the Yokohama criteria [11] were fulfilled because it was uncertain that the patient had suffered from persistent widespread pain for more than 3 months, even though the patient had suffered from occasional back pain for more than a few months. Although she had mild sleep disturbance, the chronic fatigue and autonomic symptoms such as inappropriate sweating, cyanosis, and peripheral coldness that are reportedly observed in JFM were not evident. Furthermore, she had no symptoms of photophobia, irritable bowel syndrome, or an eating disorder. She did not refuse to attend school. We could not therefore confirm the diagnosis of JFM, but a probable early-stage JFM as oppressive pain was evident in 13 of the 18 points, and pain was not detected 1 inch away from the point of tenderness. A recent review describes that representative symptoms in JFM may not present at once in the early stages [2], which supports our notion.

JFM most frequently affects children at approximately 10 years of age (4th - 5th grade in elementary school) and predominantly female children [11]. The patient matched the age and sex criteria. In JFM, elevated emotional distress, especially elevated anxiety, is not uncommon [2]. We did not observe heightened levels of emotional distress but she showed character tendencies such as being serious-minded, uncompromising, and having excessive concern for others, which is reportedly observed in patients with JFM. She might have had some problems associated with pain, including a fraught mother-child relationship and stressful personal relationships in the classroom, which are considered causes and backgrounds of disease development [11]. With such a background, the patient's anxiety about the approaching sports day, especially the relay race and coordinated group gymnastic event might have triggered an exacerbation of JFM. Although the pain and tenderness were initially expected to be prolonged, both promptly disappeared after she completed the relay race with maximum efforts and the human pyramid with her team was successfully formed on the sports day. Patient's environment as well as psychological state may trigger onset and affect the medical condition. Parental and familial pain experiences are associated with patients' use of catastrophic thinking to cope with chronic pain [12]. Poor family functioning are evident in families of adolescents with JFM [13]. In our case, relatively healthy family functioning without parents' chronic pain might contribute to early disappearance of symptoms. Our case is likely to accord with previous literature, which describes that symptoms in some pediatric patients with JFM decrease or disappear only on reaching the correct diagnosis of JFM [14] or repeated medical interviews without prescribing any medications [15].

4. Conclusion

Our patient had both family and school problems such as a fraught mother-daughter relationship and personal relationship problems with her classmates based on the background of her character traits such as perfectionism, a strong sense of responsibility, tenacity, and a tendency to pay too much attention to other people [9]. In addition to these, she was unable to handle the pressure of the fast-approaching annual sports day. Considering these circumstances, she was likely to develop JFM. A probable diagnosis of JFM at the first visit and the explanation provided to the family that JFM is often associated with psychogenic factors relieved their anxiety. Furthermore, she overcame the challenges of the sports day, which provided relief of the symptoms in the short term. Our experience suggests that clinical suspicion of JFM and proper care, including a detailed explanation of the disease, are of critical importance in management of early-stage JFM.

References

[1] Hawkins, R.A. (2013) Fibromyalgia: A Clinical Update. *The Journal of the American Osteopathic Association*, **113**, 680-689. http://jaoa.org/article.aspx?articleid=2094606
http://dx.doi.org/10.7556/jaoa.2013.034

[2] Kashikar-Zuck, S. and Ting, T.V. (2014) Juvenile Fibromyalgia: Current Status of Research and Future Developments. *Nature Reviews Rheumatology*, **10**, 89-96.
http://www.nature.com/nrrheum/journal/v10/n2/pdf/nrrheum.2013.177.pdf
http://dx.doi.org/10.1038/nrrheum.2013.177

[3] Valente, A.M., Jain, R., Scheurer, M., Fowler, V.G.J., Corey, G.R., Bengur, A.R., Sanders, S. and Li, J.S. (2005) Frequency of Infective Endocarditis among Infants and Children with *Staphylococcus aureus* Bacteremia. *Pediatrics*, **115**, e15-e19. http://pediatrics.aappublications.org/content/115/1/e15.long

[4] Fuss, S., Page, G. and Katz, J. (2011) Persistent Pain in a Community-Based Sample of Children and Adolescents. *Pain Research & Management*, **16**, 303-309. http://www.ncbi.nlm.nih.gov/pmc/articles/PMC3206778/

[5] King, S., Chambers, C.T., Huguet, A., MacNevin, R.C., McGrath, P.J., Parker, L. and MacDonald, A.J. (2011) The Epidemiology of Chronic Pain in Children and Adolescents Revisited: A Systematic Review. *Pain*, **152**, 2729-2738. http://dx.doi.org/10.1016/j.pain.2011.07.016

[6] Uziel, Y. and Hashkes, P.J. (2007) Growing Pains in Children. *Pediatric Rheumatology Online Journal*, **5**, 5.
http://dx.doi.org/10.1186/1546-0096-5-5

[7] Yunus, M.B. and Masi, A.T. (1985) Juvenile Primary Fibromyalgia Syndrome. A Clinical Study of Thirty-Three Patients and Matched Normal Controls. *Arthritis & Rheumatology*, **28**, 138-145.
http://onlinelibrary.wiley.com/doi/10.1002/art.1780280205/pdf
http://dx.doi.org/10.1002/art.1780280205

[8] Wolfe, F., Smythe, H.A., Yunus, M.B., Bennett, R.M., Bombardier, C., Goldenberg, D.L., Tugwell, P., Campbell, S.M., Abeles, M., Clark, P., *et al*. (1990) The American College of Rheumatology 1990 Criteria for the Classification of Fibromyalgia. Report of the Multicenter Criteria Committee. *Arthritis & Rheumatology*, **33**, 160-172.
http://onlinelibrary.wiley.com/doi/10.1002/art.1780330203/pdf
http://dx.doi.org/10.1002/art.1780330203

[9] Yokota, S. (2009) Juvenile Fibromyalgia. In: Nishioka, K., Ed., *Guidance for Diagnosis and Management*, Medical Review, Tokyo, 75-82.

[10] Wolfe, F., Clauw, D.J., Fitzcharles, M.A., Goldenberg, D.L., Katz, R.S., Mease, P., Russell, A.S., Russell, I.J., Winfield, J.B. and Yunus, M.B. (2010) The American College of Rheumatology Preliminary Diagnostic Criteria for Fibromyalgia and Measurement of Symptom Severity. *Arthritis Care & Research* (*Hoboken*), **62**, 600-610.
http://onlinelibrary.wiley.com/doi/10.1002/acr.20140/full
http://dx.doi.org/10.1002/acr.20140

[11] Yokota, S., Kikuchi, M. and Miyamae, T. (2013) Juvenile Fibromyalgia: Guidance for Management. *Pediatrics International*, **55**, 403-409. http://onlinelibrary.wiley.com/doi/10.1111/ped.12155/full

http://dx.doi.org/10.1111/ped.12155

[12] Schanberg, L.E., Anthony, K.K., Gil, K.M., Lefebvre, J.C., Kredich, D.W. and Macharoni, L.M. (2001) Family Pain History Predicts Child Health Status in Children with Chronic Rheumatic Disease. *Pediatrics*, **108**, E47. http://pediatrics.aappublications.org/content/108/3/e47.long http://dx.doi.org/10.1542/peds.108.3.e47

[13] Kashikar-Zuck, S., Lynch, A.M., Slater, S., Graham, T.B., Swain, N.F. and Noll, R.B. (2008) Family Factors, Emotional Functioning, and Functional Impairment in Juvenile Fibromyalgia Syndrome. *Arthritis & Rheumatology*, **59**, 1392-1398. http://onlinelibrary.wiley.com/doi/10.1002/art.24099/full http://dx.doi.org/10.1002/art.24099

[14] Miyamae, T., Watanabe, Y. and Yokota, S. (2008) The Actual State and Clinical Features of Fibromyalgia in Our Country. *The Journal of the Japan Pediatric Society*, **112**, 1769-1777.

[15] Yokota, S., Umebayashi, H., Miyamae, T., Imagawa, T. and Mori, M. (2007) Our Experience of 3 Cases with Childhood Fibromyalgia. *The Journal of the Japan Pediatric Society*, **111**, 462-468.

29

Evaluation of the Early Age Married Girls Applying to Our Department

Bulut Kasım[1*], Uysal Cem[1], Korkmaz Mustafa[1], Sivri Süleyman[2], Bozkurt İsmail[1], Durmaz Ubeydullah[1], Tıraşçı Yaşar[1], Gören Süleyman[1]

[1]Forensic Medicine Department, Dicle University, Diyarbakır, Turkey
[2]Diyarbakır Directorate of Forensic Medicine Office, Diyarbakir, Turkey
Email: *drksmblt@hotmail.com

Abstract

Underage marriages are going on to keep their commonness in countries such as Turkey although frequencies of them are decreasing in the world. According to the law, marriages before eighteen years old are also defined as early marriages. Being married of girls at early ages makes these children deprived from education life and their vicinity. Therefore severe psychological difficulties occur in these children. In this study, 19 girls, who were being married at early ages and psychologically examined between January 1st, 2013-April 1st, 2015 in physical and mental health committee of the Dicle University, Medical Faculty, were taken to evaluate. These 19 cases were retrospectively assessed in sociodemographic data (age, education level, and relative degrees), type of marriage, state of mind, forensic reports and files. Of 410 cases, who admitted to our mental and physical committee, 19 (4.6%) were at the category of early age marriage. These 19 cases range between 13 and 17 years of age. Three of them (15.8%) were thinking of suicide and one of them (5.3%) attempted suicide. At least, one mental disorder was diagnosed in 8 (42.1%) of the cases and the most common diagnose was acute stress disorder in four (21.1%) cases. It has been stated that marriages at early ages are caused by economic and cultural reasons. As conclusion, being married of children at early ages is an important risk factor in social and mental health.

Keywords

Child Marriage, Mental Disorders, Forensic Medicine

1. Introduction

Marriage is defined as a relation which has a legal validity between an adult female and male requiring certain

*Corresponding author.

rights and liabilities [1] [2]. Although early age marriages decrease gradually worldwide, it is still common in underdeveloped countries or developing countries such as Turkey. United Nations and other international organizations define child marriages as violation of children and human rights. Universal declaration of human rights mentions that individuals should marry with their own free will in the lawful ages. Code of Child Welfare identifies the child as "the minor individual even she/he reaches the puberty in the early ages" [3]. Accordingly, marriages before 18 years of age are evaluated as "early marriages" [4] [5]. Turkish Civil Code states the earliest marriage age as 17 and 16 by decision of the judge for extraordinary circumstances [6]. When girls are noted to be espoused before 15 years of age, penalty is predicted for the crime of "sexual abuse of the child" for the spouse and taking part in the crime for parents of both the girl and his spouse [7]. No penalty codes are involved in our law system for early marriages. Since existing penal codes are focused on sexual abuse, some problems are faced [4].

A study conducted detected that marriage over 60 million among all existing marriages worldwide consist of minor children. These marriages include approximately 30 million in Southern Asia, 14 million in African Sahara and 6.6 million in Latin America and Caribbean. Furthermore, 50% of the girls marry in the early ages in some regions of India [8]. Early age pregnancies which appear as a result of these marriages are defined as a serious healthcare problem in the world since 1960 [9]. In Turkey, child marriages are observed as one of the four marriages as well as one of three marriages in some regions [4]. Research of Turkish Population and Health Research (TPHR) performed on 8867 women between the ages of 20 and 49 in 2008 determined 40.3% of women married before 20 years, 22.2% married until 18 years and 4.4% married before 15 years. Marriages before 15 years of age which was 7.6% in 1998 were detected as 5.0% in 2003 and 4.4% in 2008 in our country [10]. Despite significant decrease in the very early marriage, they still exist. Number of early marriages is predicted to increase especially in the Southeastern Anatolia region and in many other regions by asylum of the individuals running away from the civil war in Syria in particular and there is not any study conducted on this topic yet.

Early marriages before completion of biopsychosocial maturity of the girls may lead severe traumas. Children are overwhelmed by severe burden of the marriage as well as deprived of the environment and education life with their peers. These children, as a result, feel rejected, ineligible and consequently unhappy. Severe mental problems appear on these children accordingly [3] [4].

The aim of the present study was to evaluate sociodemographic characteristics of the girls who were referred our department for evaluation of physical and mental health and were below 18 years of age when they married, and also mental disorder diagnoses.

2. Materials & Methods

In the present study, through request of the courts, 410 victims who were exposed to sexual assault were assessed in Dicle University Medical Faculty Hospital between January, 1st, 2013 and April, 1st, 2015. Since 19 cases meet the early marriage criteria among 410 cases, our manuscript was limited by 19 cases. Sociodemographic data (age, educational level, kinship level etc.), form of the marriage, pregnancy status, mental status of the child after the assault were evaluated retrospectively. Categorical variables were presented in number of the cases and (%). Since no mental retardation was considered on the cases included clinically, intelligence test was not deemed necessary. This study was approved by the local Ethics Committee of Dicle Univesity, Medical School. The objective of our committee is to evaluate if mental health of the cases who were exposed to sexual assault have disrupted (post-traumatic stress disorder, acute stress reaction, incident-induced depression). Concerning courts request this evaluation from us. The case is questioned to detect this disorder. The cases voluntarily answer these questions. Therefore, this included the informed consent.

SPSS for Windows 16.0 package program was used for statistical analysis of the study. Categoric data were analyzed by ki-square test. Frequency distribution and mean values were calculated. The significance level of 95% ($p < 0.05$) was adopted in the study.

3. Results

Age range of marriage of 19 cases (4.6%) included were found between 13 and 17. Most common age of our cases was 13 with 6 (31.6%) cases. Eight (42.1%) cases were observed as not literate, 6 (31.6%) cases were elementary school graduate and 5 (26.3%) cases were high school graduate. Mental retardation was not detected in any of the cases clinically.

Before marriage, 10 (52.6%) cases were from extended families, 8 (42.1%) were from elementary families and 1 (5.3%) was from broken families. After marriage, 10 (52.6%) cases started to live in an elementary family whereas 9 (46.4%) started to live in an extended family.

Eight (42.1%) cases were observed to be married off to close relatives (cousin) and 11 (57.9%) married with individuals without any kinship. No early marriage with distant relative was detected in our study.

It was detected that 8 (42.1%) cases married with their own free will and within their parents' knowledge, 6 (31.6%) cases married with the accused after eloping, 2 (10.5%) cases were forced into marriage with the accused by their parents without their own free will and 2 (10.5%) cases were forced into marriage involuntarily after being raped and 1 (5.3%) married with the accused with her own free will after being kidnapped.

Detection form of early marriages in our study included the following; most common appearance of the event by reflection of domestic violence to judicial authorities with 6 (31.6%) cases, 4 (21.1%) cases were detected after delivery in the hospital, 3 (15.8%) cases during pregnancy follow-up of the child and 3 (15.8) cases by referring to the court because of sexual intercourse and 2 (10.5%) cases by referring to the court because of eloping of the child.

Girls enrolled into the study were observed with history of one and multiple pregnancy in 7 (36.8%) cases, pregnant during the examination in 3 (15.7%) cases and not pregnant in 9 (47.4%) cases.

At least one mental disorder has been diagnosed in 8 (42.1%) cases; the most common diagnosis was Acute Stress disorder by 5 (26.3%) cases and Major depressive Disorder, Post-traumatic Stress Disorder and Anxiety have also been diagnosed. Three (15.8%) cases were understood to have a thought of suicide and 1 (5.3%) case have attempted to suicide. All of these 3 cases (100%) with thought of suicide consisted of the cases who have married involuntarily.

The situation between mental health disorder status and kinship of the victim and the accused, the age and educational level of the victim, age difference between the victim and the accused, type of marriage formation and pregnancy status of the victim are presented in **Table 1**. Situation of the kinship of the victim and accused means that the accused is cousin of the victim before marriage.

4. Discussion

The most common causes of early marriages were reported as economical and cultural [3] [4]. Age during the first marriage is higher in line with the higher welfare of the household. Women at the highest welfare level marry after more than three years than those at the lowest welfare level. A positive relation has been detected between educational level and mean age of marriage in a study. The differences between women who had education at least at high school level and others are noticed. Age average of marriage for women who are high school graduate and over was found 24.1; this was 3 years more than the age average of women who have not completed secondary school and 5 years more than the age average of women who have been uneducated or have not graduated from elementary school [10]. Previous studies detected that families of the girls exposed to early marriage have poor economic level and majority of these girls were uneducated or quit the school before completion of the elementary school [3] [4] [11]. In the present study, income level of the families was observed poor and 42.1% of the girls were not literate and had low educational level. Majority of the girls were observed to live in expanded families because of social and economical reasons and continued to live in expanded families after marriage. Early age marriages lead many risks and problems. The women interviewed expressed that they have perceived marriage as a game and struggled to fulfill roles and tasks expected from them [2]. Unless the financial status allows, responsibilities of the marriage almost make the children to continue on education impossible. Actions to be taken to make the girls to continue on school were determined as to provide financial support to the family, to give meal to the children whose families have a low income and to assure a job after completion of the school. This study is important to indicate prevention of early marriage for the girls [12].

Early marriage also means early pregnancy. A study conducted in our country reported that 9.6% of women between 15 and 19 years of age are married and ratio for at least one live birth was 40.7% for these women [10]. Another study determined 6.4% of the girls between 15 and 19 years of age were married in Denizli, Turkey and 76.7% of them got pregnant. Majority of the women enrolled into the research was elementary school graduate (65.5%); 19.5% was secondary school graduate and 12.3% were high-school graduate. [9]. Low educational level of the adolescent pregnant women and their husbands was found as a risk factor for adolescent pregnancy. As a result of risk factor research for early pregnancy in many studies, higher educational level of the partner causes a decrease in the frequency of early pregnancy [9]. Early pregnancies lead to many risks. Children who

Table 1. Characteristics of early married girls.

	MHD None n (%)	MHD Present n (%)	Total n (%)
Kinship			
None	8 (72.7)	3 (37.5)	11 (57.9)
Present	3 (27.3)	5 (62.5)	8 (42.1)
Age			
13	4 (36.4)	2 (25)	6 (31.6)
14	1 (9.1)	3 (37.5)	4 (21.1)
15	3 (27.3)	1 (12.5)	4 (21.1)
16	2 (18.2)	2 (25)	4 (21.1)
17	1 (9.1)	0 (0)	1 (5.3)
Educational Level of the Victim			
Not literate	6 (54.5)	2 (25)	8 (42.1)
Primary education	1 (9.1)	5 (62.5)	6 (31.6)
High school	4 (36.4)	1 (12.5)	5 (26.3)
Age Difference			
Accused is younger than the victim	1 (9.1)	1 (12.5)	2 (10.5)
Accused is 0 - 5 years older	4 (36.4)	4 (50.0)	8 (42.1)
Accused is 6 - 10 years older	5 (45.5)	1 (12.5)	6 (31.6)
Accused is 11 years and more older	1 (9.1)	2 (25.0)	3 (15.8)
Type of Marriage Formation			
Married voluntarily	8 (72.7)	0 (0)	8 (42.1)
Married involuntarily	0 (0)	2 (25.0)	2 (10.5)
Eloped voluntarily	3 (27.3)	3 (37.5)	6 (31.6)
Forced to marriage by kidnapping	0 (0)	1 (12.5)	1 (5.3)
Married after rape	0 (0)	2 (25.0)	2 (10.5)
Pregnancy			
None	4 (36.4)	5 (62.5)	9 (47.4)
Present	7 (63.6)	3 (37.5)	10 (52.6)
Total	11 (57.9)	8 (42.1)	19 (100)

MHD: Mental Health disorder.

get pregnant before 18 years of age have a risk of premature birth or low birth weight babies by a rate of 35% - 55% when compared with those who get pregnant after 19 years of age. Death rate of the infants of mothers who are below 18 years is 60% more [3]. People believe that early marriage of their girls protects them from HIV/AIDS disease. However, studies presented marriages before 20 years of age are risk factor for HIV infection. In Kenya, married girls are more likely to be infected with HIV when compared to singles by 50%. They are infected by their husbands. Because, girls have frequent and unprotected sexual intercourse with their husbands to get pregnant as soon as possible and prove that they are fertile. Pregnant women in endemic malaria regions have a higher risk for infection. The highest risk is observed during the first pregnancy. Pregnancy is not a sole risk factor for malaria; however, incidence of malaria was found more in pregnant women below 19 years when compared with those older than 19 years of age [3]. Unintended pregnancies are observed more in early age marriages [4] [13]. In the present study, 52.6% of the cases were detected pregnant or previously pregnant.

In a study, mental disorder was detected in 45.8% of the cases as a result of mental evaluation of the girls who had early marriage [4]. Similarly, at least one mental disorder was observed in 42.1% of these children in the present study. Our study detected that the victim had higher mental disorder rate especially in involuntary marriage of the victim.

Studies conducted found that suicidal ideation and attempt significantly increases in the cases who had early marriage [4]. In our research, suicidal ideation and attempt was observed higher in the children who had involuntary marriage in particular.

Outcomes indicate that these children who were exposed to early marriage have a significant risk for social and mental disorder. In a study, it is reported that physical and emotional violence/abuse in addition to sexual abuse, to undertake responsibilities such as home, family and children, to separate from the family, to have conflicts with the spouse's family, to live in a large family after marriage, to be forced for marriage develop mental disorders more. Therefore, consideration of sexual assault only would be deficient for the early age marriage cases; all factors that are considered to affect the child's mental health should be discussed together [4].

5. Conclusion

We concluded that social, educational and legal solutions to prevent early marriages should be sought; girls and their families should be trained accordingly and mental therapies of the victim girls should be performed rigorously.

References

[1] Bozkurt, V. (2004) Sociology in the Changing World. Alfa Publishing, Istanbul.

[2] Çoban, A.İ. (2009) Adolescent Marriages. *Family and Community Education Culture and Research Journal*, **16**, 37-50.

[3] Nour, N.M. (2009) Child Marriage. A Silent Health and Human Rights Issue. *Reviews in Obstetrics Gynecology*, **2**, 51-56.

[4] Soylu, N. and Ayaz, M. (2013) Sociodemographic Characteristics and Psychiatric Evaluation of Girls Who Were Married at Younger Age and Referred for Criminal Evaluation. *Anatolian Journal of Psychiatry*, **14**, 136-144. http://dx.doi.org/10.5455/apd.36694

[5] Child Protection Code (2005) T.R. Official Gazette, 15, 5395. http://www.resmigazete.gov.tr/eskiler/2005/07/20050715-1.htm

[6] Turkish Civil Code. Code: 4721. (2001) T.R. Official Gazette, 8, 24607. http://www.resmigazete.gov.tr/eskiler/2001/12/20011208.htm#1

[7] Resolution of Penal Department no. 2007/1609K of Supreme Court Dated 28.02.2007 https://www.tbmm.gov.tr/komisyon/kefe/docs/komisyon_rapor.pdf

[8] Vasanth, C., Ilayaraja, B.S. and Ramya, S. (2015) Assessing Parents Awareness on Health Impacts of Early Marriage: A Study in Selected Villages of Moradabad. *International Journal of Basic Medicine and Clinical Research*, **2**, 98-102.

[9] Özşahin, A., Zencir, M., Gökçe, B. and Acimis, N. (2006) Adolescent Pregnancy in West Turkey. Cross Sectional Survey of Married Adolescents. *Saudi Medical Journal*, **27**, 1177-1182.

[10] Turkish Population and Health Research. Hacettepe University, Institute for Population Survey, General Directorate of Mother and Child Care and Family Planning, Secreteriat of the State Planning Organization and TUBITAK, Ankara, Turkey, 2008.

[11] Noah, G. (2007) Uganda: Early Marriage as a form of Sexual Violence. *Forced Migration Review*, **27**, 51-55. http://www.fmreview.org/en/FMRpdfs/FMR27/full.pdf

[12] Mathur, S., Greene, M. and Malhotra, A. (2003) Too Young to Wed: Thelives, Rights and Health of Young Married Girls. International Center for Research on Women, Washington DC, 1-5.

[13] Santhya, K.G. (2011) Early Marriage and Sexual and Reproductive Health Vulnerabilities of Young Women: A Synthesisof Recent Evidence from Developing Countries. *Current Opinion in Obstetrics and Gynecology*, **23**, 334-339. http://dx.doi.org/10.1097/GCO.0b013e32834a93d2

30

Acute Chest Syndrome in Children with Sickle Cell Anaemia: An Audit in Port Harcourt, Nigeria

Innocent O. George*, Chika N. Aiyedun

Department of Paediatrics, University of Port Harcourt Teaching Hospital, Port Harcourt, Nigeria
Email: *geonosdemed@yahoo.com

Abstract

Background: Acute chest syndrome (ACS) is a leading cause of death from sickle cell disease worldwide accounting for about 25% of all deaths. The aim of this study was to determine the prevalence, clinical features and outcome in Port Harcourt, Nigeria. Materials and Methods: A retrospective cohort study during a five year period. Records of all patients with sickle cell anaemia (SCA) admitted into the Wards were examined. Those enrolled for the study satisfied two criteria: 1) lower respiratory tract symptoms and 2) new pulmonary infiltrates on the chest radiograph. Sociodemographics, genotype, clinical and laboratory features, treatment given and outcome were obtained. Data were analysed by descriptive statistics. Variables were compared by students' t-test. P value ≤ 0.05 was regarded as significant. Results: A total of 345 children with sickle cell anaemia were admitted during the 5 year period. Twelve of them had acute chest syndrome (3.5%). Majority 7 (58.3%) of them were under 5 years. There were more males 8 (66.7%) than female 4 (33.3%). The most common clinical features were fever 12 (100%), cough 10 (83.3%), chest pain 5 (41.7%), pulmonary consolidation 12 (100%), and respiratory distress 12 (100%). The admitting diagnosis were bronchopneumonia 6 (50%), severe malaria 3 (25%) and vaso-occlusive crises 3 (25%). There were very high levels of leukocyte. Received ceftriaxone or ampicillin + gentamicin ± oral erythromycin), paracetamol 12 (100%), ibuprofen 8 (66.7%), tramadol 3 (25.0%), pentazocine 8 (66.7%) and blood transfusion 9 (75%). The average length of stay was 7 days (range 4 - 14 days). One patient died (8.3%). Conclusion: ACS is not uncommon in children with SCA in Port Harcourt. Education of parents on the need to recognize early symptoms of the disease is essential. Clinicians must be trained to correctly diagnose and manage it promptly and efficiently to avoid its related disastrous consequences.

*Corresponding author.

Keywords

Acute Chest Syndrome, Clinical Features, Treatment, Outcome, Port Harcourt

1. Introduction

Sickle cell anemia is one of the most prevalent genetic diseases worldwide [1] [2]. It frequently poses a task to health care providers for whom the disease can be considered one of the most significant haemoglobinopathies. Amid a diverse range of complications of varying complexity, none can become as rapidly disastrous as acute chest syndrome (ACS) [2]. It is the leading cause of death from sickle cell disease (SCD) worldwide accounting for about 25% of all deaths.

ACS is defined as a new pulmonary infiltrate on chest X-ray, combined with one or more manifestations such as fever, cough, sputum production, tachypnoea, dyspnoea, or new onset hypoxia [3]. It has a varied pathogenesis that includes occlusion of the pulmonary vascular bed by sickle erythrocytes, infection, embolized marrow fat, and lung infarction. It often follows a painful event, particularly in adults and although many pathologic processes may coexist establishing a specific cause is often difficult. Infections due to bacteria like *Mycoplasma*, *Chlamydia*, *Legionella*, *Streptococcus pneumoniae*, *Haemophilus influenzae* and viruses are more likely in children [4].

ACS is a frequent cause of hospitalization for patients with SCD. In the cooperative study of sickle cell disease (CSSCD), the mortality rate in patients with ACS was 1.1% in children [5]. In another multicenter study in the USA [3], the national ACS study group analyzed 671 episodes of ACS in 538 patients, with a mortality rate of 3%. In a 5-year study on the impact of seasonal variation of climatic factors on morbidities associated with vaso-occlusive crisis (VOC) among patients with sickle cell anaemia (SCA) in Maiduguri and Kano Teaching Hospitals, Nigeria, Ahmed *et al.* [6] found 56 episodes of ACS out of 2652 patients of VOC, giving a proportion of 2.11%.

Treatment for ACS is largely supportive in most cases. Early detection and supportive treatment may limit its severity and prevent death. Treatment includes continuous pulse oximetry and delivery of supplemental oxygen to patients with hypoxemia, adequate pain management, empiric antimicrobial therapy, monitoring of the haemoglobin concentration, blood transfusion, and maintenance of good hydration [7].

There are limited data on ACS in Nigeria and none has been reported in Port Harcourt, the capital city of Rivers state, Nigeria. In view of this, we decided to retrospectively audit all children with sickle cell anaemia with diagnosis of ACS. We hope to establish the prevalence, common clinical features and outcome of treatment in Port Harcourt, Nigeria.

2. Materials and Methods

A retrospective cohort study during a five year period beginning January 2009 and ending December 2014 was done. The records of all patients with sickle cell anaemia who were admitted to the Children Emergency and Paediatric Wards of the University of Port Harcourt Teaching Hospital (UPTH), Port Harcourt, Nigeria, during the period stated by the study were carefully examined. Ethical clearance was obtained from the Ethical Committee of UPTH. Those admitted to the study satisfied two criteria: 1) lower respiratory tract symptoms and 2) new pulmonary infiltrates on the chest radiograph. Information obtained included age, gender, haemoglobin genotype, clinical features, laboratory parameters (full blood count, chest X-ray and thick and thin film for malaria parasite), treatment given and outcome. Data were spread in excel sheets and analysis done by descriptive statistics in form of means and percentages. Variables were compared by student t test. P value ≤ 0.05 was regarded as significant.

3. Results

A total of 345 children with Sickle cell anaemia were admitted during the 5 year period. Twelve of them satisfied being diagnosed for acute chest syndrome (3.5%). They were aged 3 - 15 years with 7 (58.3%) of them under 5 years. There were more males 8 (66.7%) than female 4 (33.3%) (**Table 1**).

The presenting symptoms are reported in **Table 2**. The most common presenting symptoms were fever 12 (100%), cough 10 (83.3%), and chest pain 5 (41.7%). Two (16.7%) of the patients had wheeze/rhonchi. The most common physical findings were pulmonary consolidation 12 (100%), fever 12 (100%) and signs of respiratory distress 12 (100%). The admitting diagnosis were bronchopneumonia 6 (50%), severe malaria 3 (25%) and vaso-occlusive crises 3 (25%) but subsequently developed ACS during their hospital stay.

Table 1. General characteristics of the study group.

Characteristics	Number (12)	Percentage (%)
Age group (years)		
<5	7	58.3
>5	5	41.7
Gender		
Male	8	66.7
Female	4	33.3
Regular follow up		
Yes	3	25
No	9	75
On antibiotics prophylaxis		
Yes	0	0
No	12	100

Table 2. Clinical features of ACS.

Clinical features	Number	Percentage (%)
Initial symptoms		
Fever	12	100
Cough	10	83.3
Chest pain	5	41.7
Bone pains	3	25
Weakness	4	33.3
Abdominal pains	3	25
Vomiting	2	16.7
Wheeze	2	16.7
Clinical signs		
Anaemia	11	91.7
Jaundice	5	41.7
Haemoglobinuria	1	8.3
Respiratory distress	12	100
Bone tenderness	2	16.7
Rhonchi	2	16.7
Chest X-ray findings		
Lobar consolidation	4	33.3
Diffuse consolidation	8	66.7
Malarial parasitaemia		
Negative	2	16.7
Positive	10	83.3

ACS = Acute chest syndrome.

Laboratory test results showed very high levels of leukocytes, neutrophils and relatively high packed cell volume (**Table 3**). CRP and LDH results were not available. Chest X-ray mainly showed diffuse pulmonary consolidations 8(66.7%).

Patients were placed on two to three antibiotics: ceftriaxone or ampicillin + gentamicin ± oral erythromycin) (**Table 4**). Analgesics in the form of paracetamol 12 (100%), ibuprofen 8 (66.7%). tramadol 3 (25.0%) and pentazocine 8 (66.7%) were administered. Nine (75%) had blood transfusion. The average length of stay (LOS) was 7 days (range 4 - 14 days). One patient died giving a mortality rate of 8.3%.

4. Discussion

This study showed that ACS accounted for 3.5% of SCA children admitted in our hospital. This rate is lower than the 10% - 20% rate of hospital admissions reported by Miller and Gladwin in their review [8]. Also, Alkali and Ambe [9] in their retrospective study reported that of the 120 cases of SCA admitted 80 were found to have ACS. This lower rate of ACS in this study may be underestimated as some unknown SCA patients may have

Table 3. Laboratory parameters of children with ACS.

Laboratory parameters	Steady state	At presentation	P-value
Packed cell volume	21 ± 2.1	23 ± 3.4	>0.05
Leucocytes mm^3	12,541 ± 3.8	27,437 ± 5.1	<0.05
Neutrophil	45 ± 2.8	48 ± 3.2	>0.05
Platelet	180 ± 5.8	182.4.3	>0.05
Eosinophil	2.3 ± 0.3	3.4 ± 0.8	>0.05

ACS = Acute chest syndrome.

Table 4. Treatment and outcome of children with ACS.

Treatment and outcome	Number	Percentage (%)
Antibiotics therapy		
Ceftriaxone	8	66.7
Ampicillin	5	41.7
Gentamycin	7	58.3
Erythromycin	2	16.7
Antimalaria		
No	0	0
Yes	12	100
Analgesics		
Ibuprofen	8	66.7
Tramadol	3	25
Pentazocine	8	66.7
Oxygen		
No	1	8.3
Yes	11	91.7
Transfusion		
No	3	25
Yes	9	75
Duration of admission (days)		
<5	2	16.7
>5	10	83.3

ACS = Acute chest syndrome.

presented with this condition without relevant laboratory workup and diagnosis and thus missed been enrolled. Furthermore, it is also possible that due to parents' financial constraints, the only chest X-ray done during hospitalization could have been normal given that radiographic findings in some case of ACS may progress over time [5].

We observed a male predominance in line with previous studies [8] [10] [11]. Fever (100%), cough (83.3%) and chest pains (41.7%) were the main symptoms among our patients. This is in keeping with previous reports [5] [12].

There was significantly high leukocyte counts 27,437 mm^3 compared with steady state leukocyte count of 12,541 mm^3 [$P \leq 0.05$]. This may suggest that infection may precipitate the development of ACS among our patients, validating previous reports elsewhere [11] [13] [14]. It also has been reported in the literatures that microorganisms such as *Streptococcus pneumonia, Chlamydiae pneumonia, Mycoplasma pneumonia, influenza virus* A H1N1, *parainfluenza virus, respiratory syncytial virus* and *coronavirus* among others have been associated with ACS [5]. The predominant radiological finding in our study was diffuse lung involvement, in form of bronchopneumonia. This has been reported by Alkali and Ambe [9].

All of our patients were initially diagnosed as bronchopneumonia, severe malaria and vaso-occlusive crisis but subsequently developed ACS. Several studies [5] [8] have shown that ACS may develop 1 - 3 days after admission for VOC as there may exist a close relationship between ACS and VOC.

In line with the literatures [15] [16], our management of ACS included broad-spectrum antibiotics, analgesics, supplemental oxygen and transfusion. Early transfusion of SCA patients presenting with ACS should be encouraged, especially transfusion of packed red blood cells [17].

The average duration of hospitalization of 7 days is comparable to the 7 days-duration reported by Bertholdt *et al.*, [14] but lower than what has been reported by Vichinsky *et al.* [5]. Introduction of other supportive care in our practice like bronchodilators and incentive spirometry as elsewhere, along with systematic oxygen supplementation and early blood transfusion could substantially reduce the duration of hospital stay [8] [17].

One of our patients died, hence a mortality rate of 8.3% which is higher than the 4% percentage obtained by Bertholdt *et al.* in Belgium [14].

5. Conclusion

ACS is not an uncommon complication among children with SCA in Port Harcourt, Nigeria. There is need to educate parents on the need to recognize early symptoms of the disease, and seek help promptly. More so, clinicians must be trained to correctly diagnose ACS, and manage it promptly and efficiently to avoid its related disastrous consequences.

References

[1] Taylor, I.C., Carter, F., Poulose, J., Rolle, S., Babu, S. and Crichlow, S. (2004) Clinical Presentation of Acute Chest Syndrome in Sickle Cell Disease. *Postgraduate Medical Journal*, **80**, 346-349. http://dx.doi.org/10.1136/pgmj.2003.012781

[2] Thomas, A.N., Pattison, C. and Serjeant, G.R. (1982) Causes of Death in Sickle Cell Disease in Jamaica. *British Medical Journal*, **285**, 633-635.

[3] Vichinsky, E.P., Neumayr, L.D., Earles, A.N., Williams, R., Lennette, E.T., Dean, D., *et al.* (2000) Causes and Outcomes of the Acute Chest Syndrome in Sickle Cell Disease. National Acute Chest Syndrome Study Group. *The New England Journal of Medicine*, **342**, 1855-1865. http://dx.doi.org/10.1056/NEJM200006223422502

[4] Lal, A. and Vichinsky, E.P. (2005) Sickle cell disease. In: Hoffbrand, A.V., Catovsky, D. and Tuddenham, E.G., Eds., *Postgraduate Haematology*, 5th Edition, Blackwell Publishing, Hoboken, 104-118. http://dx.doi.org/10.1002/9780470987056.ch7

[5] Vichinsky, E.P., Styles, L.A., Colangelo, L.H., Wright, E.C., Castro, O. and Nickerson, B. (1997) Acute Chest Syndrome in Sickle Cell Disease: Clinical Presentation and Course. Cooperative Study of Sickle Cell Disease. *Blood*, **89**, 1787-1792.

[6] Ahmed, S.G., Kagu, M.B., Abjah, U.A. and Bukar, A.A. (2012) Seasonal Variations in Frequencies of Acute Vaso-Occlusive Morbidities among Sickle Cell Anaemia Patients in Northern Nigeria. *Journal of Blood Disorders & Transfusion*, **3**, 120. http://dx.doi.org/10.4172/2155-9864.1000120

[7] Yusuf, B.J., Abba, A.A. and Tasiu, M. (2014) Acute Chest Syndrome. *Sub-Saharan African Journal of Medicine*, **1**, 111-118. http://dx.doi.org/10.4103/2384-5147.138930

[8] Miller, A.C. and Gladwin, M.T. (2012) Pulmonary Complications of Sickle Cell Disease. *American Journal of Respiratory and Critical Care Medicine*, **185**, 1154-1165. http://dx.doi.org/10.1164/rccm.201111-2082CI

[9] Alkali, M.B. and Ambe, J.P. (2015) Acute Chest Syndrome in Paediatric Patients with Sickle Cell Disease in Northeastern, Nigeria. *Direct Research Journal of Health and Pharmacology*, **3**, 45-50.

[10] Bernard, A.W., Yasin, Z. and Venkat, A. (2007) Acute Chest Syndrome of Sickle Cell Disease. *Hospital Physician*, **44**, 5-23.

[11] Castro, O., Brambilla, D.J., Thorington, B., Reindorf, C.A., Scott, R.B., Gillette, P., Vera, J.C. and Levy, P.S. (1994) The Acute Chest Syndrome in Sickle Cell Disease: Incidence and Risk Factors. The Cooperative Study of Sickle Cell Disease. *Blood*, **84**, 643-649.

[12] Lamarre, Y., Romana, M., Waltz, X., Lalanne-Mistrih, M.L., Tressières, B., Divialle-Doumdo, L., Hardy-Dessources, M.D., Vent-Schmidt, J., Petras, M., Broquere, C., *et al.* (2012) Hemorheological Risk Factors of Acute Chest Syndrome and Painful Vaso-Occlusive Crisis in Children with Sickle Cell Disease. *Haematologica*, **97**, 1641-1647. http://dx.doi.org/10.3324/haematol.2012.066670

[13] Sprinkle, R.H., Cole, T., Smith, S. and Buchanan, G.R. (1996) Acute Chest Syndrome in Children with Sickle Cell Disease. A Retrospective Analysis of 100 Hospitalized Cases. *Journal of Pediatric Hematology/Oncology*, **8**, 105-110.

[14] Bertholdt, S., Lê, P.Q., Heijmans, C., Huybrechts, S., Dedeken, L., Devalck, C., Schifflers, S. and Ferster, A. (2012) Respiratory Complications of Sickle Cell Anemia in Children: The Acute Chest Syndrome. *Revue Médicale de Bruxelles*, **33**, 138-144.

[15] Miller, S.T. (2011) How I Treat Acute Chest Syndrome in Children with Sickle Cell Disease. *Blood*, **117**, 5297-5305. http://dx.doi.org/10.1182/blood-2010-11-261834

[16] Elenga, N., Cuadro, E., Martin, E., Cohen-Addad, N. and Basset, T. (2014) Associated Factors of Acute Chest Syndrome in Children with Sickle Cell Disease in French Guiana. *International Journal of Pediatrics*, **2014**, Article ID: 213681. http://dx.doi.org/10.1155/2014/213681

[17] Nansseu, J.R., Noubiap, J.J., Ndoula, S.T., Zeh, A.F. and Monamele, C.G. (2013) What Is the Best Strategy for the Prevention of Transfusion-Transmitted Malaria in Sub-Saharan African Countries Where Malaria Is Endemic? *Malaria Journal*, **12**, 465. http://dx.doi.org/10.1186/1475-2875-12-465

31

"Inverse Type" Apple-Peel Syndrome Is Associated with Type III Colonic Atresia in a Neonate with Gastroschisis—A "New" Subtype of Colonic Atresia

Ralf-Bodo Tröbs[1*], Micha Bahr[1], Ralf Schulze[2], Matthias Neid[3], Wolfgang Pielemeier[4], Claudia Roll[4]

[1]Department of Pediatric Surgery, St. Mary's Hospital, St. Elisabeth Group, Ruhr-University of Bochum, Herne, Germany

[2]Department of Obstetrics and Gynecology, St. Vincenz' Hospital, Datteln, Germany

[3]Institute of Pathology, Ruhr-University of Bochum, Georgius-Agricola-Foundation, BG-Clinics Bergmannsheil, Bochum, Germany

[4]Center of Perinatology, Department of Neonatology and Pediatric Intensive Care, Vest Children's Hospital, University of Witten-Herdecke, Datteln, Germany

Email: [*]ralf-bodo.troebs@elisabethgruppe.de, micha.bahr@elisabethgruppe.de, r.schulze@vincenz-datteln.de, matthias.neid@rub.de, w.pielemeier@kinderklinik-datteln.de, c.roll@kinderklinik-datteln.de

Abstract

The colon is an unusual site of intestinal atresia. Colonic atresia is subdivided into three phenotypes. Type III is the most common phenotype, where the proximal and distal blind sacs are not connected. Here, we report on the presence of colonic atresia with an "inverse apple-peel" appearance in a neonate with gastroschisis. The lack of mesenteric fixation of the entire small intestine, including the proximal colon, and the twisting around the vascular axis of the superior mesenteric artery led to intrauterine volvulus and hemorrhagic infarction of the ileocolic bowel at 34 weeks of gestation. According to the current nomenclature for small bowel atresia, we introduce type IIIB into the current colonic atresia classification. The occurrence of type IIIB has been mentioned in the literature, but no single cases have been reported until now. Patients with this type of atresia are predisposed to the loss of the ileocecal region.

[*]Corresponding author.

Keywords

Apple-Peel Syndrome, Colonic Atresia, Volvulus, Gastroschisis

1. Introduction

Colonic atresia (CA) is a very rare congenital malformation with a prevalence of 1 in 20,000 live births [1]. Prenatal ultrasonography typically shows enlarged loops of the small and large bowel. CA can be associated with anomalies of the heart, gastrointestinal tract, abdominal wall, and musculoskeletal system. Clinically, a newborn with CA develops signs of complete obstruction. Distension of the abdomen within 24 to 48 hours and delayed feculent vomiting are the leading symptoms. According to the recent literature, three different types are described. Type III is characterized by the complete interruption of the colonic continuity and the presence of a gap in the mesocolon [1]-[4]. For the more common types of small bowel atresia, the nomenclature encompasses four types, and type III is subdivided into two subtypes [5] [6]. According to the clinical phenotype, subtype IIIB is referred to as "*apple-peel*" or "*Christmas tree*" atresia. The term "apple-peel" was first introduced in 1961 [7] for a special type of jejunal atresia with a discontinuity of the small bowel and a wide mesenteric gap. It describes a shortened and coiled small bowel around a retrograde perfusing artery, suggestive of a coiled apple peel. This retrograde perfusing artery of the apple-peel predominately compensates for the interrupted superior mesenteric artery [8]. Infants with complex gastroschisis carry an increased risk for small bowel atresia or CA [9] [10]. To the best of our knowledge, this is the first detailed report on the association of CA with an apple-peel phenotype affecting the small gut in combination with the ileocolic region.

2. Case Report

A prenatal ultrasound at 14 weeks of gestation revealed the extrusion of the fetal bowel out of the coelom associated with extra-abdominal bowel dilatation. At 34 weeks of gestation, the boy was delivered by Cesarean section (CS) due to fetal compromise. An ultrasound revealed pathological thickening of the bowel wall and an impaired cardiotocogram. The birth weight was 1820 g (10th percentile), and the Apgar scores were 6, 8 and 9 at 1, 5 and 10 minutes, respectively. The umbilical arterial pH was 7.35, and the amniotic fluid was stained with blood and meconium. Gastroschisis with the eventration of nearly the entire bowel and the stomach was confirmed. The lower parts of the infant's body were immediately placed in a "bowel bag". The infant was then stabilized with intubation, mechanical ventilation and intravenous fluid administration. A gastric tube was inserted, and aspiration revealed the presence of large amounts of bloody gastric content. The postnatal laboratory investigations revealed anemia with a hemoglobin (Hb) level of 12.8 g/dL, and an erythrocyte transfusion was required preoperatively. A surgical evaluation and primary closure of the abdominal wall were performed at the local neonatal intensive care unit (NICU). The abdominal defect was approximately 3 cm in diameter, and there was no fibrous coating over the extra-abdominal bowel. The protruded, non-fixed and twisted bowel was adherent to only a very small mesenteric pedicle. It consisted of the entire small bowel, the ileocecal region and 4 cm of the blind end of the cecum with the appendix vermiformis, and the ascending colon (**Figure 1**). There was a broad gap between the proximal colon and the tiny, non-used distal colon. The latter was densely adhered to the base of the mesentery (**Figure 2**). The derotation of the twisted mesenterial pedicle revealed the presence of a common ileocolic mesentery containing the blood supply to the small and the ileocecal bowels (**Figure 3**). In addition to the apple-peel deformity, the terminal portion of the extra-abdominal bowel was twisted at least 180° with a resulting hemorrhagic infarction. The resection of the proximal and atretic portion of the colon (15-cm length), including the terminal ileum, was required, and a temporary terminal ileostomy was created. The postoperative course was prolonged due to the inability for full enteral feeding for several weeks. Under parenteral nutrition, the infant tolerated increasing amounts of oral feeding. At 8 weeks of age, a temporary end-to-side anastomosis with a stoma of the proximal bowel according to Santulli was established [7]. During surgery, the relation of the bowel diameter was determined to be 6 to 1. The passage of increasing amounts of stool occurred after two weeks and allowed the closure of the enterostomy after five months with a body weight of 4520 g (below 3rd percentile). Oral nutrition by breastfeeding was tolerated increasingly, and weight gain 1.5 month after surgery was 1.45 kg. During a follow up of 11 moths a slow catch up growth occurred.

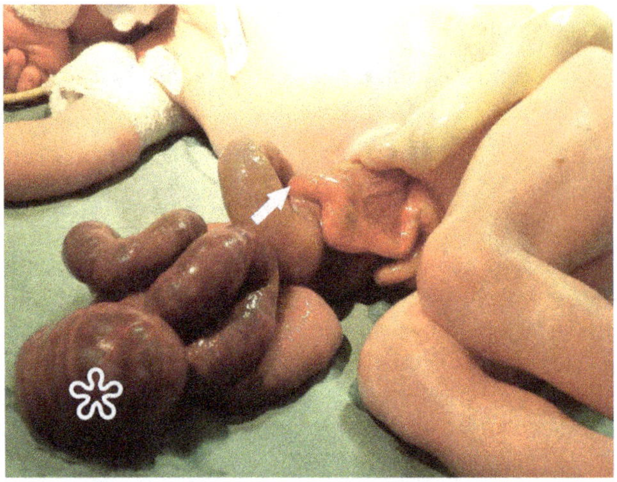

Figure 1. The appearance of the dilated and blind-ending colonic atresia (asterisk). The unused colon is fixed to the base of the mesenteric stalk (arrow).

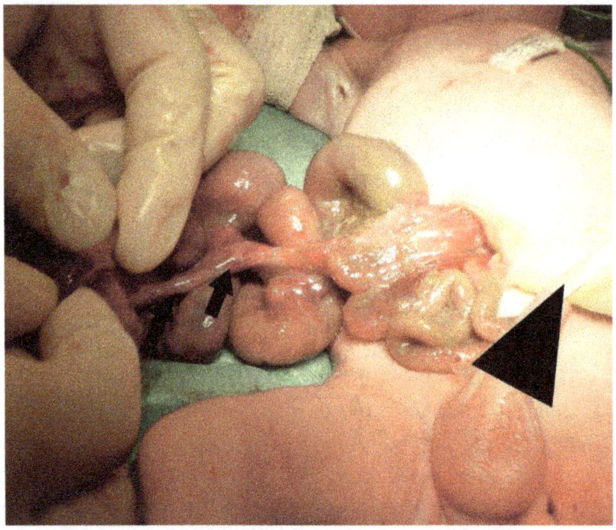

Figure 2. The vascular axis of the small bowel (arrows) together with the ileocecal region after detorsion.

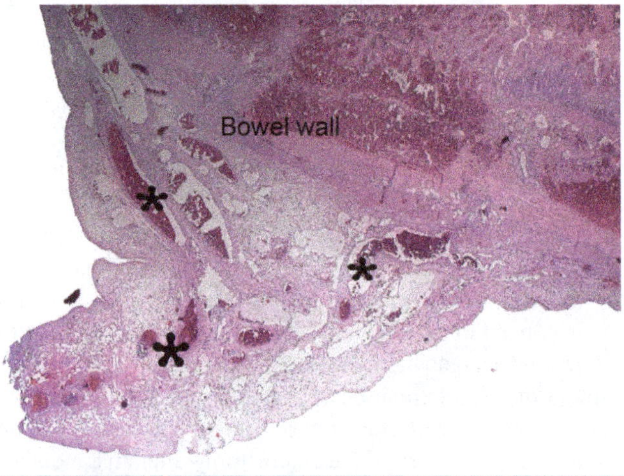

Figure 3. The histology of the adherent small mesenteric rim with dilated blood (asterisks) and lymphatic vessels (hematoxylin/eosin, ×50).

3. Discussion

Colonic atresias account for 1.8% to 15% of all intestinal atresias, and they are subdivided into three phenotypes [1] [2] [5] [6] [11]-[13]. Type I is characterized by complete obstruction by a diaphragm, and in type II, the two blind ends are connected by a fibrous band. Type III is the most common phenotype, where the proximal and distal blind sacs are not connected. *The occurrence of type IIIB has been mentioned in the literature, but no cases have been reported until now* [5] [6] [12].

It has been shown that intrauterine events or "catastrophes", such as volvulus, intussusception, herniation and snaring of the bowel during the fetal time period, may be responsible for the development of bowel atresia below the duodenum [2] [7] [11] [12] [14]. This "vascular theory" for the pathogenesis of bowel atresia was confirmed via animal experiments. In fetal puppies, the interruption of the blood supply to the bowel was able to induce the entire spectrum of different types of intestinal atresia or stenosis [14]. Therefore, with the exception of duodenal atresia, vascular disruption is responsible for the majority of the cases with bowel atresia.

The presence of nonrotation of the entire gut together with a narrow mesenteric pedicle predisposes patients with gastroschisis to develop intestinal atresia during the intrauterine period. Approximately 5% to 25% of these neonates are affected with intestinal atresia, and in 2.5% of the infants with gastroschisis, a CA can be expected [1] [10]. The coincidence of gastroschisis and the associated intestinal pathologies, such as intestinal atresia, perforation or volvulus (complex gastroschisis), is associated with an elevated risk for postsurgical morbidity and mortality [9] [13]. Early elective delivery for suspected complex cases of gastroschisis is normally advocated in order to prevent the development of bowel necrosis secondary to the abdominal events. However, a recently published multi-institutional study did not reveal any benefit to the elective delivery at <37 weeks of gestation [15].

In this case report, we present a "new" subtype of apple-peel malformation associated with CA in an infant with gastroschisis. In its classic form, apple-peel syndrome is associated with complete jejunal atresia with a broad gap between both blindly ending parts of the intestine and twisting of the distal small bowel (type IIIB) [5]. According to the vascular hypothesis, the occlusion of the superior mesenteric artery causes the absence of part of the jejunum, and the perfusion of the distal small intestine is maintained in a retrograde manner by the collateral vessels originating from the ileocolic artery [8].

In this "inverse" case of apple-peel syndrome, the atresia was located distally in the ascending colon and the "inverse" apple-peel affected the proximal small bowel and included the ileocolic region. The vascular supply of the entire small and ileocolic intestines was maintained by the completely preserved superior mesenteric artery. The described malformation can be explained by the interruption of the ileocolic, right, and middle colonic arteries. The disappearance of the middle portion of the colon, the tiny, non-used distal colon, and the absence of any bile stained content in the distal colon indicate that the atresia developed during early fetal development.

Fetal compromise at 34 weeks of gestation led to an emergency CS. In our case, the bowel infarction was not the result of a tight or closing abdominal wall defect [2]. Additionally, the volvulus was facilitated by the presence of only a small mesenteric stalk in the extracoelomic gut. The colonic atresia together with a broad mesenteric defect led to failed fixation and a perpendicular predisposition to the torsion of the gut. Concordant with the presented course, it has been described that the presence of meconium or blood-stained amniotic fluid and either prenatal or postnatal gastrointestinal complications is associated with an older age to reach full enteral feeds [16]. Therefore, the reported infant suffered from type 2 intestinal failure, requiring >28 days of parenteral nutrition [15].

4. Conclusion

In contrast to the classical type of apple-peel syndrome, the "inverse type" of apple-peel syndrome is associated with a high risk to the loss of the ileocecal region.

References

[1] Aguayo, P. and Ostlie, D.J. (2010) Duodenal and Intestinal Atresia and Stenosis. In: Holcomb III, G.W. and Murphy, J.P., Eds., *Ashcraft's Pediatric Surgery*, 5th Edition, Saunders, Elsevier, Philadelphia, 413-415. http://dx.doi.org/10.1016/b978-1-4160-6127-4.00031-8

[2] Baglaj, M., Carachi, R. and MacCormack, B. (2010) Colonic Atresia: A Clinicopathological Insight into Its Etiology. *European Journal of Pediatric Surgery*, **20**, 102-105. http://dx.doi.org/10.1055/s-0029-1242735

[3] von Schweinitz, D. (2013) Angeborene fehlbildungen und obstruktionen des dünndarms. In: von Schweinitz, D. and Ure, B., Eds., *Kinderchirurgie*, 2nd Edition, Springer, Berlin, Heidelberg, 344-345. http://dx.doi.org/10.1007/978-3-642-29779-3_26

[4] Wester, T. (2011) Colonic and Rectal Atresias. In: Puri, P., Ed., *Newborn Surgery*, 3rd Edition, Hodder Arnold, London, 505-511. http://dx.doi.org/10.1201/b13478-59

[5] Grosfeld, J., Ballantine, T. and Shoemaker, R. (1979) Operative Management of Intestinal Atresia and Stenosis Based on Pathological Findings. *Journal of Pediatric Surgery*, **14**, 595-599. http://dx.doi.org/10.1016/S0022-3468(79)80502-3

[6] Veccia, L.K.D., Grosfeld, J.L., West, K.W., Rescorla, F.J., Scherer, L.R. and Engum, S.A. (1998) Intestinal Atresia and Stenosis. A 25-Year Experience with 277 Cases. *Archives of Surgery*, **133**, 490-497.

[7] Santulli, T.V. and Blanc, W.A. (1961) Congenital Atresia of the Intestine: Pathogenesis and Treatment. *Annals of Surgery*, **154**, 939-948.

[8] Holmes, L.B. (2012) Common Malformations. Oxford University Press, Oxford, New York, Auckland, 37-44, 109-115.

[9] Bergholz, R., Boettcher, M., Reinshagen, K. and Wenke, K. (2014) Complex Gastroschisis Is a Different Entity to Simple Gastroschisis Affecting Morbidity and Mortality. A Systematic Review and Meta-Analysis. *Journal of Pediatric Surgery*, **49**, 1527-1532. http://dx.doi.org/10.1016/j.jpedsurg.2014.08.001

[10] Fleet, M.S. and de la Hunt, M.N. (2000) Intestinal Atresia with Gastroschisis. *Journal of Pediatric Surgery*, **35**, 1323-1325. http://dx.doi.org/10.1053/jpsu.2000.9324

[11] Lynn, H.B. and Espinas, E.E. (1959) Intestinal Atresia. An Attempt to Relate Location to Embryologic Process. *Archives of Surgery*, **79**, 357-361. http://dx.doi.org/10.1001/archsurg.1959.04320090005001

[12] Menardi, G. (1987) Congenital Colonic Atresias. *European Journal of Pediatric Surgery*, **42**, 31-35. http://dx.doi.org/10.1055/s-2008-1075549

[13] Snyder, C.L., Miller, K.A., Sharp, R.J., Murphy, J.P., Andrews, W.A., Holcomb III, G.W., Gittes, G.K. and Ashcraft, K.W. (2001) Management of Intestinal Atresia in Patients with Gastroschisis. *Journal of Pediatric Surgery*, **36**, 1542-1545. http://dx.doi.org/10.1053/jpsu.2001.27040

[14] Louw, J. (1964) Investigation into the Etiology of Congenital Atresia of the Colon. *Diseases of the Colon & Rectum*, **7**, 741-748. http://dx.doi.org/10.1007/BF02616944

[15] Carnaghan, H., Pereira, S., James, C.P., Charlesworth, P.B., Ghionzoli, M., Mohamed, E., Cross, K.M.K., Kiely, E., Patel, S., Desai, A., Nicolaides, K., Curry, J.I., Ade-Ajayi, N., de Coppi, P., Davenport, M., David, A.L., Pierro, A. and Eaton, S. (2014) Is Early Delivery Beneficial in Gastroschisis? *Journal of Pediatric Surgery*, **49**, 928-933. http://dx.doi.org/10.1016/j.jpedsurg.2014.01.027

[16] Bucher, B.T., Mazotas, I.G., Warner, B.W. and Saito, J.M. (2012) Effect of Time to Surgical Evaluation on the Outcomes of Infants with Gastroschisis. *Journal of Pediatric Surgery*, **47**, 1105-1110. http://dx.doi.org/10.1016/j.jpedsurg.2012.03.016

32

Emergency Surgical Intervention by Mobile Surgical Team in the NICU

R.-B. Tröbs[1*], A. Stein[2], U. Felderhoff[2], L. Hanssler[2]

[1]Department of Pediatric Surgery, Catholic Foundation Marienhospital Herne, Ruhr-University of Bochum, Herne, Widumer, Germany

[2]Department of Pediatrics I, University Hospital Essen, Hufelandstr, Essen, Germany

Email: *ralf-bodo.troebs@marienhospital-herne.de, anja.stein@uk-essen.de, ursula.felderhoff@uk-essen.de, anja.stein@uk-essen.de

Abstract

The objective of this study was to describe our NICU's (neonatal intensive care unit) experience with mobile surgical team and to demonstrate its effectiveness. Method: We analyzed the data of 17 consecutive very low birth weight and extremely low birth weight infants over 3 years who underwent 22 procedures (19 emergency and 3 elective). The gestational age at birth was a median of 25 weeks (range 24 - 39), and the median birth weight was 613 g (range from 340 g to 1100 g). The infants received their operations during their first 2 weeks of life (median 7 days, range from 1 to 14). Results: The spectrum of primary surgical diagnoses included spontaneous intestinal perforations (n = 8), gastric perforations (n = 3), necrotizing enterocolitis (n = 2), meconium ileus (n = 2), and miscellaneous (n = 2). An emergency laparotomy with either a bowel or a gastric procedure was performed in 16 cases. Postoperatively, all infants required mechanical ventilation from 1 to 43 days (median 6.5 days). Complications included a metachronous small bowel perforation, an ileostomy retraction, a prolapsed stoma, and impaired wound healing; we had one postoperative death. Two infants died later in the NICU (mortality 3 of 16; 19%). Conclusion: Off-site surgery for preterm infants in the NICU is feasible. This approach prevents the risks of transportation, and parents and neonatologists alike feel comfortable with this regimen. However, biases may exist regarding the surgeon's decision to operate, the choice of procedure, and the follow-up.

Keywords

Off-Site Surgery, NICU, Extremely Low Birth Weight Infants, Necrotizing Enterocolitis, Spontaneous Bowel Perforation, Gastric Perforation

*Corresponding author.

1. Introduction

In many centers, "*in-situ surgery*" (ISS) in the neonatal intensive care unit (NICU) is selected for specific emergency procedures on critically ill and unstable neonates. It is *performed on the incubator without transporting the baby outside.* Preoperative assessment, surgery, and immediate postoperative surveillance are provided by the local pediatric surgery service.

In contrast, "*off-site surgery*" (*OSS*) is provided by a surgical team from a distant hospital. *OSS is not a common practice worldwide.* Close cooperation and good communication between the neonatology and the surgical teams are essential. Adequate decision-making requires rapid communication if problems arise, and in some cases, the surgeon's intuition is required.

Recent medical developments and technical improvements have facilitated the care of very low birth weight (VLBW, birth weight ≤1500 g) and extremely low birth weight (ELBW, birth weight ≤1000 g) infants with excellent results [1]. These developments present the pediatric surgeon with the challenging group of very delicate and extremely stress-sensitive infants.

In this study, our goal was to examine the benefits and limitations of OSS in an NICU located 20 km from the pediatric surgery department within a congested area. This surgery was performed to provide a pediatric surgical care service for the NICU, which lacks its own pediatric surgery department.

Surgery under the described circumstances was performed transitionally until the introduction of a high quality local neonatal surgery service.

2. Material and Methods

A retrospective, IRB approved analysis of all infants undergoing neonatal emergency surgery between March 2007 and March 2010 was performed. Our investigation focused on the feasibility, short-term morbidity and mortality during a hospital stay. After the reported period an "onsite" surgeon started his work. The decision to admit a patient to the NICU was determined by telephone consultations or by the submission of abdominal X-rays via the internet. In cases with a high probability for intervention, a team consisting of a surgeon, a pediatric surgical resident, a scrub nurse, and an assistant nurse were sent to the NICU. Ordinarily, we used a public taxi to reach the NICU. Depending on road traffic volume, 20 to 50 minutes was allotted for team transportation, and the neonatology team used this time period to prepare the infant for surgery. In each case, the decision for surgery was made at the infants' incubator.

Anesthesia in these very premature babies was performed by an experienced neonatologist in close cooperation with a pediatric anesthesiologist.

During surgery, the regular activities of the NICU were not suspended. The staff working in the unit wore caps and masks, and only the operating team wore surgical clothes. The operation was performed in an open incubator or warmer with a radiant heating system (Giraffe Omnibed®, GE Healthcare, Germany) in a separate area of the NICU.

For anesthesia, all patients were prepared for intubation and ventilation. Venous access was achieved by a percutaneously placed central venous line (silicone catheter) for the administration of fluid, analgesics, blood products, and vasopressors. Furthermore, a second peripheral venous catheter was used. An arterial line in the posterior tibial, radial or ulnar artery was used for invasive blood pressure monitoring. For anesthesia and sedation, a combination of propofol, fentanyl and the non-depolarizing muscle relaxant vecuronium was given intravenously. Titration of anesthetics, fluid, vasopressors and blood transfusions were determined by the neonatologist and anesthesiologist.

Monitoring during surgery included pulse oxymetry, electrocardiography, transcutaneous pCO_2 measurement and oscillometric and invasive blood pressure measurements, with an umbilical or peripheral arterial access and a transcutaneous or rectal temperature measurement. Transurethral catheterization was used to empty the bladder in order to monitor the urine output and avoid urinary retention after fentanyl administration.

The postoperative surgical follow-up was routinely performed with telephone calls, and visits were performed on request.

The following variables were extracted from the records: (1) biometric data and age; (2) prenatal application of betamethasone, postnatal medical treatment with surfactants, and treatment of patent ductus arteriosus (PDA) with indomethacin; (3) application of catecholamines and duration of artificial ventilation; (4) diagnosis and type of surgery; and (5) presence of intraventricular hemorrhage (IVH), as well as postoperative morbidity and mortality. Postoperative mortality was defined as death either during surgery or within 7 days after surgery, and the overall mortality was related to the length of the hospitalization.

Statistics: The data are expressed as medians and ranges. Furthermore, the arithmetic mean and standard deviation were estimated.

3. Results

Seventeen patients receiving 22 procedures in the NICU were included. In one additional engagement, an operation was not performed because of the lack of an indication for surgery, and the team left without performing an operation. There was a predominance of female infants (12). Four infants were from two twin births, and two were from a triplet birth. Patient characteristics are given in **Table 1**. The median gestational age at birth was 25 weeks (24 - 39 weeks). The median weight at birth was 613 g (340 - 1100 g). Five infants had a birth weight below 500 g, and 7 infants weighed between 500 and 750 g (**Figure 1**). The prenatal induction of lung maturation with betamethasone was started in 16 cases and completed in 12 cases. A porcine surfactant was substituted postnatally in 11 infants who each received one (n = 6), two (n = 1) or three doses (n = 4) (Curosurf®). Furthermore, the medical closure of patent ductus arteriosus (PDA) with indomethacin was attempted preoperatively in 8 infants. However, a subsequent surgical PDA ligature was required in 3 infants. Seven infants were ventilated mechanically prior to the intervention due to abdominal distension, failure to pass meconium or recurrent apnea. Three infants received catecholamines immediately prior to the operation. Pneumoperitoneum on a preoperative X-ray was found in patients with spontaneous intestinal perforation (SIP), except for one infant with a covered perforation. In two infants with NEC, pneumatosis intestinalis was the leading radiological symptom.

Table 1. Biometric data and age at operation, diagnoses, and mortality (n = 17).

Parameter	Median (min/maximum)
Birth weight [g]	613 (340 - 1100)
Gestational age [weeks]	25 (24 - 39)
Postnatal age at operation [days]	7 (1 - 14)
Primary diagnosis	8 SIP 3 Gastric perforation 2 NEC 2 Meconium ileus 2 Necrosis of forefood, skin
Postoperative ventilation [days]	6.5 (1 - 43)
Mortality	3 (12 h, 12 days postop.; 4 months)

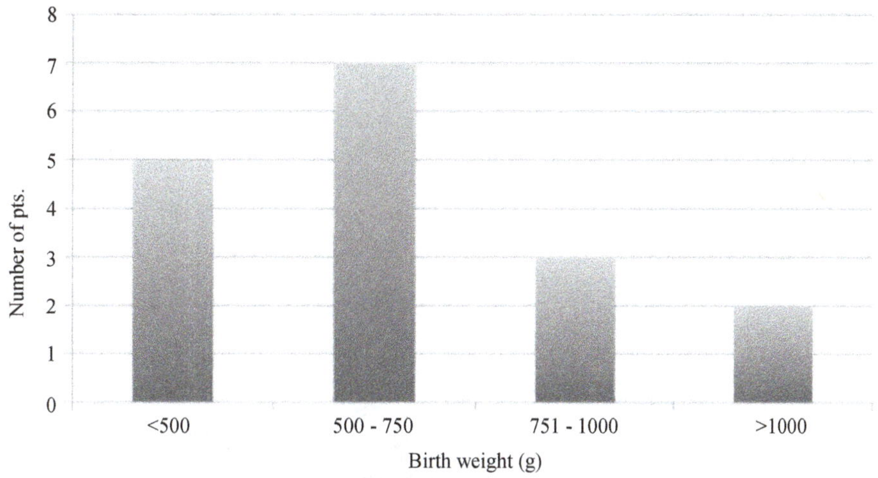

Figure 1. Distribution of birth weights.

The surgical diagnoses were established as follows: SIP (n = 8), gastric perforation (n = 3), necrotizing enterocolitis (n = 2), meconium ileus (n = 2), anorectal malformation with prostatic fistula (n = 1), secondary necrosis of the forefoot (n = 1), and extended skin necrosis (n = 1). The procedures performed included the following: single double-barreled enterostomies (n = 8), two separate double-barreled enterostomies (n = 4), gastrostomies (n = 3), and double barreled descending colostomy for anorectal malformation, skin debridement, and forefoot necrectomies. **Figure 2** presents the postnatal ages at surgery. The mean age at initial intervention was 7 days (range 1 - 14). The early repair of stomas was performed during surgery in 2 infants with jejunostomy at body weights of 1040 g and 1200 g and postnatal ages of 2 and 3 months, respectively. The remaining stomas were closed electively in the surgical theatre of the pediatric surgical unit. Postoperatively, all infants required mechanical ventilation from 1 to 43 days (median 6.5 days). The following 16 urgent or emergency neonatal surgery emergency cases were born during the observation time span in the cooperating hospital and subsequently operated upon in our pediatric surgical department:

SIP (n = 3), NEC (n = 1), small bowel atresia (n = 3; 1 multiple, 1 jejunum, 1 ileum), gastroschisis (n = 2); meconium peritonitis after intrauterine perforation (n = 1); meconium plug (n = 1; conservative treatment), esophageal atresia with tracheoesophageal fistula (TEF) of the lower segment (n = 1); anorectal malformation with perineal fistula (n = 1); congenital diaphragmatic hernia (n = 1); cloacal extrophy (n = 1); and mesoblastic nephroma (n = 1). No mortality was observed in these cases.

Preoperatively, an intraventricular hemorrhage (IVH) was present in 5 infants (1 grade I, 3 grade II, and 1 grade IV). Postoperative ultrasound examinations did not reveal any progressive or new bleeding in these infants. In one triplet infant weighing 400 g, a postoperative cerebellar hemorrhage with the subsequent atrophy of the affected cerebellar hemisphere was diagnosed postoperatively by ultrasound.

Two infants required a second procedure. One had a metachronous small bowel perforation, and the other required the repair of a retracted ileostomy. One infant developed a severe stoma prolapse requiring an urgent laparotomy and a segmental bowel resection, which was performed in the NICU. Impaired wound healing occurred in 3 immature infants. One infant developed septicemia and subsequent ischemic necrosis of one forefoot with mummification.

There was one early postoperative death due to septic shock 12 hours postoperatively in an infant weighing 490 g following gastric perforation and segmental ileal necrosis. Two infants died during the latter course; one triplet infant with SIP died due to septicemia on the 12th postoperative day. In the second case, the infant died 4 months after the initial laparotomy due to respiratory insufficiency caused by bronchopulmonary dysplasia.

4. Discussion

Surgical interventions in very small infants carry a high potential for morbidity and mortality. Perioperative management is characterized by an interdisciplinary approach; however, the pediatric surgeon is predominantly responsible for the decision to operate and for the supervision of the postoperative course.

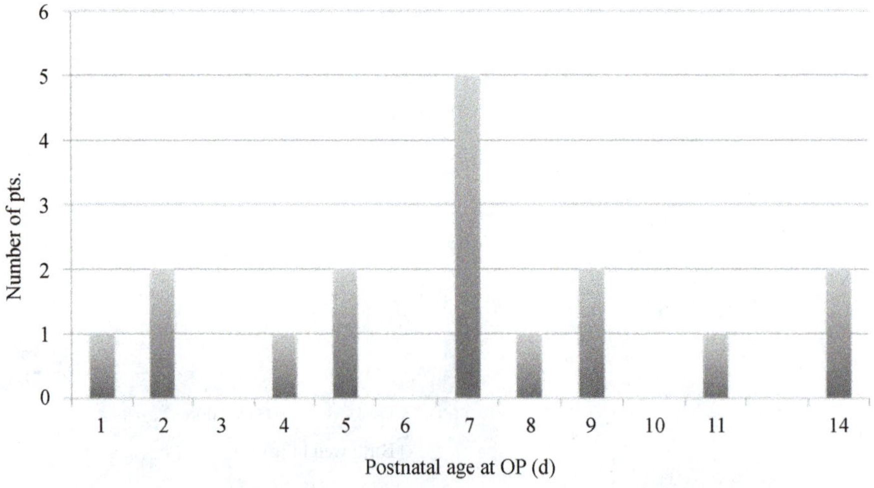

Figure 2. Postnatal age at operation.

The mortality rates for ELBW infants have been decreasing compared to those a decade ago; this improvement has been the most prominent for infants with birth weights from 450 to 700 g, among whom mortality rates remain the highest [1]. Routine manipulations in VLBW infants, such as the heel-prick blood test, the insertion of naso-gastric tubes, and venipuncture, increase oxygen consumption and contribute to cardiovascular destabilization and energy loss. If transport and surgical intervention are required, such a situation is obviously a severe form of stress. Stress induces short-term problems, such as hypertension, hyperglycemia, and poor peripheral perfusion [2]. In addition, long-term stress-related sequel, such as neurodevelopmental and cognitive problems, may occur. Given this knowledge, avoiding transportation may reduce stress and therefore benefit the infant.

However, surgical treatment at an off-site department may be associated with specific risks and limitations.

To limit transport of patients to an offsite facility, a distance of 20 km in the congested Ruhr Area had to be traveled by the surgical team, which is time-consuming and personally intensive.

Transportation of the surgical team by public taxi was practicable, cost-effective, and safe. Alternatively, an ambulance would be able to penetrate the congested traffic, which could shorten the transportation duration but is more expensive.

Despite the fact that transporting the infants was avoided, off-site pediatric surgery has some further limitations:

1) The decision to operate may be subject to bias if the pediatric surgeon and a complete operation team have to be transported to the infant.

2) The personal resources of the department of pediatric surgery are limited, and the team is not always available for outside activities.

3) In some instances, elective procedures in the pediatric surgery unit would have to be postponed.

Generally, operations in the NICU are (irregularly) performed on preterm, very sick and critically ill infants. These operations comprise a spectrum of pediatric surgical procedures that can be performed successfully in the NICU (**Table 2**). Surgical *in-situ* PDA ligation has been reported previously by two groups [3] [4] and is now well established in many centers. Finer and coworkers [5] compared the outcomes for infants who received operations within an NICU with the results obtained from patients who underwent operations within the theater. They found a higher mortality in babies receiving operations in an NICU. However, the latter infants had lower birth weights, lower gestational ages and greater illness severity [5]. Our series has shown that OSS on the NICU even in extremely immature infants can be performed without elevated infection rates and minimal mortality.

With the introduction of surfactants, the increased viability at lower gestational ages has led to the presence of a number of infants susceptible to bacterial overgrowth, some of whom develop surgical intestinal disease [6]. The series presented here focuses on emergency bowel and gastric surgeries in this special group of ELBW and VLBW infants.

Our series is characterized by a very low gestational age (median 25 weeks), very or extremely low birth

Table 2. Spectrum of neonatal ISS procedures from 3 series.

Type of surgery	Finer *et al.* (1993)	Gavilanes *et al.* (1997)	Fanning *et al.* (1998)	Presented series
Abdominal, bowel, and gastric	40	12	5	17 emergency + 2 elective
Peritoneal drain	0	0	4	0
CDH repair	10	2	2	0
Omphalocele, Gastroschisis	2	0	0	0
Esophageal atresia/TEF	1 TEF	0	2 TEF + gastrostomy	0
Inguinal hernia	2	0	1	0
Orchidopexy bilaterally	10	0	0	0
CSF-reservoir	0	14	0	0
PDA-Ligation	3	16	0	0
Miscellaneous	13	1	4	2

weights (median 613 g) and a predominance of infants undergoing operations for SIP. The induction of prenatal lung maturation using betamethasone was begun in the majority of our patients. Surfactants were substituted in more than one half, and in one half of the analyzed group of infants, a medical closure of the PDA was attempted. Three pediatric surgical series exist within the English literature that concern abdominal *in-situ* surgery in NICUs (5, 7, 11). These series include a high number of emergency bowel surgeries in cases of neonatal acute abdomens. Other important indications for ISS in NICUs included the repair of congenital diaphragmatic hernias and the ligation and dissection of a TEF or inguinal hernia. In addition, Gavilanes and coworkers showed that the implantation of cerebrospinal fluid reservoirs can be performed in NICUs [7].

Mortality rates from NEC are generally high, ranging from 15% to 30% [8]. However, necrotizing enterocolitis is an umbrella diagnosis for the different defined entities that are called acquired intestinal disease. This group of entities comprises NEC, viral enteritis of infancy and SIP. In addition, the food intolerances of premature babies must be considered [6].

Infants with spontaneous intestinal perforation (SIP) represented the majority of our patients. This entity is characterized by the focal perforation of the ileum or jejunum, the presence of pneumoperitoneum, and the absence of pneumatosis intestinalis. SIP typically occurs within the first 2 weeks of life in infants below 1,000 g [6]. Compared with genuine NEC, infants with SIP are more likely to have received surfactants, more likely to have patent ductus arteriosus requiring treatment, and more likely to require vasopressors [6]. The early use of indomethacin solely or in combination with steroids is one of the main risk factors for the development of SIP [9]. In our series, indometacine for the treatment of PDA was applied preoperatively in 8 infants: 5 who developed SIP; two who developed gastric perforations; and one who had a meconium ileus. Bowel perforations occurred on days 7 and 14, and gastric perforations, on days 7 and 11. The infant with meconium ileus underwent an operation on day 9 after birth.

In contrast, preterm infants with NEC are commonly older than 2 weeks. Intestinal pneumatosis and/or a perforation on X-ray and/or ultrasound indicate advanced NEC. At surgery, a multifocal pattern predominately affecting the terminal ileum and ascending colon is typically observed [6].

It has been shown that NEC is associated with a significantly poorer neurodevelopmental outcome than prematurity alone. The presence of advanced NEC and the need for surgery increase the risk of neurological impairment [10]. Surgery for NEC further impairs this relationship. However, none of the infants in our series developed postoperative IVH, although one case of unilateral cerebellar hemorrhage was detected by postoperative ultrasound. According to the literature, there is reason to believe that a SIP survivor may be capable of better neurodevelopmental outcomes than survivors of surgical preterm NEC [6].

Perioperative mortality in our series occurred in one infant (6%). Despite the immaturity of our patients and the special operative settings, a mortality of 3 of 17 (18%) did not exceed the mortality rates reported in comparable reports, which range from 4% to 33% [5] [7] [11].

Most commonly, we had to perform a laparotomy with a resection of the affected bowel and the creation of small bowel stomas. Peritoneal drainage for unstable infants, introduced by Ein *et al.* in 1977, and primary anastomoses were avoided in our series [12]. In a meta-analysis, Henry and Moss (2008) were unable to identify differences in the survival between infants treated with a laparotomy and those treated with primary peritoneal drainage for NEC [8]. However, peritoneal drainage requires a significant number of secondary surgical procedures. With respect to the circumstances of off-site surgery, we preferred the most definitive form of surgical emergency treatment, *i.e.*, the creation of a stoma.

In three infants in our series, gastric perforation was observed. In these cases, we inserted a catheter into the perforation and created a temporary gastrostomy. After the removal of the gastrostomy in the two surviving infants, a spontaneous closure of the gastric stoma occurred, and no further interventions were required. In a critical appraisal of the literature, Leone and Krasna (2000) noted that gastric perforations are rare, predominantly occur in immature infants and are associated with other contributing factors. The mortality rates from the published series fell between one- and two-thirds of patients [13].

Some technical details should be noted. Surgery within a closed incubator, with light reflecting off of the surfaces and restricted access, should be reserved for simple procedures. In our series, we only worked in an open incubator to provide almost unlimited access to the infant. Vital factors for surgery include proper illumination by one, or preferably two, procedure lamps. Alternatively, portable fiberoptic heat lamps give very good lighting; however, they are uncomfortable. Loupe magnification and suture materials of 6 or 7 × 0 are appropriate for this very delicate type of surgery. For hemostasis, we used bipolar diathermia, which is safer than monopolar electrocautery.

5. Conclusion

In conclusion, OSS in a NICU can be performed with excellent results; transportation and unnecessary stress for the infant can be avoided. However, its routine use is limited as an interim proceeding to bridge period of time. In cases of very unstable and extremely immature infants with bowel perforation avoiding of transportation should be the preferable advance.

Conflicts of Interest

None.

References

[1] Meadow, W., Lee, G., Lin, K. and Lantos, J. (2004) Changes in Mortality for ELBWI in the 1990s. *Pediatrics*, **113**, 1223-1229. http://dx.doi.org/10.1542/peds.113.5.1223

[2] Currie, J.M. (2008) Stress and Pain Relief in the Care of the Surgical Neonate. *Seminars in Pediatric Surgery*, **17**, 285-289. http://dx.doi.org/10.1053/j.sempedsurg.2008.07.007

[3] Taylor, R.L., Grover, F.L., Harman, P.K., Escobedo, M.K., Ramamurthy, R.S. and Trinkle, J.K. (1986) Operative Closure of Patent Ducus Arteriosus in Premature Infant in the Neonatal Intensive Care Unit. *The American Journal of Surgery*, **152**, 704-708. http://dx.doi.org/10.1016/0002-9610(86)90453-8

[4] Hubbard, C., Rucker, R.W., Realyvasquez, F., Sperling, D.R., Hicks, D.A., Worcester, C.C., *et al.* (1986) Ligation of the Patent Ductus Arteriosus in Newborn Respiratory Failure. *Journal of Pediatric Surgery*, 3-5. http://dx.doi.org/10.1016/S0022-3468(86)80639-X

[5] Finer, N.N., Woo, B.C., Hayashi, A. and Hayes, B. (1993) Neonatal Surgery. Intensive Care Unit versus Operating Room. *Journal of Pediatric Surgery*, **28**, 645-649. http://dx.doi.org/10.1016/0022-3468(93)90021-C

[6] Gordon, P.V., Swanson, J.R., Attridge, J.T. and Clark, R. (2007) Emerging Trends in Acquired Neonatal Intestinal Disease: Is It Time to Abandon Bell's Criteria. *Journal of Perinatology*, **27**, 661-671. http://dx.doi.org/10.1038/sj.jp.7211782

[7] Gavilanes, A.W.D., Heinemann, E., Herpers, M.J. and Blanco, C.E. (1997) Use of Neonatal Intensive Care Unit as a Safe Place for Neonatal Surgery. *Archives of Disease in Childhood*, **76**, F51-F53. http://dx.doi.org/10.1136/fn.76.1.F51

[8] Henry, M.C.W. and Moss, R.L. (2008) Neonatal Necrotizing Enterocolitis. *Seminars in Pediatric Surgery*, **17**, 98-109. http://dx.doi.org/10.1053/j.sempedsurg.2008.02.005

[9] Gordon, P.V. and Attridge, J.T. (2009) Understanding Clinical Literature Relevant to Spontaneous Intestinal Perforations. *American Journal of Perinatology*, **26**, 309-316. http://dx.doi.org/10.1055/s-0028-1103514

[10] Rees, C.M., Pierro, A. and Eaton, S. (2007) Neurodevelopmental Outcomes of Neonates with Medically and Surgically Treated Necrotizing Enterocolitis. *Archives of Disease in Childhood. Fetal and Neonatal Edition*, **92**, F193-F198. http://dx.doi.org/10.1136/adc.2006.099929

[11] Fanning, N.F., Casey, W. and Corbally, M.T. (1998) *In-Situ* Emergency Paediatric Surgery in the Intensive Care Unit. *Pediatric Surgery International*, **13**, 587-589. http://dx.doi.org/10.1007/s003830050410

[12] Ein, S.H., Marshall, D.G. and Girvan, D. (1977) Peritoneal Drainage under Local Anesthesia for Perforations from Necrotizing Enterocolitis. *Journal of Pediatric Surgery*, **12**, 963-967. http://dx.doi.org/10.1016/0022-3468(77)90607-8

[13] Leone, R.J. and Krasna, I.H. (2000) "Spontaneous" Neonatal Gastric Perforation: Is It Really Spontaneous? *Journal of Pediatric Surgery*, **35**, 1066-1069. http://dx.doi.org/10.1053/jpsu.2000.7773

33

Pathophysiology of Hypertrophic Pyloric Stenosis Revisited: The Use of Isotonic Fluid for Preoperative Infusion Therapy Is Supported

Ralf-Bodo Troebs

Klinik für Kinderchirurgie, Marien Hospital Herne, Ruhr University of Bochum, Bochum, Germany
Email: ralf-bodo.troebs@web.de

Abstract

Background: The aim of this study was to elucidate the preoperative clinical and biochemical profile of infants with IHPS to optimize infusion therapy. Patients and Method: We retrospectively analyzed data from 56 infants who were operated for IHPS. Our study includes growth and laboratory data prior to the initiation of therapy. Results: Median duration of propulsive vomiting was 4 d; the median age was 37 d (18 - 108), and the median body weight was 3840 g (2760 - 5900). Metabolic alkalosis (MAlk) with a pH of 7.45 ± 0.06 and an st HCO_3^- of 28.7 ± 4.5 mmol/l was found. In a subgroup of the infants, negative base excess (BE) was observed. The sodium concentration was normal or reduced (mean/median of 137 mmol/l). There was a strong negative correlation between st HCO_3^- and K^+. The carbon dioxide partial pressure tended to increase (5.72 ± 0.84 kPa). Calculations of osmolality revealed a normal osmolarity. Hypoglycemia did not occur. The creatinine clearance according to the Schwartz formula remained at a normal level (85.3 ± 24.3 ml/min/1.73 m^2). Discussion: The presented case series is characterized by a short duration of preoperative vomiting. MAlk can be classified as a chloride deficiency syndrome. It is accompanied by normo- or hyponatremic dehydration with normal osmolality. Partial respiratory compensation occurred. A normal creatinine clearance indicated good glomerular renal function. Conclusion: The presented study supports the use of an isotonic infusion fluid with a low glucose concentration for preoperative infusion therapy.

Keywords

Infantile Pyloric Stenosis, Metabolic Alkalosis, Dehydration, Osmolality, Glucose, Lactate, Creatinine Clearance, Infusion Therapy

1. Introduction

Infantile hypertrophic pyloric stenosis (IHPS) is the most common abdominal surgical condition in infants. The prevalence in Germany is 2.29 per 1000 live births [1]. IHPS is characterized by hypertrophy of the pyloric muscle, which results in gastric outlet obstruction. The typical presentation involves progressive, projectile, and nonbilious vomiting immediately following feeding. Palpability of the pylorus ("olive") and ultrasound imaging confirm the diagnosis [2]. The homeostasis is mainly disrupted by dehydration, metabolic alkalosis (MAlk), and catabolism [3] [4].

The pathogenesis of the pylorus tumor remains enigmatic. There is good evidence that the inherited hyperacidity caused by an immature feedback mechanism in gastric production is the predominant factor [5]. However, whether the elevation of serum gastrin is a primary or secondary phenomenon remains unclear.

Our study was designed to elucidate the clinical and biochemical characteristics of IHPS patients who received an early diagnosis. The aim was to analyze the acid-base status and electrolyte levels together with the glucose, lactate, and renal parameters. In particular, this study was performed to determine the type of dehydration that accompanied IHPS. These data were provided to define the baseline for optimized preoperative fluid management [6].

2. Material and Methods

Records of 66 infants who underwent an extramucosal pyloromyotomy between 2007 and 2010 were identified. The inclusion criteria were a clinical presentation, conformation of IHPS by ultrasound (100% of cases), and surgical treatment for IHPS. Data from 10 infants with IHPS were excluded from further analysis (lack of acid-base analysis at admission [n = 8], hydrops fetalis, and history of previous operation).

Data from 56 infants (45 male, 11 female) met the criteria for further investigation. The gestational age (GA), birth weight, age at admission, body weight (BW), and length (BL) were extracted from the records. Any infant born before 37 weeks (wk) of gestation was defined as preterm. The gain of weight (GW) was estimated as the difference between the BW at admission and the birth weight. For biochemical investigations, we used the results of the routine laboratory assessment prior to the initiation of therapy. The biochemical spectrum included the hemoglobin concentration (Hb), hematocrit (Hct), acid-base status (pH, base excess [BE], partial pressure of carbon dioxide [pCO_2], and standard bicarbonate [HCO_3^-]), and ion concentrations (sodium [Na^+], potassium [K^+], calcium [Ca^{++}], and chloride [Cl^-]). In addition, data on the serum concentrations of glucose, lactate, creatinine, and urea were collected. For reference, we used the values from age matched-patients in our hospital in accordance with the literature [7]-[8]. The data are expressed in SI units.

Calculated parameters. The anion gap (AG) was defined as the difference between the anions and cations:

$$AG = \left(Na^+ + K^+\right) - \left(Cl^- + HCO_3^-\right) \quad [9].$$

The theoretical serum osmolality (OSM) was calculated according the equation OSMc = 2 Na^+ + glucose + urea [mmol/l] [7], and for a more detailed estimation, we used the following formula: OSMc = 1.86 ($Na^+ + K^+$) + 1.15 glucose + urea + 14 [mosm/kg] [10].

The creatinine clearance (C_{cr}) was estimated using the Schwartz formula [11]:

C_{cr} [ml/min/1.73m^2] = 0.45 × BL [cm]/creatinine [mg/dl] (creatinine [mg/dl] = μmol/l/88.4).

2.1. Limits

The presented study has some limits. It is based on a retrospective chart review and data analysis. Furthermore, some data were missing, and some terms (e.g., propulsive vomiting) were not precisely defined. Blood samples were tested. The laboratory results are based on the analysis of capillary blood (CB) in 4/5 of the infants and venous blood (VB) in 1/5. The gold standard for blood gas analysis is the use of arterial blood. However, CB samples are routinely used to estimate the acid-base balance and the levels of ions, glucose, and lactate with commercially available blood gas analyzers [12]. All analyzers underwent sequential calibrations and quality controls by the "Ring Trial". For the acid-base analysis (pCO_2, pH, and BE), evidence suggests a good correlation between arterial and capillary or venous samples. However, in arterialized CB or VB, the pH is lower by an average of 0.05, and the pCO_2 may be higher [7].

2.2. Statistics

Data are expressed as the arithmetic mean ± standard deviation (SD), the median value, and/or the minimum/maximum (noted in parentheses). A significant difference between the median and mean indicates a skewed distribution. For the statistical analysis, we used linear regression analysis and Pearson's correlation coefficient (**Table 4**). The significance level for the correlation coefficient was tested for (n-2) degrees of freedom.

3. Results

3.1. Biometrics (Table 1)

The male to female ratio was 4:1. The median BW was 3200 g (1990 - 4300), and we found a median gestational age of 38 weeks (33 - 41). Fourteen infants were preterm, with a GA between 33 and 36 wk. The median GW from birth to admission remained at 578 g (−160 - 2160). However, 19 infants had a GW less than 500 g (including 4 with BW below birth weight). The series included three sets of twins, and both partners were affected in one twin set. The median duration of propulsive vomiting was 4 days (1 - 28 d). At the time of the operation the median age was 37 d (18 - 108), and the median BW at admission was 3840 g (2760 - 5900). The median body length was 54 cm (49 - 61).

3.2. Biochemical Profile (Table 2 and Table 3)

Acid-base balance. As expected, the majority of the IHPS patients showed an elevated st HCO_3^- of 28.7 ± 4.5 mmol/l (27.9; 21 - 41), and the pH was 7.45 ± 0.06 (7.45; 7.32 - 7.65). In the majority of patients, MAlk was partially compensated by a pCO_2 increase to 5.72 ± 0.84 kPa (5.73; 3.27 - 8.36). Hypercapnia with $pCO_2 > 6.5$ kPa occurred in 6 infants. The BE was >3 mmol/l in 58% of the patients. A negative BE was found in a subgroup of 5 infants (*i.e.*, BE values of −0.1, −0.2, −1, −4, −4 mmol/l). These patients were characterized by the following median parameters: st HCO_3^- of 22.9 mmol/l, pCO_2 of 5.0 kPa, pH of 7.36, anion gap of 16.3 mmol/l, and lactate level of 3.4 mmol/l.

Hemoglobin and hematocrit. The Hb and Hct values were 13.1 ± 2.4 (12.8; 9.1 - 17.8) and 37.9 ± 6.52 mmol/dl (36.5; 27 - 54.7), respectively.

Electrolytes. The range of the blood cations was mainly within normal limits: the Na^+ concentration was 137 ± 2.49 mmol/l (137; 130 - 144). Six infants had a slightly reduced Na^+ concentration: <135 mmol/l. The infants presented with a K^+ concentration of 4.7 ± 0.83 mmol/l (4.8; 3.1 - 7.2); 19 infants had $K^+ > 5$ mmol/l, but no infants had levels below 3 mmol/l. Ca was estimated as the total Ca of 2.8 ± 0.68 mmol/l (2.7; 2.4 - 5.2) and the Ca^{++} of 1.29 ± 0.14 mmol/l (1.34; 0.87 - 1.42).

The Cl^- level was estimated in 22 infants with a value of 98 ± 7.56 mmol/l (101; 83 - 108). From the difference between the cations and anions, we derived a mean AG of 13.1 ± 3.5 mmol/l (12.8; 5.8 - 19.9). In 6 infants, the AG was below 12 mosm/l, and in 2 infants, it was above 17 mosm/l.

Glucose and lactate levels, and creatinine clearance. The glucose level was 5.11 ± 0.62 mmol/l (5.05; 4 - 6.72). We found a serum lactate of 2.0 ± 0.95 mmol/l (1.8; 0.8 - 9.8). Seven infants had an elevated serum lactate of >2.5 mmol/l. The creatinine remained at 0.32 ± 0.08 mg/dl (0.30; 0.17 - 0.52), and the C_{cr} calculated from the Schwartz formula was 85.3 ± 24.3 ml/min/1.73m^2 (85.2; 54 - 161.5).

Table 1. Biometric data.

Parameter	Median	Min-Max	Mean	SD
Birth weight [g]	3200	1990 - 4300	3253	547
Gestat. age [weeks]	38	33 - 41	38	2.5
Duration of vomiting [days]	4	1 - 28	6	19
Weight gain since birth	578	(−260 - 2160)	767	438
Age at OP [days]	37	18 - 108	39	20.2
Body weight at OP [g]	3840	2760 - 5900	3992	757
Body length [cm]	54	49 - 61	55	3.27

Table 2. Acid-base status, ion concentrations, anion gap, and osmolarity.

Parameter	N	Med	Min-Max	Mean	SD	Reference Values (RV)
pH	55	7.45	7.32 - 7.65	7.45	0.06	7.33 - 7.45
BE [mmol/l]	55	3.8	−4.0 - 17.9	5.2	4.98	−3 to +3
St HCO_3^- [mmol/l]	51	27.9	21.0 - 41.0	28.7	4.48	18.2 - 25
pCO_2 [kPa]	53	5.73	3.72 - 8.36	5.72	0.84	4.5 - 6.5
Hb [mmol/l]	53	7.95	5.65 - 11.05	8.14	1.27	Age dependent
Hct [%]	53	36.5	27.0 - 54.7	37.9	6.52	31 - 59
Na^+ [mmol/l]	53	137	130 - 144	137	2.49	135 - 145
K^+ [mmol/l]	53	4.8	3.1 - 7.2	4.7	0.83	3.5 - 5.0
Ca^{++} [mmol/l]	24	1.34	0.87 - 1.42	1.29	0.14	1.1 - 1.3
Ca total [mmol/l]	27	2.7	2.4 - 5.2	2.8	0.68	2.2 - 2.7
Cl^- [mmol/l]	22	101	83 - 108	98	7.56	95 to 108
Anion gap [mmol/l]	21	12.8	5.8 - 19.9	13.1	3.5	<12 - 17
Osmol* [mosm/l]	14	280	269 - 290	280	9.2	270 - 295
Osmol** [mosm/kg]	14	285	274 - 295	283	10.4	282 - 302

*according to [7]; **according to [10].

Table 3. Serum concentrations of metabolites and renal parameters.

Parameter	N	Median	Min-Max	Mean	SD	Reference Values
Glucose [mmol/l]	50	5.05	4.00 - 6.72	5.11	0.62	2.6 - 6.60
Lactate [mmol/l]	27	1.8	0.8 - 3.9	2.0	0.95	<2.5
Creatinine [µmol/l]	27	26.52	15.03 - 45.97	28.29	7.07	<44.2
Crea-Clearance [ml/min/1.73 m^2]	22	85.2	54 - 161.5	85.3	24.3	41 - 91*
Urea [mmol/l]	16	2.91	0.83 - 4.80	2.86	1.01	1.35 - 2.33

*according to [13].

Osmolality (*OSM*). We found normal or slightly elevated levels of urea: (n = 16) 2.86 ± 1.01 mmol/l (2.91; 0.83 - 4.80). The OSM calculated using the standard formula was 280 ± 9.19 mmol/l (280; 269 - 290). Using the improved formula, which is described elsewhere [15], we found 283 ± 10.4 mosm/kg.

3.3. Ethics

The Research Ethics Board of the Ruhr-University of Bochum (4271-12) approved the study.

4. Discussion

The pathogenesis of IHPS is multifactorial and includes hypergastrinemia, abnormal pyloric innervation, genetic mutations, and environmental influences [5] [14]. This study was performed in Nordrhein-Westfalen (NRW). In this area, the prevalence of IHPS declined from 3.88 to 2.30 per 1000 live births from 2000 to 2008 [1]. We found a predominance of males with a 4:1 ratio, which was consistent with the literature [2] [13] [15] [16]. Most of the IHPS infants were mature with a normal gestation and age-appropriate birth weight [10] [17] [18]. However, up to 1/4 of the patients were premature [9] [13] [14] [16]. The median duration of propulsive vomiting was 4 d, which was shorter than that in previous clinical series [2] [14]-[16]. In concordance with the literature, the vast majority of infants presented to the hospital at the age of 5 to 6 wk. Due to a lack of data on the body weight before the initiation of propulsive vomiting, we were not able to estimate the weight loss for the period prior to admission. In our cohort, the median GW since birth was 585 g, with significant variability. As a rule, the BW in healthy infants increases 200 g per week in the first trimester [19], *i.e.*, 1000 g in the first 5 wk. Thus, the majority of our patients showed a marked weight deficiency.

Preoperative replacement of water and electrolytes is the main step in the preoperative therapy for IHPS. Under the condition of perioperative stress, non-osmotic stimulation with antidiuretic hormone (ADH) may result in water intoxication and hyponatremia. Thus, it has been shown that the use of hypotonic fluids is associated with an elevated risk of hyponatremia. To prevent this rare but serious complication, the use of isotonic solutions has been recommended for perioperative fluid substitution in surgically ill infants [12] [20].

According to the Henderson-Hasselbalch equation, the blood pH is determined by the ratio between HCO_3^- and pCO_2. An elevation of HCO_3^-, and therefore alkalemia, are the hallmarks of MAlk. We found a strong positive correlation between st HCO_3^- and pH (**Table 4**).The present study confirms the decreased Cl^- levels that result from vomiting. Our results are consistent with previous investigations reporting 10 to 49% of infants with Cl^- concentrations of <90 to 98 mmol/l [2]. The chloride concentration correlated negatively with st HCO_3^- (p = 0.001, **Table 4**), indicating increasing alkalosis with the progressive loss of Cl^-. The alkalosis associated with IHPS can be classified as the type that accompanies Cl^- deficiency syndrome, [7] *i.e.*, Cl^- is lost from the transcellular compartment with an accompanying loss of H^+ and K^+, and to a lesser extent, Na^+.

In our series, the infants presented with st HCO_3^- > 25 mmol/l, and 46% of the infants showed enhanced alkalemia: >28 mmol/l. Thus, our rate seems to be higher than that in a recent meta-analysis in which an initial severe alkalosis with HCO_3^- > 28 to 30 mmol/l was reported in 9% to 37% of infants [2]. Hypovolemia and hypochloremia are two additional factors leading to increased HCO_3^- levels via renal mechanisms.

IHPS typically presents with a positive BE. Surprisingly, we found a subgroup of 5 infants with a negative BE, indicating a lack of buffer bases. This subgroup showed compensated pH and HCO_3^- at the low end of the normal range, low Hb, and elevated lactate levels. The Hb-OxyHb system is one of the most powerful buffer systems; thus, the negative BE may be enhanced by anemia.

In this investigation, we used the *in vitro* generated "artificial" parameters for st HCO_3^- and BE. Both are often used in clinical practice. However, BE may be misleading in some instances. For atypical ABA results, a differential diagnosis must account for gastroesophageal reflux (GER), and in rare cases, for an inborn error of metabolism and salt loss from adrenogenital syndrome [21] [22].

All infants with IHPS lose potassium due to vomiting and enhanced renal excretion [23]. Compared with blood, gastric juice contains lower amounts of Na^+ (51 mmol/l) and higher amounts of K^+ (11.7 to 25 mmol/l). Thus, vomiting mainly results in the loss of fluid that is rich in both K^+ and Cl^-. The compensatory shift of

Table 4. Regression (y = Ax + B) and correlation analysis of biochemical parameters.

Correlation	N	A	r	p
Hb - age	50	−0.06	−0.53	0.001
Hct - st bicarb	47	0.452	0.32	0.05
pCO_2 - st bicarb	47	0.616	0.42	0.01
Na - Cl	22	#	0.31	n.s.
Na - st bicarb	47	#	−0.20	n.s.
K - st bicarb	47	−0.108	−0.59	0.001
Ca^{++} - pH	24	−0.862	−0.42	0.05
Cl - st bicarb	21	−1.259	−0.88	0.001
pH - st bicarb	47	0.009	0.71	0.001
Lact - st bicarb	27	−0.084	−0.39	0.05
Lact - pH	27	#	−0.19	n.s.
AG - pH	21	−25.04	−0.457	0.05
AG - BE	21	#	0.076	n.s.
Urea - st bicarb	15	#	−0.02	n.s.
Urea - pH	16	#	0.27	n.s.

n.s.—no significance; #—useless.

intracellular H^+ into the extracellular space and the reverse shift of K^+ favors the hypokalemia that is characteristic of MAlk. In addition, the reduced circulation volume may activate the renin-angiotensin-aldosterone system, resulting in Na^+ reabsorption and renal K^+ loss. However, these mechanisms appear to be less important in infants [24]. In concordance with the results of a previous study [15], a correlation analysis confirmed a strong negative correlation between st HCO_3^- and K^+ ($p = 0.001$, **Table 4**). In our cohort, we predominantly found a highly normal serum K^+ concentration, and less than 10% of the infants had values below 3.5 mmol/l. To explain our results, the bias when using capillary blood to estimate K^+ must be taken into account. Compared with VB, CB tends to have a higher K^+ concentration. This difference is caused by the difficulty in collecting blood from dehydrated infants, the influence of the K^+-rich cytosol of hemolytic red cells, and the addition of interstitial fluid, which contains 7% - 8% more K^+ as a result of the Gibbs-Donnan equilibrium [19]. In previous investigations, a low K^+ concentration was associated with a high HCO_3^- concentration [16], and a highly significant trend of reduced K^+ was observed as the duration of the symptoms and the dehydration increased [13].

Calcium is another important cation. In the case of MAlk, a shift from Ca^{++} to the protein-bound form is expected. Accordingly, we found a weak negative influence of pH on the plasma Ca^{++} ($p = 0.05$) [7].

Water and electrolyte disturbances result from the loss of fluid and electrolytes and from the movement of water and electrolytes between body compartments. The weak correlation between Hct and st HCO_3^- ($p = 0.05$) indicated increased Hct with an elevation of HCO_3^- due to water loss (**Table 4**). In our patients, Hct was not helpful for determining the degree of dehydration.

Sodium plays a key role in extracellular fluid (ECF) volume regulation. An increased sodium concentration indicates that the ECF is becoming concentrated. In our cohort, we found a normally distributed Na^+ concentration around the mean/median of 137 mmol/l with a trend toward hyponatremia. The sodium concentration did not correlate with the Cl^- concentration. The Na^+ and st HCO_3^- concentrations were inversely related (n.s.; **Table 4**). These results correspond to those of a previous study [16]. Others described a slow decline in Na^+ concentration as the symptoms persisted [13] and a negative correlation between the Na^+ and HCO_3^- levels [15]. In a recent Chinese study, hyponatremia was found in 54% of infants with IHPS [8]. In rare instances, IHPS can be associated with dehydration and severe hyponatremia due to pseudo Bartter's syndrome [7].

Osmolality is defined as the molar concentration of all of the solutes in a given weight of water. The most important solute for the OSM is sodium salts, whereas other ions, glucose, and urea contribute to a lesser extent. In clinical practice, OSM is measured per liter of solution (molar) rather than per kg of solvent (molal). In our investigation, we used two different formulas to calculate the OSM. In infants with IHPS, we found a theoretical OSM of 280 ± 92 mmol/l or 283 ± 10.4 mosm/kg (iso-osmolar). Thus, these results indicate the presence of normotonic-normonatremic/hyponatremic dehydration in IHPS.

The anion gap provides important information for further differentiation of the underlying acid-base disturbance [7]. AG reflects the unmeasured anions and cations. Correlation analysis revealed a negative correlation between pH and AG ($p = 0.05$; **Table 4**). It can be assumed that the AG in IHPS is mainly influenced by the increase in HCO_3^-, the loss of Cl^-, and the production of organic acids (lactate, acetoacetate, and β-hydroxybutyrate). Ketonuria in IHPS has been reported previously [16].

In some patients, lactate was present in elevated amounts. This finding might result from tissue hypoperfusion and anaerobic metabolism. Lactate may serve as a fuel for gluconeogenesis in the liver and kidney and thus stabilize glucose levels. In our study, the correlation between lactate and either HCO_3^- or pH was weak or non-existent (**Table 4**). Whether the combination of stress, low Hb, and the left shift of the oxygen-hemoglobin dissociation curve caused by alkalosis contributed to the elevated lactate levels remains unknown. As expected, we found low Hb concentrations and a negative correlation between age and Hb.

The physiological respiratory compensatory mechanism for MAlk is clinically important. The decreased H^+ results in a decrease in ventilation and hypercapnia. This effect is most often neutralized by the physiological stimulation of chemoreceptors in response to the increased pCO_2 and decreased pO_2; this stimulation restores the ventilatory drive. However, clinical reports have described life-threatening respiratory depression in IHPS, with symptoms including apnea, desaturation, and bradycardia [25] [26]. The majority of our patients presented with pCO_2 values that were elevated to the high end of the normal range. We found a good positive correlation between st HCO_3^- and pCO_2 ($p = 0.01$; **Table 4**). Feng *et al.* reported elevated HCO_3^- and pCO_2 in a late-onset group (2014). However, serious respiratory problems in IHPS are rare. Nonetheless, pulse oximetry is advised for IHPS patients.

The kidney is extraordinarily important for regulating the ECF volume and acid-base balance. For clinical purposes, the glomerular filtration rate (GFR) can be quantified by estimating the creatinine clearance. Physiological maturation of the kidney is accompanied by a threefold increase in GFR during the first trimester. The Schwartz formula value of C_{cr} provides good information on glomerular function in children [11]. We only found normal C_{cr} values, which indicated a normal, age-appropriate GFR.

Urea is a product of protein catabolism. Ammonia is incorporated into urea, and it is excreted by the kidney. Theoretically, the increased blood pH in alkalosis increases urea synthesis within the liver and leads to increased filtration of HCO_3^- [18]. In a previous study, the urea level was elevated in the IHPS group but not in the GER group [27]. In our small series, a regression analysis did not reveal any correlation between urea and either pH or HCO_3^- (**Table 4**). In a previous investigation, neither the creatinine nor the urea concentration reflected the degree of dehydration in IHPS [4].

Hypoglycemia as a result of hepatic glucose depletion has been described postoperatively in IHPS [22] [28]. However, none of our patients presented with a blood glucose level below 4.0 mmol/l. The glycogen stores of a fasting neonate will be exhausted within 12 to 24 hours. In infants, energy is mainly stored as fat, and the fat reserves of a term infant may be sufficient for a 21-day fast [29]. Thus, fatty acid oxidation is the most important provider of energy to support gluconeogenesis and stabilize blood glucose levels in fasting infants [18]. In exceptional cases, severe hypoglycemia as a result of neonatal hyperinsulinism in association with IHPS has been reported [30]. Early postoperative feeding with continuous intravenous electrolyte and glucose supplementation is effective at preventing hypoglycemia and the subsequent adverse neurodevelopment [9].

5. Conclusion

In conclusion, we presented a series of IHPS patients with a short duration of vomiting. MAlk, hypochloremia, increased pCO_2 iso- or mild hypotonic dehydration, and normoglycemia were the most important findings at admission. These data support the use of an isotonic solution with a low glucose concentration for preoperative fluid substitution in infants with IHPS.

References

[1] Laffolie, J., Turial, S., Heckmann, M., *et al.* (2012) Decline in Infantile Hypertrophic Pyloric Stenosis in Germany in 2000-2008. *Pediatrics*, **129**, e901-e906. http://dx.doi.org/10.1542/peds.2011-2845

[2] Glatstein, M., Carbell, G., Boddu, S.K., *et al.* (2011) The Changing Clinical Presentation of Hypertrophic Pyloric Stenosis: The Experience of a Large, Tertiary Care Pediatric Hospital. *Clinical Pediatrics*, **50**, 192-195. http://dx.doi.org/10.1177/0009922810384846

[3] Clark, R.G. and Norman, J.N. (1964) Metabolic Alkalosis in Pyloric Stenosis. *Lancet*, **1**, 1244-1245. http://dx.doi.org/10.1016/S0140-6736(64)91869-0

[4] Dawson, K.P. and Graham, D. (1991) The Assessment of Dehydratation in Congenital Pyloric Stenosis. *The New Zealand Medical Journal*, **104**, 162-163.

[5] Rogers, I.M. (2006) The True Cause of Pyloric Stenosis Is Hyperacidity. *Acta Paediatrica*, **95**, 132-136. http://dx.doi.org/10.1111/j.1651-2227.2006.tb02197.x

[6] Foster, B.A., Tom, D. and Hill, V. (2014) Hypotonic versus Isotonic Fluids in Hospitalized Children: A Systematic Review and Meta-Analysis. *The Journal of Pediatrics*, **165**, 163-169. http://dx.doi.org/10.1016/j.jpeds.2014.01.040

[7] Bianchetti, M.G. and Bettinelli, A. (2008) Differential Diagnosis and Management of Fluid, Electrolyte, and Acid-Base Disorders. In: Geary, D.F. and Schaefer, F., Eds., *Comprehensive Pediatric Nephrology*. Mosby/Elsevier, Philadelphia. http://dx.doi.org/10.1016/B978-0-323-04883-5.50033-7

[8] Fox, G., Hoque, N. and Watts, T. (2010) Oxford Handbook of Neonatology. Oxford University Press, Oxford, New York.

[9] Graham, D.A., Mogride, N., Abbott, G.D., *et al.* (1993) Pyloric Stenosis: The Christchurch Experience. *The New Zealand Medical Journal*, **106**, 57-59.

[10] Khajuria, A. and Krahn, J. (2005) Osmolality Revisited—Deriving and Validating the Best Formula for Calculated Osmolality. *Clinical Biochemistry*, **38**, 514-519. http://dx.doi.org/10.1016/j.clinbiochem.2005.03.001

[11] Hogg, R.J., Furth, S., Lemley, K.V., *et al.* (2003) National Kidney Foundation's Disease Outcomes Quality Initiative Clinical Practice Guidelines for Chronic Kidney Disease in Children and Adolescents: Evaluation, Classification and Stratification. *Pediatrics*, **111**, 1416-1421. http://dx.doi.org/10.1542/peds.111.6.1416

[12] Tan, S. and Campbell, M. (2008) Acid-Base Physiology and Blood Gas Interpretation in the Neonate. *Paediatrics and*

Child Health, **18**, 172-177. http://dx.doi.org/10.1016/j.paed.2007.12.013

[13] Beasley, S.W., Hudson, I., Hok Pan, Y., *et al.* (1986) Influence of Age, Sex, Duration of Symptoms and Dehydration of Serum Electrolytes in Hypertrophic Pyloric Stenosis. *Australian Paediatric Journal*, **22**, 193-197.

[14] Feng, Z., Nie, Y., Zhang, Y., *et al.* (2010) The Clinical Features of Infantile Hypertrophic Pyloric Stenosis in Chinese Han Population: Analysis from 1998 to 2010. *PloS ONE*, **9**, e88925. http://dx.doi.org/10.1371/journal.pone.0088925

[15] Shanbhogue, L.K.R., Sikdar, T., Jackson, M., *et al.* (1992) Serum Electrolytes and Capillary Blood Gases in the Management of Hypertrophic Pyloric Stenosis. *British Journal of Surgery*, **79**, 251-253. http://dx.doi.org/10.1002/bjs.1800790322

[16] Touloukian, R.J. and Higgins, E. (1983) The Spectrum of Serum Electrolytes in Hypertrophic Pyloric Stenosis. *Journal of Pediatric Surgery*, **18**, 394-397. http://dx.doi.org/10.1016/S0022-3468(83)80188-2

[17] Czeizel, A. (1972) Birthweight Distribution in Congenital Pyloric Stenosis. *Archives of Disease in Childhood*, **47**, 978-980. http://dx.doi.org/10.1136/adc.47.256.978

[18] Doenecke, D., Koolman, J., Fuchs, G., *et al.* (2005) Karlsons Biochemie und Pathobiochemie. Georg Thieme Verlag, Stuttgart, New York.

[19] Muntau, A.C. (2007) Intensivkurs Pädiatrie. Urban & Fischer, München.

[20] Saba, T.G., Fairbairn, J., Houghton, F., *et al.* (2011) A Randomized Controlled Trial of Isotonic versus Hypotonic Maintenance Intravenous Fluids in Hospitalized Children. *BMC Pediatrics*, **11**, 82. http://dx.doi.org/10.1186/1471-2431-11-82

[21] Lehnert, W., Schenck, W. and Niederhoff, H. (1979) Isovaleric Acidemia Combined with Hypertrophic Pyloric Stenosis. *Klinische Pädiatrie*, **191**, 477-482.

[22] Shumake, L.B. (1975) Postoperative Hypoglycemia in Congenital Hypertrophic Pyloric Stenosis. *Southern Medical Journal*, **68**, 223-224. http://dx.doi.org/10.1097/00007611-197502000-00024

[23] Roman, A. and Burmeister, W. (1978) Hypokalemia in Infants Due to Disturbed Salt, Water and Acid-Base Balance. *Klinische Pädiatrie*, **190**, 108-117.

[24] Lorenz, J.M. (2008) Potassium Metabolism. In: Oh, W., Guignard, J.P. and Baumgart, S., Eds., *Nephrology and Fluid/Electrolyte Physiology: Neonatal Questions and Controversies*, 2nd Edition, Saunders/Elsevier, Philadelphia, 54-65. http://dx.doi.org/10.1016/B978-1-4160-3163-5.50009-9

[25] Pappano, D. (2011) Alkalosis-Induced Respiratory Depression from Infantile Hypertrophic Pyloric Stenosis. *Pediatric Emergency Care*, **27**, 124. http://dx.doi.org/10.1097/PEC.0b013e318209af50

[26] Tigges, C.R. and Bigham, M.T. (2012) Hypertrophic Pyloric Stenosis: It Can Take Your Breath Away. *Air Medical Journal*, **1**, 45-48. http://dx.doi.org/10.1016/j.amj.2011.06.009

[27] Smith, G.A., Mihalov, L. and Shields, B.J. (1999) Diagnostic Aids in the Differentiation of Pyloric Stenosis from Severe Gastroesophageal Reflux during Early Infancy: The Utility of Serum Bicarbonate and Serum Chloride. *The American Journal of Emergency Medicine*, **17**, 28-31. http://dx.doi.org/10.1016/S0735-6757(99)90009-8

[28] Henderson, B.M., Schubert, W.K., Hug, G., *et al.* (1968) Hypoglycemia with Hepatic Glycogen Depletion: A Post-operative Complication of Pyloric Stenosis. *Journal of Pediatric Surgery*, **3**, 309-316. http://dx.doi.org/10.1016/0022-3468(68)90016-X

[29] Pierro, A., De Coppi, P. and Eaton, S. (2012) Neonatal Physiology and Metabolic Considerations. In: Coran, A.G., Adzik, N.S., Krummel, T.M., *et al.*, Eds., *Pediatric Surgery*, 7th Edition, Elsevier/Saunders, Philadelphia, 89-107. http://dx.doi.org/10.1016/B978-0-323-07255-7.00006-4

[30] Dutta, S., Lodha, R., Kabra, M., *et al.* (2000) Persistent Hypoglycemia with Pyloric Stenosis. *Indian Pediatrics*, **37**, 890-893.

Permissions

All chapters in this book were first published in OJPED, by Scientific Research Publishing; hereby published with permission under the Creative Commons Attribution License or equivalent. Every chapter published in this book has been scrutinized by our experts. Their significance has been extensively debated. The topics covered herein carry significant findings which will fuel the growth of the discipline. They may even be implemented as practical applications or may be referred to as a beginning point for another development.

The contributors of this book come from diverse backgrounds, making this book a truly international effort. This book will bring forth new frontiers with its revolutionizing research information and detailed analysis of the nascent developments around the world.

We would like to thank all the contributing authors for lending their expertise to make the book truly unique. They have played a crucial role in the development of this book. Without their invaluable contributions this book wouldn't have been possible. They have made vital efforts to compile up to date information on the varied aspects of this subject to make this book a valuable addition to the collection of many professionals and students.

This book was conceptualized with the vision of imparting up-to-date information and advanced data in this field. To ensure the same, a matchless editorial board was set up. Every individual on the board went through rigorous rounds of assessment to prove their worth. After which they invested a large part of their time researching and compiling the most relevant data for our readers.

The editorial board has been involved in producing this book since its inception. They have spent rigorous hours researching and exploring the diverse topics which have resulted in the successful publishing of this book. They have passed on their knowledge of decades through this book. To expedite this challenging task, the publisher supported the team at every step. A small team of assistant editors was also appointed to further simplify the editing procedure and attain best results for the readers.

Apart from the editorial board, the designing team has also invested a significant amount of their time in understanding the subject and creating the most relevant covers. They scrutinized every image to scout for the most suitable representation of the subject and create an appropriate cover for the book.

The publishing team has been an ardent support to the editorial, designing and production team. Their endless efforts to recruit the best for this project, has resulted in the accomplishment of this book. They are a veteran in the field of academics and their pool of knowledge is as vast as their experience in printing. Their expertise and guidance has proved useful at every step. Their uncompromising quality standards have made this book an exceptional effort. Their encouragement from time to time has been an inspiration for everyone.

The publisher and the editorial board hope that this book will prove to be a valuable piece of knowledge for researchers, students, practitioners and scholars across the globe.

List of Contributors

C. M. Essomo Megnier-Mbo
Service de Réanimation Néonatale et Néonatologie HIAOBO, Libreville, Gabon

C. M. Essomo Megnier-Mbo and S. Mayi
Departement Mère Enfant HIAOBO, Libreville, Gabon

Y. Vierin, J. Koko, A. Moussavou and C. M. Essomo Megnier-Mbo
Département de Pédiatrie, Faculté de Médecine, Libreville, Gabon

A. Ndjoyi Biguino
Laboratoire de Microbiologie, Faculté de Médecine, Libreville, Gabon

Wubishet Lakew
Department of Pediatrics and Child Health, University of Gondar, Gondar, Ethiopia

Bogale Worku
Department of Pediatrics and Child Health, Addis Ababa University Medical Faculty, Addis Ababa, Ethiopia

Konstantinos Tsoumakas, Marsela Tanaka, Konstantinos Petsios, Georgios Fildisis and Ioanna Pavlopoulou
Faculty of Nursing, National and Kapodistrian University of Athens, Athens, Greece

Athanasios Gkoutzivelakis
University General Hospital of Alexandroupoli, Alexandroupoli, Greece

Ellen van der Gaag and Miriam Münow
Department of Pediatrics, Hospital Group Twente, Hengelo, The Netherlands

Wendy C. W. Wang, Loana Tovar Suinaga, Klenise S. Paranhos and Sang-Choon Cho
Ashman Department of Periodontology and Implant Dentistry, New York University College of Dentistry, New York, USA
Shibata RVGE Study Group

Tomohiro Oishi
Department of Pediatrics, Niigata University Medical and Dental Hospital, Niigata City, Niigata, Japan

Shinya Tsukano
Pediatric Department, Niigata Prefectural Shibata Hospital, Shibata City, Niigata, Japan

Tokushi Nakano
Nakano Children's Clinic, Shibata City, Niigata, Japan

Shoji Sudo
Sudo Pediatric Clinic, Shibata City, Niigata, Japan

Hiroaki Kuwajima
Pediatric Department, Kuwajima Clinic, Shibata City, Niigata, Japan

Clare Skerritt, Saira Haque and Erica Makin
Department of Pediatric Surgery, The Royal London Hospital, London, UK

Manoj Gupta and Christopher S. Snyder
Division of Pediatric Cardiology, Department of Pediatrics, Rainbow Babies and Children's Hospital, Cleveland, OH, USA
School of Medicine, Case Western Reserve University, Cleveland, OH, USA

Walter Hoyt
Division of Pediatric Cardiology, Department of Pediatrics, School of Medicine, University of Virginia, Charlottesville, VA, USA

Carmen Madrigal Díez
Primary Paediatric Health Care, Centro de Salud Bezana, Servicio Cántabro de Salud, Spain

Sara Rodríguez Prado
Department of Opthalmology, Hospital de Sierrallana, Torrelavega, Cantabria, Spain

José Héctor Fernández Llaca
Department of Dermatology, Hospital Universitario Marqués de Valdecilla, Santander, Cantabria, Spain

Caroline Yonaba, Angel Kalmogho and Ludovic Kam
Department of Pediatric, Yalgado Ouedraogo University Teaching Hospital, Ouagadougou, Burkina Faso

Fla Koueta, Diarra Yé, Aïssata Ouedraogo, Sylvie Armelle Pingwende Ouédraogo and Bourama Ouattara
Department of Pediatric, Charles de Gaulle Pediatric University Teaching Hospital, Ouagadougou, Burkina Faso

Wietse P. Zuidema and Jan W. A. Oosterhuis
Department of Surgery, VU University Medical Center, Amsterdam, The Netherlands

Alida F. W. van der Steeg, Wietse P. Zuidema, Christien Sleeboom and Hugo A. Heij
Pediatric Surgical Center of Amsterdam, Emma Children's Hospital AMC and VU University Medical Center, Amsterdam, The Netherlands

Alida F. W. van der Steeg
Center of Research on Psychology in Somatic Diseases (CoRPS), Tilburg University, Tilburg, The Netherlands

Stefan M. van der Heide
Department of Cardio-Thoracic Surgery, Radboud University Medical Center, Nijmegen, The Netherlands

Elly S. M. de Lange-de Klerk
Department of Epidemiology and Biostatistics, VU University Medical Center, Amsterdam, The Netherlands

Ayelet Rimon, Amit Hess, Oren Tavor and Miguel Glatstein
Pediatric Emergency Medicine, Dana-Dwek Children's Hospital, Tel-Aviv, Israel

Ayelet Rimon, Amit Hess, Oren Tavor, Miguel Glatstein and Shirley Friedman
Sackler School of Medicine, Tel Aviv University, Tel-Aviv, Israel

Dennis Scolnik
Divisions of Pediatric Emergency Medicine and Clinical Pharmacology and Toxicology, Department of Pediatrics, The Hospital for Sick Children, University of Toronto, Toronto, Canada

Shirley Friedman
Pediatric Intensive Care, Dana-Dwek Children's Hospital, Tel-Aviv, Israel

Maryam Saboute, Mandana Kashaki and Arash Bordbar
Department of Pediatrics, Akbarabadi Hospital, Iran University of Medical Sciences, Tehran, Iran

Nasrin Khalessi
Department of Pediatrics, Ali Asghar Hospital, Iran University of Medical Sciences, Tehran, Iran

Zahra Farahani
Maternal Fetal and Neonatal Research Center, Tehran University of Medical Sciences, Tehran, Iran

Shristi Shakya and Zhongyue Li
Department of Gastroenterology, Children's Hospital of Chongqing Medical University, Chongqing, China

Sumisti Shakya
Department of Obstetrics and Gynaecology, The Second Affiliated Hospital of Chongqing Medical University, Chongqing, China

Caroline Yonaba, Aichatou Djibo, Chantal Zoungrana, Angèle Kalmogho, Ousseine Diallo
Patrice Tapsoba, Noufounikoun Méda and Ludovic Kam
Centre Hospitalier Universitaire Yalgado Ouedraogo, Ouagadougou, Burkina Faso

David Green
School of Medicine, University of Mississippi Medical Center, Jackson, USA

Nina Dave
Division of Pediatric Allergy-Immunology, University of Mississippi Medical Center, Jackson, USA

Hua Liu and Michael J. Nowicki
Division of Pediatric Gastroenterology, University of Mississippi Medical Center, Jackson, USA

Charu Subramony
Department of Pathology, University of Mississippi Medical Center, Jackson, USA

Norman E. Buroker
Department of Pediatrics, University of Washington, Seattle, USA

Merav Goldblatt, Rivka Yahav and Tsameret Ricon
Faculty of Social Welfare & Health Sciences, University of Haifa, Haifa, Israel

Ahmed Ezzat Rozeik
Pediatric Surgery Unit, Zagazig University, Al Sharqia Governorate, Egypt

Radi Elsherbini
Pediatric Surgery Unit, Mansoura University, Mansoura, Egypt

Hamdi Almaramhy
Faculty of Medicine, Taibah University, Medina, KSA

Muhammad Rehan Khan, Shakeel Ahmed, Syed Rehan Ali, Prem Kumar Maheshwari and Muhammad Saad Jamal
Department of Pediatrics and Child Health, The Aga Khan University Hospital, Karachi, Pakistan

Shakeel Ahmed
Department of Paediatrics, Medical & Dental College, Bahria University, Islamabad, Pakistan

Fla Kouéta, Sonia Kaboret, Aïssata Kaboré, Lassina Dao, Diarra Yé, Caroline Yonaba and Emile Bandré
Training and Research Unit of Health Sciences, University of Ouagadougou, Ouagadougou, Burkina Faso

Sak-Wend-Tongo Daïla, Hamidou Savadogo, Fla Kouéta, Sonia Kaboret, Aïssata Kaboré, Lassina Dao and Diarra Yé
Service of Medical Pediatrics, Charles de Gaulle Pediatric University Teaching Hospital, Ouagadougou, Burkina Faso

Caroline Yonaba
Department of Pediatrics, Yalgado University Teaching Hospital, Ouagadougou, Burkina Faso

Emile Bandré
Pediatric Surgery Service, Charles de Gaulle Pediatric University Teaching Hospital, Ouagadougou, Burkina Faso

Yoshihiko Sakurai
Department of Pediatrics, Matsubara Tokushukai Hospital, Matsubara, Japan

Séraphin Nguefack, Andréas Chiabi, Jacob Enoh, Evelyn Mah, Karen Kengne Kamga and Elie Mbonda
Departement of Pediatric Neurology, Yaounde Gynaeco-Obstetric and Pediatric Hospital, Yaounde, Cameroon

Sandra Tatah, El Hadji Djouberou, Elie Mbonda, Evelyn Mah, Séraphin Nguefack and Andréas Chiabi
Faculty of Medicine and Biomedical Sciences, University of Yaounde I, Yaounde, Cameroon

Jacob Enoh
Departement of Pediatric, University of Cocody-Abidjan, Abidjan, Côte d'Ivoire

Jean Koko, Daniel Gahouma and Armelle Pambou
General Pediatrics Service, Owendo Peditric Hospital (OPH), Libreville, Gabon

Cathérine Seilhan
Laboratory of Medical Biology, Owendo Pediatric Hospital (OPH), Libreville, Gabon

André Moussavou, Simon Ategbo, Jean Koko and Daniel Gahouma
Pediatrics Department, Faculty of Medicine, Health Sciences University (USS), Libreville, Gabon

Vincenzo Domenichelli, Simona Straziuso, Maria Domenica Sabatino and Silvana Federici
Pediatric Surgical Unit, "Infermi" Hospital, AUSL Romagna, Rimini, Italy

Concepción Míguez, Mercedes Fariñas Salto and Rafael Marañón
Pediatric Emergency Department, Hospital General Universitario Gregorio Marañón, Madrid, Spain

Sevgi Yavuz and Aydin Ece
Division of Pediatric Nephrology, Dicle University, Diyarbakir, Turkey

Yoshihiko Sakurai
Department of Pediatrics, Matsubara Tokushukai Hospital, Matsubara, Japan

Bulut Kasım, Uysal Cem, Korkmaz Mustafa, Bozkurt İsmail, Durmaz Ubeydullah, Tıraşçı Yaşar and Gören Süleyman
Forensic Medicine Department, Dicle University, Diyarbakır, Turkey

Sivri Süleyman
Diyarbakır Directorate of Forensic Medicine Office, Diyarbakir, Turkey

Innocent O. George and Chika N. Aiyedun
Department of Paediatrics, University of Port Harcourt Teaching Hospital, Port Harcourt, Nigeria

Ralf-Bodo Tröbs and Micha Bahr
Department of Pediatric Surgery, St. Mary's Hospital, St. Elisabeth Group, Ruhr-University of Bochum, Herne, Germany

Ralf Schulze
Department of Obstetrics and Gynecology, St. Vincenz' Hospital, Datteln, Germany

Matthias Neid
Institute of Pathology, Ruhr-University of Bochum, Georgius-Agricola-Foundation, BG-Clinics Bergmannsheil, Bochum, Germany

Wolfgang Pielemeier and Claudia Roll
Center of Perinatology, Department of Neonatology and Pediatric Intensive Care, Vest Children's Hospital, University of Witten-Herdecke, Datteln, Germany

R.-B. Tröbs
Department of Pediatric Surgery, Catholic Foundation Marienhospital Herne, Ruhr-University of Bochum, Herne, Widumer, Germany

A. Stein, U. Felderhoff and L. Hanssler
Department of Pediatrics I, University Hospital Essen, Hufelandstr, Essen, Germany
Ralf-Bodo Troebs
Klinik für Kinderchirurgie, Marien Hospital Herne, Ruhr University of Bochum, Bochum, Germany

www.ingramcontent.com/pod-product-compliance
Lightning Source LLC
Chambersburg PA
CBHW080520200326
41458CB00012B/4279
9781632414090